Statistical Methods
in Cancer Research
Volume IV
Descriptive Epidemiology

International Agency for Research on Cancer

The International Agency for Research on Cancer (IARC) was established in 1965 by the World Health Assembly, as an independently financed organization within the framework of the World Health Organization. The headquarters of the Agency are at Lyon, France.

The Agency conducts a programme of research concentrating particularly on the epidemiology of cancer and the study of potential carcinogens in the human environment. Its field studies are supplemented by biological and chemical research carried out in the Agency's laboratories in Lyon and, through collaborative research agreements, in national research institutions in many countries. The Agency also conducts a programme for the education and training of personnel for cancer research.

The publications of the Agency are intended to contribute to the dissemination of authoritative information on different aspects of cancer research. A complete list is printed at the back of this book.

Authors

Jacques Esteve

Adviser on Biostatistics, International Agency for Research on Cancer

Ellen Benhamou

Epidemiologist, Gustave Roussy Institute, Paris, France

Luc Raymond

Epidemiologist, Geneva Cancer Registry and Department of Social and Preventive Medicine, University of Geneva, Switzerland

Translator

Mary Sinclair

Scientific Editor, Alpha Biomedical Communications, Sydney, Australia

WORLD HEALTH ORGANIZATION

INTERNATIONAL AGENCY FOR RESEARCH ON CANCER

Statistical Methods
in Cancer Research
Volume IV
Descriptive Epidemiology

Jacques Estève, Ellen Benhamou, Luc Raymond

Translated from French by Mary Sinclair

IARC Scientific Publications No.128

International Agency for Research on Cancer

Lyon

1994

Published by the International Agency for Research on Cancer
150 cours Albert Thomas, 69372 Lyon Cedex 08, France

IARC Library Cataloguing in Publication Data

Statistical methods in cancer research /
  Jacques Esteve, Ellen Benhamou, Luc Raymond

  Contents: v. 4. Descriptive epidemiology

  (IARC scientific publications; 128)

  1. Neoplasms epidemiology 2. Statistics
  I. Esteve, Jacques II. Benhamou, Ellen III. Raymond, Luc
  IV. Series

  ISBN 92 832 2128 1 (NLM Classification: QZ 206)

ISSN 0300-5085

Printed in France

Contents

Preface

As the authors of this book remind us in their introduction, classical descriptive epidemiology was long regarded as simply a first, rather crude, step in the exploration of an epidemiological problem. Based essentially on comparisons between populations, it could do no more than stimulate ideas and hypotheses. Instead, it was up to analytical epidemiology, a more precise science since it involves measurements at the individual level, to produce firm evidence on risk factors, and it is mainly on the methodology of this area that various books have focused over the last thirty years.

Nevertheless, I can recall a number of major successes of descriptive epidemiology. For example, simply mapping the distribution of mortality rates for oesophageal cancer and of alcoholic cirrhosis enabled us, with Daniel Schwartz and Odile Lasserre, to demonstrate a relationship between alcohol consumption and oesophageal cancer. Likewise, comparison between the rising curve of lung cancer mortality and that of cigarette consumption certainly played a decisive role in focusing the attention of Richard Doll on the link between tobacco and cancer.

In recent years, the establishment of numerous cancer registries has encouraged many researchers to attempt to draw the maximum advantage from the data collected on cancer incidence and mortality. This has led to many original ideas and raised many important questions. Some biostatisticians entered this arena and they have gradually been able to lay the necessary statistical and mathematical foundations that were lacking. Problems such as those posed by the study of risks when the denominator is unknown, competing risks, and autocorrelation have led to the development of solid methodological concepts.

The great merit of this volume is that it brings together and reviews in one coherent text the different techniques needed for a modern approach to descriptive epidemiology. With the help of this compilation, researchers in this field will henceforth be able to tackle the study of their data armed with a methodological arsenal giving them the optimal chance of success. Other readers such as doctors and public health specialists will be able to obtain guidance, without having to enter into all the mathematical details, on how to avoid the many pitfalls that confront those who have to interpret collections of numerical data. The authors make extensive use of examples of analysis of real data sets and show how these can be treated and interpreted, so that the reader can follow in detail the development of the methods described and better comprehend the range of their applications.

I have known Jacques Estève, Ellen Benhamou and Luc Raymond for very many years, as a productive team with complementary capabilities. I am certain that this book that they have co-authored will provide an indispensable guide for numerous researchers and for decision-makers in public health who are concerned with epidemiology. Personally, as an epidemiologist and oncologist, I have found it to be of the greatest interest.

Professor Robert Flamant
Director of the Gustave Roussy Institute,
Villejuif, France

Foreword

This monograph presents and discusses some methods used in descriptive epidemiology which are relevant to cancer research. In presenting the fundamental concepts, we have tried to keep the mathematical formulation at a level which is compatible with an elementary knowledge of statistics and probability, but which nevertheless enables the logical relationships between the concepts currently used in epidemiology to be understood.

With the above objective in mind. Chapter 1 describes briefly the epidemiological context in which the methods will be used and devotes some space to their mathematical formulation. An elementary knowledge of statistics and probability as well as some familiarity with mathematical reasoning is expected from the reader of this chapter.

Chapter 2 describes how, in practice, the analysis and comparison of incidence and mortality can be carried out. Most attention is given to the multiplicative model and to the concept of proportional hazards, which is particularly relevant to cancer research. The exposition of these notions relies on many numerical examples, but no great mathematical sophistication is needed.

Chapter 3 is devoted to geographical analysis, ecological studies and analysis of time trends. These fields are at present subjects of interesting methodological research, and we have tried to show from several examples how modern statistical tools can considerably improve the interpretation of geographical and temporal data in epidemiology.

Chapter 4 describes the methods of analysis of survival probability at an elementary mathematical level, and the emphasis is placed on the interpretation of such data when they are collected in the context of routine cancer registry operations. Much space is therefore given to the concept of relative survival and many examples are presented to show the difficulty of interpretation when the procedures for data collection may imply several types of bias.

We have tried to give the reader sufficient understanding to use the methods which are presented by giving the details of calculations whenever possible and some examples of the use of the GLIM software, which is cheap, widely available and enables many methods presented in this book to be readily implemented.

This text was first written in French and was translated by Mary Sinclair, whom we gratefully acknowledge for her careful work. With the exception of the correction of known errors and some inevitable adaptation of French to English style, no effort has been made to update the content which was essentially written before 1991; this is why some recent references which would have been relevant are not included.

The finalization of the manuscript of this monograph benefited from the careful reading of John Cheney. We gratefully acknowledge his help.

Acknowledgements

This book was originally conceived as the proceedings of two seminars on statistical methods organized by the group of cancer registries in Latin countries. However, the absence in the French scientific literature of an up-to-date text on methods in descriptive epidemiology led us to write a manual on the key concepts and statistical methods in this area.

We hope that this manual will be of value to those working in, or with cancer registries, for whom it was originally intended. We trust that the mathematical nature of some parts of the book will not be an obstacle to its use and that the inclusion of numerous examples will serve to establish the link between the theoretical development and its epidemiological interpretation.

Many people have contributed to the development of this book: most notably the participants at the seminars mentioned above, whom we gratefully acknowledge. We are especially indebted to those who have made unpublished data available to illustrate the procedures presented in this book.

We are especially grateful to Catherine Com-Nougue and Agnes Laplanche who carefully read the manuscript and assisted us with pertinent advice and suggestions; to Annick Rivoire for her invaluable contribution in the preparation and production of the book; and to Aude Jaccard for organizing the bibliography. Finally, we thank Nicholas Day for his encouragement and help when initiating this project.

St Just et Vacquières, April 1992

Chapter 1

Fundamental concepts

Introduction

It has long been acknowledged that descriptive epidemiology is primarily characterized by its exploratory goals. It is seen as a first approach aimed at defining the scope of a research problem, at best generating hypotheses without aspiring to verify them. When descriptive epidemiology is seen in this light, the fact that no important developments in methodology had taken place until recently is less surprising. Its basic techniques were borrowed from demography: mortality and morbidity rates were seen as the key descriptive tools, with their comparison and standardization being the only methodological sophistication required. Statistical variability was rarely taken into account, sometimes producing serious errors in interpretation.

Several factors seem to have inspired the development of the techniques which make up modern descriptive epidemiology. The first is probably the proliferation and improvement of epidemiological data. In the area of cancer research these developments have undoubtedly been greater for incidence data than for mortality data. Cancer registries have multiplied and worked to standardize their definitions and registration procedures. The collection of demographic data, which provides the denominators of rates, has also seen a marked improvement, notably in the frequency of their publication.

The accumulation of incidence and mortality data over time has led to a focus on the analysis of time series. New techniques, mainly based on mathematical modelling, have been developed to distinguish between the different factors that underlie changes in rates. These methods have had both explanatory as well as predictive goals.

Descriptive epidemiology have also benefited from a more rigorous definition of its concepts, and from a more satisfactory incorporation in its methodology of the basic ideas developed in the context of stochastic process analysis. Appropriate mathematical and statistical methods have been developed, largely due to the contribution of epidemiologists. These advances follow a similar development of statistical methods in other areas of medicine. It is significant that published reports of epidemiological investigations now have a readership which includes specialists from other areas of research. The new approaches have led to better solutions to the

1

problems posed, in particular through more appropriate definition of hypotheses and the construction of suitable models for their evaluation.

The integration into descriptive epidemiology of spatial analysis and a more critical consideration of ecological studies are two examples of the increasing interaction between the improvement in data collection and the need for more sophisticated methods. Thus, the collection of increasingly detailed morbidity and mortality data, and the creation of data systems which allow cases and deaths to be located in time and space, have provided a basis for evaluating real or supposed environmental hazards, requiring in turn the development of appropriate statistical methods.

In the same way, when suspected exposures are easier to define at a group level rather than at an individual level, it is the role of descriptive epidemiology to assess the relationship between these exposures and the risk of cancer. Techniques to better control for potential confounding factors have thus been added to the classical methods of geographical correlation.

Traditionally, epidemiology is defined as the study of the distribution of diseases over time and place and according to individual characteristics. For the purpose of this book, descriptive epidemiology can be defined by replacing this last term with 'group characteristics'. This definition encompasses the intended contribution of descriptive epidemiology to etiologic research, as well as emphasising that data known only at a group level are the basis of the discipline. Inference is made from the group to the individual, in contrast to analytical epidemiology, in which risk is studied in groups formed a posteriori from data collected at an individual level. Throughout this text, it will be seen that the formation of groups on which the analysis is ultimately based is one of the crucial problems confronting descriptive epidemiology.

Apart from the methods of data collection, both for defining populations at risk and identifying risk factors, descriptive epidemiology utilizes exactly the same methodology as that of cohort studies in analytical epidemiology. Moreover, it will be seen that the concepts used are exactly the same. This resemblance is especially obvious when descriptive epidemiology has the task of describing the survival of cancer patients according to group characteristics. In this situation, data are available for individuals and the distinction between analytical and descriptive epidemiology becomes somewhat artificial. Survival studies have progressively found their place as an activity appropriate to cancer registries, and their goals are mainly descriptive in this context. Presentation of the methods of incidence analysis and then of survival analysis in the same text is in any case justified both mathematically and statistically. These two forms of analysis both concern the occurrence of an event (diagnosis or death respectively) in the presence of competing risks which lead to incomplete observation (also known as censoring). The estimation and modelling of the probability of occurrence of such an event leads to analytical methods requiring mathematical concepts rarely taught in medical schools.

In this first chapter, our goal will be primarily to convince the reader of the need for such ideas, then to present them as simply as possible through examples, while also providing the appropriate theoretical background. The subsequent chapters offer a more user-oriented description of the methods, so that the reader can carry out the calculations and tests presented. It should be emphasized that the reader who does not wish to become involved in the theoretical developments of the first chapter can by-pass them, without compromising an understanding of the rest of the book.

Basic concepts of descriptive epidemiology

Time and the concept of incidence

While no-one would dispute that cancer incidence varies with time, there is less agreement over the causes of its evolution. Public opinion readily seizes upon the idea that the disease is a modern-day plague. Some people maintain that the increase in the incidence of cancer is simply due to the ageing of Western populations and to the fact that the other diseases from which people used to die are being controlled. On the other hand, there are others who will state that it is a curse, linked to atmospheric pollution, nuclear energy or the use of new chemicals. Epidemiology allows us to establish that, in any given age group, the frequency of cancer (apart from those associated with tobacco) is remaining almost constant or, in some countries, is even decreasing (see Chapter 3, page 174).

These contradictory statements may seem to be an illustration of the saying that statistics are a sophisticated form of lying. In fact, they result from the difficulty of differentiating between the effects of many variables which are acting simultaneously on the phenomenon being studied: at the end of the twentieth century, the 'educated layman' does not necessarily have available the tools needed to make an objective analysis of the effects of these variables. The first step towards an understanding of the problem is an accurate definition of the concept of incidence.

In epidemiology as in demography, time can be located by two indices: date and age. Cancer incidence can only be described properly by taking into account both of the indices which play parallel roles and are in fact measures of time with respect to two different origins.

Figure 1.1 (the Lexis diagram) illustrates this duality: a segment of oblique line in this graph represents the observable fraction of an individual's life, that is, the interval of time and age during which an event of interest (e.g., incidence of cancer or complications of diabetes or AIDS in a seropositive patient) can occur. The left extremity of the segment is the start of observation: it is for example the date of birth in the descriptive study of cancer incidence, or the date of first employment in an industrial cohort aimed at measuring the risk of a suspected exposure. It could also be the date of the start of treatment in a study designed to measure the risk of relapse after illness or the chance of survival after the occurrence of a serious disease. The other extremity is the end of observation, characterized by the date and age at which either the event under study took place or the individual stopped being observed. This second possibility can be due to death (when we are interested in the incidence of some other event), loss to follow-up of the subject or the end of the study. In these three situations, it is said that the observation is *censored* because the event had not yet taken place at the end of the observation period. It is only known that the time necessary for the event to happen to the individual is greater than the duration of the observation period.

In some studies it is the death from a given disease which is the event of interest, either because incidence data are not available or because the probability of surviving from this diseases is the subject of the analysis. The censored observations comes in this context from subjects who died from other causes, who were lost to follow-up or for whom the diagnostic of the disease was too recent.

Depending on the point of view adopted, we can look at different segments of an individual's trajectory on the Lexis diagram. In a study of survival, the origin of the time scale is most often the date of diagnosis or of first treatment. The duration of *time at risk of death* is therefore measured as the time elapsed from this date, age being considered as an additional prognostic variable. Conversely, in an industrial cohort study, the basic measure of time is usually age, the time since the first entry being taken as an explanatory covariate. But, in both situations, the time

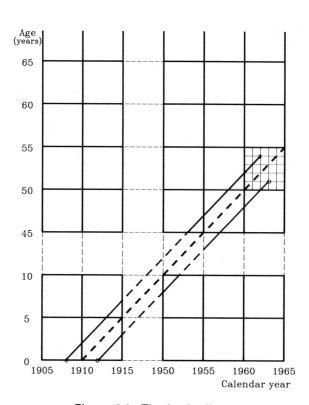

Figure 1.1   The Lexis diagram

origin is specific to each individual in the study; for a correct statistical analysis, we must 'synchronize the clocks' governing each individual's life events.

The aim of the epidemiologist is to draw conclusions about the different levels of risk to which groups of individuals are subjected. This requires well defined measures of risk in order to make objective comparisons between one situation and the next, or between one country and another. These measures might take the form of the probability of developing cancer or of dying from it, or they might be the survival rate or the probability of relapse. In all cases, the measures are based on a ratio between the number of observed events (the numerator) and the number of individuals at risk within a given period of time (the denominator). Alternative choices of the latter can lead to widely divergent results.

A few simple analogies will show how important the problem is. For example, if we want to compare the safety of different types of transport, should we measure the number of passenger deaths per kilometre travelled, per passenger x kilometre, or per passenger x time travelled? It is obvious that the definition of risk depends on the method of calculation. To compare the incidence of cancer in two cohorts, should we base our results on the observed proportion of cancer in each group, or should we take into account the number of years for which each individual was actually observed and at risk of developing cancer? If the two cohorts have the same average age and have been observed for the same time period and if the only reason for stopping observation was the onset of cancer (or, more generally, the event under study), the proportion is a good index of comparison. If, as more often happens, other events prematurely bring some individual observations to an end and if, in addition, these events do not occur in the same way in the two cohorts, it is likely that more cancers will be seen in the group which has, on average, been observed for longer. Conversely, if we take the duration of employment as an approximate measure of exposure in a study of lung cancer mortality in an asbestos mine, we should be aware that remaining employed for a given duration means having survived this number of years. Thus, if we want to assess the risk of people employed for more than twenty years, only the period beginning after twenty years of employment and the corresponding cases of cancer would be taken into account for the evaluation of this risk.

These examples lead to the following principles:

- the calculation of the denominator should take into account the number of years of observation relevant to the proposed study; it should take into account the continuous modification of the population actually 'at risk' throughout the duration of the study. By definition, a subject is no longer at risk after the occurrence of the event or after the censoring time.[1]

- incidence rate should be defined as the number of events per *person-year*, that is, per person and per year of observation relevant to the risk being analysed.

---

[1] Note however that cancer registries record second primary cancers. Strictly speaking, the period at risk starts in this situation immediately after the first tumour as if a new subject was added to the population at risk at this point.

• A given period of observation of a subject will contribute to the person years in the denominator only if this subject would have been counted in the numerator had he experienced the event being studied over that period of time.

Here it is appropriate to introduce *the instantaneous rate*, a concept which is crucial to epidemiology. Intuitively, this parameter measures the probability that an individual in a defined population becomes a victim of the event at a specified time point, given that the individual is still living and under observation at that time. In the same way that the speed at a given moment can be approximated by an average speed, so an instantaneous rate can be approximated by an average rate. In Figure 1.1, the squared cell shows individuals who were 50 to 55 years old between the years 1960 and 1965, that is, individuals who were born between 1905 and 1915. If the asterisk represents the end of observation due to the occurrence of cancer and the point represents the termination of observation for all other reasons, the risk of developing cancer between 50 and 55 years of age for individuals born around 1910 is then measured by the number of asterisks observed in the square divided by the number of years accumulated in the same space by the individuals born between 1905 and 1915. Only individuals born in 1910 will be able to accumulate five years of observation; the further the birth date is from this date, in either direction, the smaller the individual's contribution to the calculation of the denominator in this square. The resulting ratio, generally called the *average annual rate* of cancer between 50 and 55 years for the generation born around 1910, or else the *specific rate* for the age group 50-55 years, is an approximation to the instantaneous rate.

Figure 1.2 shows the evolution with age of lung cancer mortality in France; it can be seen that, for successive generations, those born more recently have suffered the highest lung cancer mortality. In such a situation, the cross-sectional curve obtained by plotting age-specific rates at a given time point (for example, the curve obtained by joining the points corresponding to the period 1950-1954) would be an incorrect description of the phenomenon if it was interpreted as a representation of the effect of age. Actually, the observed decrease in risk for higher ages corresponds to a *generation effect*: it has been shown that the lung cancer risk in the older French population is lower only because the corresponding generation has had less exposure to tobacco. The phenomenon is clearly seen in Figure 1.3, where the evolution of mortality from cancers of the lung, the oesophagus and the larynx in France is shown for successive generations. The lung cancer risk increases regularly with date of birth, whereas the risk of cancers of the oesophagus and larynx, which are much more dependent on alcohol consumption, have both been smaller for those generations subjected to rationing related to the second world war.

Group characteristics and place

By revealing the large variability in cancer incidence throughout the world, descriptive epidemiology has shown that the prevention of cancer is, at least partially, possible; differences observed, particularly within the same ethnic groups, have

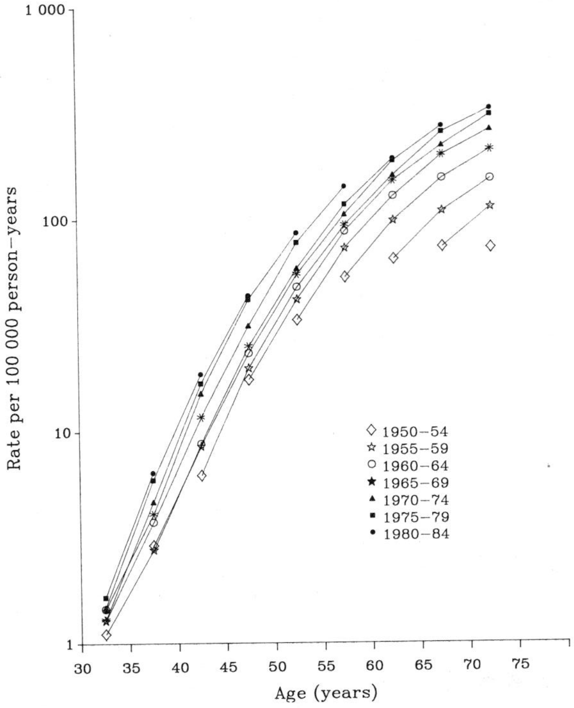

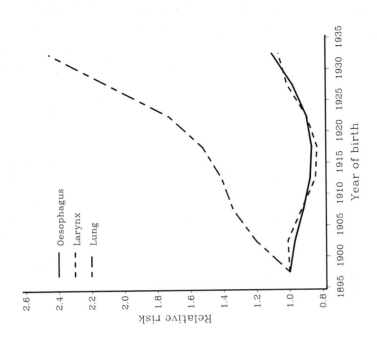

Figure 1.3 Relative risk of death from lung, larynx and oesophageal cancers for successive male birth cohorts in France compared to the cohort born around 1897

Figure 1.2 Evolution of lung cancer mortality in France, men; age-effect in successive birth cohorts drawn from cross-sectional mortality in successive time periods

unambiguously established that environmental factors play a determining role in the development of cancer. The most striking example is probably that of oesophageal cancer for which the risk is 300 times more elevated in the north-east of Iran than it is in Nigeria. The reasons for this difference have only been partially identified, and it is quite likely that multiple factors are responsible [1]. In Europe, the risks in the regions most affected by oesophageal cancer are about a factor of 30 greater than in the regions least affected; the incidence of this cancer is highest, where the highest average alcohol consumption is reported, notably in the west of France.

Given this large variability, it is extremely tempting to try to establish causal relationships by analysing the correlation between the variation of incidence and environmental factors in different populations, and in fact many such analyses have been attempted. On the whole, however, these attempts have been rather unsuccessful: on an international scale, no substantial correlation has been demonstrated between oesophageal cancer and alcohol consumption. Undoubtedly, one of the reasons for this failure is that cancer is a multifactorial disease and that the determining factors need not be the same in two regions with very different cultural traditions. Another reason is that the degree of exposure to the factor can be distributed unequally among the individuals in the regions being compared, even if the average rate of exposure in the regions is similar. For example, it is conceivable that a country with a minority of heavy drinkers and a majority of teetotallers would report more cancer than another area with more widespread consumption at a lower level.

An absence of correlation can also be observed for less obvious methodological reasons. For example, studies on individuals show that tobacco is responsible for 85% of the lung cancer observed in populations where smoking is widespread [2]. However, if we restrict ourselves to Europe, a group of seventeen countries that is reasonably homogeneous for other factors, the correlation for the period 1970-74 between lung cancer risk (cumulative up to 80 years) and the consumption of cigarettes for the same period is only 0.56. A correlation of this size means that the variation in the consumption of tobacco explains barely a third of the variation in mortality, which is hardly compatible with the above number of 85%.

In fact, the correlation between tobacco consumption and lung cancer is slightly more impressive if we look at it correctly [3]. The first mistake in the preceding discussion is to have considered the cumulative risk cross-sectionally, thereby adding together risks over generations that had radically different tobacco exposure. The second mistake is to have considered the consumption of tobacco contemporaneously with the mortality when the latent period between exposure and the occurrence of cancer should have been taken into account. Comparing the cumulative risk for lung cancer for the seventeen countries between the ages of 35 and 50 years for people born around 1925, and cigarette consumption between 1955 and 1964 (Table 1.1 and Figure 3.9), we obtain a correlation between the two variables equal to 0.75, a much more reasonable value for data limited by substantial imprecision.

Conversely, these remarks hold true when a factor is correlated positively with a disease on a geographical level; the correlation is not always found in studies

Table 1.1   National cigarette sales and mortality from lung cancer in selected European countries

	Cumulative risk from 35 to 50 years Generation born in 1925 ([a])	Number ([b]) of cigarettes (Rank) — 1955-64	
Portugal	0.69	905	(2)
Sweden	0.75	1 147	(4)
Norway	0.86	533	(1)
Spain	0.98	1 112	(3)
Germany ([c])	1.30	1 571	(9)
France	1.32	1 318	(6)
Iceland ([d])	1.35	1 736	(13)
Greece	1.38	1 714	(11)
Austria	1.44	1 647	(10)
Switzerland	1.54	2 281	(15)
Denmark	1.57	1 375	(7)
Netherlands	1.73	1 716	(12)
Finland	1.77	1 975	(14)
Ireland	1.88	2 600	(16)
Italy	1.95	1 265	(5)
Belgium	2.09	1 539	(8)
UK	2.83	2 672	(17)

([a]) Average risk (per thousand) for both sexes combined; source: WHO (WHO Mortality Data Bank).
([b]) Average annual cigarette sales per adult above 15 years (1955-1964) [8].
([c]) Former Federal Republic of Germany.
([d]) Risk estimated from 14 cases, and therefore of limited reliability.

involving individuals. This situation can be illustrated by the correlation found between beer consumption and mortality from cancer of the rectum [4,5] and also the correlation between consumption of fat and breast cancer mortality [6,7].

A technical presentation of this approach and other examples will be given in Chapter 3 (see page 141), where the usefulness of this methodology will be discussed. The above examples were presented to show that the interpretation of descriptive data requires the same attention as data coming from an analytical study. Only a combined analysis of results obtained at a group and an individual level will provide the correct scientific interpretation.

Epidemiology is a science of observation, which means that it is limited to making use of natural events which simulate an experimental design. Seen from this point of view, studies of migrants and religious groups have been extremely successful. Table 1.2 provides a particularly attractive example based on the incidence of certain cancers observed in various Israeli communities and in selected western populations. The figures show that, for the given cancer sites, the incidences observed in Israel are consistently lower than those observed in the western countries used as reference, but their basic interest lies in the differences that they reveal between the Israeli communities. In fact, Jewish people not born in Israel have a risk half way between the risk of their country of origin and that of their adopted country. This tends to confirm that the observed change in risk was linked to a change in environment.

Table 1.2   Cancer and migration ([a]): Incidence rates ([b]) for selected cancer sites in Israel (1972-76), in Geneva (1973-77) and in Connecticut, USA (1973-77)

Population	Males			Females		
	All cancers except skin	Respiratory ICD8: 160-162	Digestive ICD8: 150-157	All cancers except skin	Respiratory ICD8: 160-162	Digestive ICD8: 150-157
Non-Jews born in Israel	117.3	35.7	22.9	62.8	12.3	9.0
Jews born in Africa or in Asia	167.1	32.0	42.2	137.3	30.4	18.5
Jews born in Israel	183.7	22.9	51.3	187.1	35.5	30.1
Jews born in Europe or in America	211.4	34.9	66.7	226.6	55.2	32.3
Connecticut	303.0	69.7	80.4	257.3	54.3	43.6
Geneva	328.6	81.2	88.8	225.2	46.3	42.5

([a]) Source: Cancer Incidence in Five Continents [9].
([b]) Rates standardized on world population.

Table 1.3   Standardized ([a]) incidence rates (T) and standardized incidence ratio (SIR) ([b]) for selected cancer sites in Utah, USA (1967-1975) ([c])

		Mormons		Non-Mormons	
		Urban	Rural	Urban	Rural
Males					
Tobacco-related sites ([d])	T	52.8	50.4	141.0	74.4*
	SIR	44⁻	43⁻	106	59⁻
Lung (ICD8: 162)	T	27.1	27.3	75.7	40.3*
	SIR	37⁻	39⁻	96	54⁻
Females					
Breast	T	63.5	55.5	90.9	80.8
	SIR	84⁻	74⁻	121⁺	97
Uterus					
Cervix, invasive	T	8.1	9.4	17.7	18.4
	SIR	54⁻	60	120⁺	111
Cervix, in situ	T	15.9	12.9	45.4	34.7
	SIR	–	–	–	–
Corpus	T	21.9	19.1	27.4	24.8
	SIR	104	91	130⁺	107

([a]) Standardized on 1970 US population, * significantly different from the urban rate.
([b]) TNCS Standard (Third National Cancer Survey), ⁻ significantly lower than the national rate, ⁺ significantly higher than the national rate, –– data not available.
([c]) Source: Utah Cancer Registry (1967-1975) [10].
([d]) ICD8: 140 (lip), 143-150 (buccal cavity, pharynx and esophagus), 161 (larynx), 162 (lung), 188 (bladder).

Table 1.3 reproduces some results from the Utah cancer registry. A significant proportion of the population comprises Mormons, who do not consume alcohol or tobacco and who individually have less sexual partners and on average more children than the rest of the population. Taken together, this behaviour has noticeable consequences on the incidence of cancer at several sites, as shown in the Table. As these figures were not derived from a controlled experiment, it is likely that the Mormon population group differs from the non-Mormon group for other characteristics which can be associated with cancer development. Nevertheless, it is noteworthy that the classic excess of incidence in urban populations, seen here in the non-Mormon group, disappears in the Mormon community. The urban-rural difference is thus very likely to be due to differences in individual behaviour between urban and rural inhabitants, rather than being explained by one of the urban risk factors (such as pollution) usually invoked as explanatory.

In practice, the possibility of establishing relationships such as those which we have just described largely depends on the use of the appropriate statistical methodology. In particular, the methodology should provide the means of evaluating the variability attributable only to chance, so that it can be taken into account in the interpretation of observed differences. The remainder of this chapter will be devoted to a discussion of mathematical concepts which are the basis of the analytical methods. A discussion of practical applications will be kept for the subsequent chapters.

Statistical concepts for the analysis of incidence data

Formal definition of the incidence rate

We have seen above that the identification of factors favouring or causing the occurrence of a disease or a death requires the measurement of the risk of developing the event. In other words, we need an unbiased estimate of the probability that an individual, in a given environment, might develop the event under study. Besides the factors under study, this probability depends on temporal variables such as age, in incidence and mortality studies, and duration of observation in survival studies. The mathematical concept which is fundamental to risk and survival assessment is the distribution of the time separating the beginning of observation from the occurrence of the event. From a knowledge of this distribution we can measure, for example, the risk of cancer before age t, or the risk of death t years after diagnosis. The date of the development of the event under study is often unknown because observation is interrupted before the event occurs; in this case it is necessary to use specific techniques to estimate the distribution from incomplete observations.

As we noted previously, the period for which an individual is followed is the result of two competing mechanisms, which results in two different types of observation; one produces the event under study and the other includes all the other causes which might be responsible for terminating observation. Our aim is now to show how, by taking into account these two types of observation, we can reconstruct the distribution that would have been seen if all observations had been completed.

In this way people dying, for example from a cardiac disease, before age t will contribute to the calculation of the probability of having cancer before this age; similarly the follow-up of patients who were only diagnosed 1, 2, 3 or 4 years ago will contribute to the calculation of the survival probability at 5 years.

The mathematical concept used for this reconstruction is the instantaneous rate, which was defined intuitively above. We now adopt a more formal approach, which will allow further mathematical developments.

Let T denote the time period between the start and the end of observation for an individual, whether terminated by the end-point under study (for example, the occurrence of cancer) or by any other circumstance which might interrupt the follow-up. Furthermore, let δ be the indicator function of the end-point: $\delta = 1$ when the event has taken place and $\delta = 0$ when the observation is censored.

The following definitions characterize the random distribution of the couple of variables (T, δ). Let

- $R(t) = \text{Prob } (T < t)$ be the probability distribution of T
- $S(t) = 1 - R(t)$ denote the probability that the subject is still under observation (surviving) at the time-point t without the event having taken place,
- $p_1 = \text{Prob } (\delta = 1)$ be the probability that the event take place and
- $R_1(t) = \text{Prob } (T < t \mid \delta = 1)$ be the conditional distribution of the event, that is the probability that the event takes place before the time t, given that it has taken place.

Thus, the probability that the event occurs before the time t may be written

$$\pi(t) = \text{Prob } (T < t, \ \delta = 1) = p_1 R_1(t).$$

The probability that the event occurs on a given date, while the subject is still being followed-up, defines the force of incidence (or mortality) at this point in time. The following expression, which is directly derived from this probability, will be referred to as the *instantaneous rate*,

$$\lambda(t) = \lim_{\Delta t \to 0} \frac{1}{\Delta t} \text{Prob} (t < T < t + \Delta t, \ \delta = 1 \mid T > t) \tag{1.1}$$

It should be noted that $\lambda(t)$ is not, strictly speaking, a probability, but a probability per unit of time, also known as a probability rate. Application of the rules of probability immediately gives

$$\lambda(t) = \lim_{\Delta t \to 0} \frac{1}{\Delta t} \frac{p_1 R_1(t + \Delta t) - p_1 R_1(t)}{1 - R(t)} \tag{1.2}$$

The numerator is the probability that the event occurs at time t of the subject's follow-up; the denominator indicates that only the subjects who have been followed-up at least until t are taken into account. Furthermore,

$$\lambda(t)\, S(t) = p_1 \lim_{\Delta t \to 0} \frac{R_1(t + \Delta t) - R_1(t)}{\Delta t} = p_1 R'_1(t) \tag{1.3}$$

where $R'_1(t)$ is defined as the conditional probability density of T, derivative of $R_1(t)$.

In this way we obtain the relationship between $\lambda(t)$, $S(t)$ and the distribution function of T when the event occurs. The probability that the event occurs before time t can be written

$$\pi(t) = \int_0^t p_1\, R'_1(u)\, du$$

that is,

$$\pi(t) = \int_0^t \lambda(u)\, S(u)\, du \tag{1.4}$$

In the situation where there are no censored observations, $p_1 = 1$ and $R_1(t) = R(t)$; this would be the case for example in a study of mortality from all causes, if every individual in the cohort was under observation until death. In this situation, formula (1.3) leads to

$$\lambda(t) = \frac{R'(t)}{1 - R(t)} \tag{1.5}$$

which is a differential equation with solution

$$\Lambda(t) = - \text{Log}\, [S(t)] \quad \text{and} \quad R(t) = 1 - e^{-\Lambda(t)} \tag{1.6}$$

where

$$\Lambda(t) = \int_0^t \lambda(u)\, du \tag{1.7}$$

When there are censored observations, the distribution function defined by formula (1.6) is in fact that which would govern the observations if they were all complete, that is, if none was censored. The probabilities generated by this distribution are called *net probabilities* as opposed to *crude probabilities* defined by $\pi(t)$ in formula (1.4).

If T is age and if the end-point is the occurrence of cancer, the following terminology is used:

- $\lambda(t)$ is the *force of incidence*,
- $\pi(t)$ is the *crude probability* of developing cancer by age t,
- $\Lambda(t)$ is the *cumulative incidence rate* at age t.

The net probability of developing cancer by age t, $R(t) = 1 - e^{-\Lambda(t)}$, is a measure of cancer risk when there are no censored observations, that is, in the absence of mortality. Therefore, the net probability is not affected by the structure of the mortality pattern in the population under study and it can be used to compare several populations. This measure of risk is known as *cumulative risk*; its properties, and methods for its calculation are presented in Chapter 2 (page 66).

If T is the interval between diagnosis and the end of follow-up, the censored observations are essentially those for which the diagnosis is too recent; in this case, $\pi(t)$ is of little interest. The net probability of survival given in formula (1.6) is usually the parameter of interest in survival analysis.

Estimation of the instantaneous incidence rate

Having established a framework in which incidence can be defined, we must now consider methods for its calculation, or rather, for its estimation. The age-specific rates are usually calculated from the number of cases observed in the different age groups and from demographic statistics which enable the person-years of observation in each age group to be evaluated. Only the justification of the method will be given at this stage; the practical details will be left until Chapter 2.

In the case of a cohort of limited size in which each individual history is known and stretches over a long time period, the estimation of the age-specific rate requires an exact calculation of the person-years of observation. The estimation would be straightforward if the rate were independent of time and if each individual observation were complete; this situation is described on page 15. When instead some observations are censored, this fact has to be taken into account in the calculation (see page 18). The discussion will lead us to explain why the random fluctuations in the number of observed cases can be described by the Poisson distribution.

An approximation useful in descriptive epidemiology

We saw in formula (1.4) that the crude probability π of developing cancer between age t_0 and age t_1 depends on the age-specific rate $\lambda(u)$ and the probability of surviving without cancer $S(u)$, that is

$$\pi = \int_{t_0}^{t_1} \lambda(u)S(u)\, du$$

In principle, this probability can be easily estimated from data on a population with a given date of birth (a *birth cohort*). In this situation, the birth date is the natural time origin for all individuals in the cohort and the variable t is simply their age. Therefore, to estimate π we simply divide the number of cases occurring between age t_0 and t_1 by the initial size of the cohort. However, the survival to age t_0 will influence the result more than the value of the age-specific rate between t_0 and t_1. Thus, this probability is of no use in estimating $\lambda(u)$; in contrast, the conditional probability π_c of having the disease between age t_0 and t_1, given that the subject was still at risk at age t_0, is obviously not influenced by survival up until that age and is very little influenced by survival between t_0 and t_1 if this interval is short. We can write

$$\pi_c = \int_{t_0}^{t_1} \lambda(u) \frac{S(u)}{S(t_0)} du \tag{1.8}$$

If $t_1 - t_0$ is sufficiently small so that $\lambda(u)$ can be considered constant in $[t_0,t_1]$ and $S(u)$ roughly equal to $S(t_0)$ in the interval, then

$$\pi_c \approx \lambda(t_0)(t_1 - t_0)$$

If on the other hand, n_{t_0} denotes the number of subjects at risk at t_0, and k is the number of cases observed between t_0 and t_1, then the estimate of π_c is

$$\hat{\pi}_c = \frac{k}{n_{t_0}}$$

and, therefore, the estimate of λ is

$$\hat{\lambda}(t_0) \approx \frac{k}{n_{t_0}(t_1 - t_0)} \tag{1.9}$$

In other words, the instantaneous rate estimated at t_0 is obtained by dividing the number of cases observed by the number m of person-years of observation for the cohort between t_0 and t_1, where $m = n_{t_0}(t_1 - t_0)$, that is

$$\hat{\lambda}(t_0) \approx \frac{k}{m}$$

Formula (1.8), which is simply the application of the definition of λ in Formula (1.1) above, shows that the approximation will not be good if $\lambda(u)$ varies sharply within the interval $[t_0, t_1]$ or when a large number of subjects die from other causes or are lost to follow-up between t_0 and t_1; in this situation, the ratio $S(u)/S(t_0)$ would become too far from unity for the approximation being valid. If there is a substantial proportion of censored observations, survival time must be explicitly taken into account for each of the n_{t_0} individuals in the interval $[t_0, t_1]$. In other words, the number of person-years of observation appearing in the denominator of formula (1.9) must be calculated exactly, by taking into account the date of the end of follow-up for each individual.

In order to understand the procedure to be used when individual observations are available, we shall first study the situation where $\lambda(u)$ remains constant and all observations are complete. Although this is rarely the case in practice, it will help us to understand the more complicated situation where observations may be censored. This simple example will also allow the principle of the maximum likelihood estimation to be introduced.

When individual observations are available and complete

Let $t_1, t_2... t_n$ be the time elapsed between the start of the observation and the occurrence of the event under study for a random sample of n individuals subject to the same constant hazard rate $\lambda = \lambda_0$. The cumulative hazard rate is then $\Lambda(t) = \lambda_0 t$ and the probability distribution of the t_i is defined by the function (see formula (1.6)):

$$P(T < t) = R(t) = 1 - e^{-\lambda_0 t} \tag{1.10}$$

This distribution known as the exponential distribution has the density

$$r(t) = R'(t) = \lambda_0 \, e^{-\lambda_0 t}$$

According to the principle of maximum likelihood, the estimate of the unknown value of λ is the value $\hat{\lambda}$ which maximizes the probability density of n observations written as a function of λ

$$V(\lambda) = \prod_{i=1}^{n} r(t_i) = \lambda^n \, e^{-\lambda \sum_{i=1}^{n} t_i} \tag{1.11}$$

It is intuitively clear that the higher the probability of the observed data for a given λ, the more likely it is that λ will be close to the unknown value λ_0.

For technical reasons, the function to be maximized is not $V(\lambda)$ but $\text{Log}\,[V(\lambda)]$, which in this example may be written:

$$L(\lambda) = \text{Log}\,[V(\lambda)] = n \, \text{Log}\,(\lambda) - \lambda \sum_{i=1}^{n} t_i \tag{1.12}$$

The value $\hat{\lambda}$ is then obtained by equating the derivative of L to zero:

$$\frac{d\,L(\lambda)}{d\lambda} = \frac{n}{\lambda} - \sum_{i=1}^{n} t_i = 0 \tag{1.13}$$

that is,

$$\hat{\lambda} = \frac{n}{\displaystyle\sum_{i=1}^{n} t_i} = \frac{1}{\bar{T}} \tag{1.14}$$

In other words, in this situation, the instantaneous rate is estimated by the number of observed events divided by the time taken to produce all of them. This estimate can also be described as the inverse of the mean duration of the n observation times. The random variable $\hat{\lambda}$ which is a function of the t_i is known as the *maximum likelihood estimator*.

It has been shown that this approach generally produces a good estimator in that $\hat{\lambda}$ becomes numerically closer to λ_0 as n increases (*consistency*).

Study of the probability distribution of the difference between the log-likelihood of $\hat{\lambda}$ and that of λ_0 has shown that:

$$2\,[L(\hat{\lambda}) - L(\lambda_0)] \rightsquigarrow \chi_1^2 \tag{1.15}$$

It is therefore possible to state that this difference will rarely (less than 1 in 20 times) exceed the critical value 3.84 of a χ^2 with one degree of freedom. More generally using the result (1.15) allows the construction of a $(1 - \alpha)\%$ confidence interval for λ_0

$$[\lambda_I, \lambda_S] = \{\lambda \mid 2[L(\hat{\lambda}) - L(\lambda)] < Z_{\alpha/2}^2\} \qquad (1.16)$$

In order to illustrate this method, 20 observations t_i of an exponential distribution with mean $\lambda_0 = 1$ were simulated. The sum of the observations was $\sum_{i=1}^{20} t_i = 19.36$. Thus $\bar{T} = 0.9680$ and $\hat{\lambda} = 1.033$. Figure 1.4 shows the function $2L(\lambda)$ in the neighbourhood of $\hat{\lambda}$ and the 95% confidence interval obtained from the above method. The quadratic approximation of $2L(\lambda)$ is also shown on the same graph as a dotted line. Since $\dfrac{dL(\hat{\lambda})}{d\lambda} = 0$, this approximation may be written according to Taylor's formula:

$$2L(\lambda) \approx 2L(\hat{\lambda}) + \frac{d^2 L(\hat{\lambda})}{d\lambda^2} (\lambda - \hat{\lambda})^2 \qquad (1.17)$$

From this expression, it can be seen that the horizontal line $Z_{\alpha/2}^2$ units (3.84 units if $\alpha = 0.05$) below the maximum of the curve will intersect the dotted line at two points defined on the x-axis by:

$$[\lambda_I^* ; \lambda_S^*] = \hat{\lambda} \pm Z_{\alpha/2} \left\{ \sqrt{-\left[\frac{d^2L(\hat{\lambda})}{d\lambda^2}\right]^{-1}} \right\} \qquad (1.18)$$

This interval provides an approximate $(1 - \alpha)\%$ confidence interval for λ_0.

It may in fact be shown that, when n is large, the probability distribution of $\hat{\lambda}$ is normal with mean λ_0 and variance equal to the quantity under the square root sign in formula (1.18). This result, which can be generalized to more complex situations, will be used later in this book. In the simpler context of the exponential distribution presented here, the derivation of (1.13) gives:

$$\frac{d^2 L(\hat{\lambda})}{d\lambda^2} = -\frac{n}{\hat{\lambda}^2} \qquad (1.19)$$

which is equal to -18.74 in the present numerical example. Then:

$$[\lambda_I^* ; \lambda_S^*] = \hat{\lambda} \pm 1.96 \frac{\hat{\lambda}}{\sqrt{n}} \qquad (1.20)$$

which is equal to $[0.58 ; 1.49]$ as shown in Figure 1.4.

The above method provides a simple means of constructing a confidence interval for an exponential distribution using a sample of independent observations. The negative of the second derivative in (1.19) may be considered as a measure

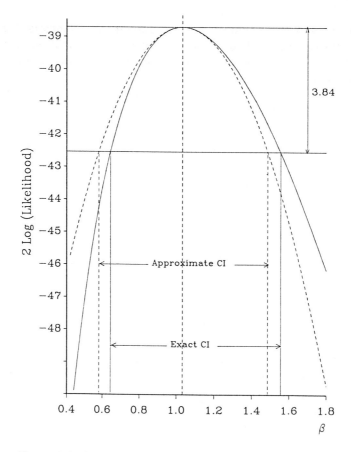

Figure 1.4   Maximum likelihood estimate of a parameter (β) and its confidence intervals (CI)

of the *information* provided by the sample with respect to the parameter λ: the larger the information, the more precise the estimate will be.

When individual observations are available but possibly censored

Let us now consider a cohort in which n individuals undergo the same force of incidence $\lambda(u)$ and the same survival $S(u)$ in the interval of observation 0, t (where the origin, 0, represents the beginning of observation, which may be, for example, the start of a five-year age interval for subjects born around the same time, see Lexis diagram Figure 1.1). Each individual observation is characterized by the value of two variables t_i and δ_i, where $\delta_i = 1$ if the event has taken place at the time t_i for individual i, and $\delta_i = 0$ if the event has not taken place at the time-point t_i when individual i ceases to be under observation, either because he has not survived or because $t_i = t$, i.e., the subject is alive at the end of observation.

If the function $\lambda(t)$ is defined by a finite number of parameters, these can be estimated from the sample of observations by choosing as previously values for the parameters which maximize their likelihood. Although the principle is the same, the situation becomes more complicated because of the presence of censored observations. The random variable (T, δ) does not have a probability density, therefore the density of complete observations $(\delta_i = 1)$ and that of censored observations $(\delta = 0)$ should be written separately.

• When $\delta_i = 1$, the contribution of the individual to the likelihood is given by formula (1.4),

$$P(t_i < T < t_i + dt, \delta = 1) = \lambda(t_i) \, S(t_i) \, dt$$

• When $\delta_i = 0$, the contribution is:

$$P(t_i < T < t_i + dt, \delta = 0) = c(t_i) \, S(t_i) \, dt,$$

where $c(u)$ is the analogue of $\lambda(u)$ for censored observations.

Thus, the likelihood may be written

$$V = \prod_{i=1}^{n} S(t_i) \, \lambda(t_i)^{\delta_i} \, c(t_i)^{1-\delta_i}$$

where $S(t)$ is the probability of still being followed up at time t without the event having occurred. Writing this probability as a function of incidence and censoring rates, we have

$$V = \prod_{i=1}^{n} e^{-\int_0^{t_i} [\lambda(u) + c(u)] \, du} \lambda(t_i)^{\delta_i} \, c(t_i)^{1-\delta_i}$$

$$V = \prod_{i=1}^{n} e^{-\Lambda(t_i)} \lambda(t_i)^{\delta_i} \, e^{-C(t_i)} \, c(t_i)^{1-\delta_i} \tag{1.21}$$

where $C(t) = \int_0^t c(u) \, du$

If the mechanism which leads to censored observations is independent of incidence, $c(t)$ does not depend on the parameters that determine $\lambda(t)$. To maximize V with respect to these parameters, we can therefore ignore the last two factors. In fact the contribution of a censored observation to the likelihood becomes the probability that T is greater than t_i in the absence of risks other than the one under consideration. Therefore, the logarithm of the function to be maximized is

$$L(\lambda) = \text{Log} \left[\prod_{i=1}^{n} e^{-\Lambda(t_i)} \lambda(t_i)^{\delta_i} \right]$$

$$L(\lambda) = -\sum_{i=1}^{n} \Lambda(t_i) + \sum_{i=1}^{n} \delta_i \, \text{Log} \, [\lambda(t_i)] \tag{1.22}$$

As an example, if $\lambda(t)$ is constant, this function becomes

$$L(\lambda) = - \sum_{i=1}^{n} \lambda\, t_i + \sum_{i=1}^{n} \delta_i \, Log\,(\lambda)$$

$$L(\lambda) = - \lambda \sum_{i=1}^{n} t_i + k\, Log(\lambda) = - \lambda m + k\, Log\,(\lambda) \tag{1.23}$$

where $k = \sum_{i=1}^{n} \delta_i$ is the number of events observed in the interval [0,t], and $m = \sum_{i}^{n} t_i$ is now the exact number of person-years of observation of the cohort within the interval [0,t]. The quantity m may also be written $n\overline{T}$ where $\overline{T}$ is the mean duration of observation.

The function reaches a maximum for

$$\hat{\lambda} = \frac{k}{\displaystyle\sum_{i=1}^{n} t_i} = \frac{k}{n\,\overline{T}} = \frac{k}{m} \tag{1.24}$$

The comparison of formulae (1.9), (1.14) and (1.24) shows that the principle governing the estimation of λ is unique. The only variation is in the way in which the mean observation time is calculated. Furthermore, as above, the precision of $\hat{\lambda}$ obtained from the second derivative of the likelihood (1.23) is:

$$Var\,(\hat{\lambda}) = \frac{\hat{\lambda}^2}{k} = \frac{\hat{\lambda}}{m}$$

At this point, it should be noted that the function to be maximized in formula (1.23) is, to within a constant, the logarithm of the likelihood of a single observation k having a Poisson distribution with parameter λm:

$$Log\left[e^{-\lambda m}\, \frac{(\lambda m)^k}{k!} \right] = L(\lambda) + M(k\,,\,m) \tag{1.25}$$

where $M(k,m) = -\,Log(k!) + k\,Log(m)$ refers to all the constant terms independent of λ.

Consequently, when estimating an instantaneous rate, although the numerator and denominator are both random variables, we are led to the same estimation procedure as if the numerator alone were random and followed a Poisson distribution. Therefore, the precision of the estimate of the incidence (or mortality) rate is judged exclusively from the variability of the numerator described by a Poisson distribution. We will use this equivalence throughout Chapter 2. The distribution of k is actually more complicated; however, there are no disadvantages and many benefits in making this approximation as long as the analytical methods are based on the likelihood. It is often stated that the true distribution of k is binomial; this would only be the case if each of n individuals exposed to a given constant risk where observed for the same duration t defined *a priori* (see formula (1.9)). In this situation, the probability that the event (disease or death) occurs in a given individual would be $R(t) = 1 - e^{-\lambda t}$ (see formula (1.10)) and the number of observed events would follow the binomial law with parameters n and R(t). Actually, when R(t) is small, this distribution is close to the Poisson distribution of parameter $n(1 - e^{-\lambda t}) \approx n\lambda t = \lambda m$. However, the argument for the binomial law has little weight in practice since the contribution of the individuals to person-years is random and varies widely from subject to subject. We shall therefore consider that the Poisson distribution is the best compromise to describe the random fluctuation of the number of cases and that it remains adequate as long as the number of events (k) is small compared to the number of individuals at risk (n).

In practice, formula (1.24) is mainly used in cohort studies [11], since its use requires knowing the time t_i for each individual in the population under study. This information is available in a survival study and the terminology traditionally used in this context will be presented in the following sections.

Conversely, in a descriptive study, individual dates are never available and, as we have previously stated, the denominators of the age-specific rates must be estimated from demographic data. The most simple method of calculation is to multiply, for each age group x, the number of individuals recorded at the mid-point of the case-registration interval, by the number of years in the interval. If the local statistical office provides annual population data, the calculation of the denominators can be made in a way which is more precise. If we know the number of cases k_x which arise in the age group x during the year t and the total number of individuals $n_x(t)$ in the age group on the 1st January of the years t and t + 1, then we can estimate λ_x by using the average of these two totals for the number of years lived during the year t by the individuals in the groups:

$$\hat{\lambda}_x = \frac{k_x}{[n_x(t) + n_x(t + 1)]/2} \qquad (1.26)$$

When the cases have been recorded between 1 January of year t and 31 December of year t + h, the sum of the annual average totals (the denominator of (1.26)) can be used to estimate the years lived for the period (see also page 27).

Statistical concepts in survival analysis

Follow-up studies

In the preceding section, basic principles for the analysis of event occurrence in the presence of censoring were discussed. These principles were illustrated by the examples of incidence or mortality where time is explicitly accounted for only in the form of age. In this context, the observation of a large number of individuals over a short period is the basis for the analysis, but it could also involve a cohort in which the individual follow-up extends over several decades; therefore the ageing of the individuals is the principal factor which modifies the instantaneous rate of occurrence of the event under study. In survival studies, on the other hand, the rate is suddenly modified by the occurrence of the disease and tends to return to normal as the time since diagnosis increases; age becomes simply a covariable which can if necessary be taken into account in comparisons of the survival of several groups. Despite the similarities of the underlying principles, each of these situations has generated its own terminology and sometimes requires specific approaches; those used in the framework of survival studies will be reviewed below.

There are three fundamental notions on which the calculation of survival depends. The first is the *group* (or *cohort*), defined by a common event whose date marks the beginning of the observation period. In the context of cancer epidemiology, this date is usually the time when the risk of death is considered to be increased by the existence of the tumour, that is, the date of diagnosis. In clinical trials, as a general rule the point chosen is the date of randomization when the force of mortality should start to decrease as a result of treatment.

The second notion is the *follow-up* of each of the individuals in the cohort, from the date of the common event which defines the cohort; this procedure enables the status (living or deceased) of cohort members to be ascertained. It ensures in particular that those for whom death has not been notified are still living and under observation.

Finally, we require the *follow-up time* of each subject, defined as the time between the date of the common event characterizing the cohort and the date at which observation ends (the variable T of page 12). There are three ways in which observation of a subject ceases: by *death*; by the subject's being *lost to follow-up*, in which case the end of observation is considered to be the date of the last information on vital status; and by *withdrawal* from the follow-up of patients who have been diagnosed recently and therefore have a duration of observation shorter than the maximum time for which survival probability will be calculated.

Any observation that terminates by death is a *complete observation*. All others are *censored observations*. Two further terms will be defined. A *closed group* consists of a group of individuals in which there are only complete observations. An *open group* is a group where observations may be incomplete. In practice, it is rare to find a closed group except in the artificial situation of the construction of a life table. In most real situations, the group is open because there are subjects either lost to follow-up or withdrawn from follow-up.

When only one cause of mortality is taken into consideration, the group should also be treated as an open group. Observations which are interrupted by death from other causes can in fact be considered, under certain conditions, in the same way as other censored observations.

A further possibility which would imply an open group is the entry into the study of subjects subsequent to the occurrence of the disease which characterizes the cohort. Such patients are by definition those who have survived at least up to their date of entry; their inclusion in the cohort would clearly lead to an overestimation of survival if this possible bias is not appropriately taken into consideration. In fact, the situation of a study cohort that accepts such subjects after the original group has been defined is rather uncommon and will not be considered further here.

In Chapter 4, we will discuss in detail different methods of follow-up which are being used at present in cancer registries.

Survival probability

If the group is closed, survival at time-point t can be calculated directly by the ratio between the total number of living subjects at time-point t and the original number of subjects, that is, n_t/n_0. In this context, the probability of survival has been termed *direct survival probability*. In this situation, survival can be estimated by the above ratio, and the statistical precision of this estimate can be assessed by noting that the numerator n_t obeys a binomial probability distribution law with index n_0, size of the cohort, and parameter $S(t)$, survival probability at time t.

In practice, as previously explained, it is rare to find a closed group for several reasons. Diagnoses occur gradually over time and information brought to the study by cases which recently join the study is useful. Alternatively, there may be a number of subjects lost to the study whose observations could contribute to the final analysis. In these circumstances, survival probability can only be properly estimated by utilizing the idea of instantaneous rate. An alternative approach, especially appropriate in dealing with discrete data, is based on the concept of conditional probabilities of death.

If $s(t)$ is the conditional probability that the subject is living at date $t + \Delta t$, given that he or she was living at t, then the probability that this subject is living at date $t + \Delta t$ is

$$S(t + \Delta t) = S(t)\, s(t) \tag{1.27}$$

Therefore, the calculation of survival depends on dividing the observation time into successive intervals $(0, t_1, t_2 ... t_k)$, and on making a separate calculation of the conditional probabilities $s(t_i)$ for each one of them.

If we know for each interval $[t_j, t_{j+1}]$ the number of subjects n_{t_j} who are at risk at the beginning of the interval t_j, as well as the number of deaths d_{t_j} occurring in the interval, we can estimate the values of $s(t_j)$ by $1 - d_{t_j}/n_{t_j}$, and, from them, we can deduce $S(t_{j+1})$ for successive intervals. Thus the probability of surviving until the end of the ith interval is

$$S(t_i) = \prod_{j=0}^{i-1} s(t_j) \tag{1.28}$$

with $t_0 = 0$.

The actuarial method and the Kaplan-Meier method described in detail in Chapter 4 are both based on this principle. These two methods actually differ only in the definition of the intervals used for calculating $s(t_j)$. The choice of intervals is linked to the assumption that we make about the instantaneous death rate. For the actuarial method, we assume that the instantaneous rate is constant in the intervals which are defined *a priori*; in the second situation, no assumption is made about the instantaneous rate, which leads us to assume that it is zero in the interval between two deaths; the dates of death are then the end-points of the intervals (Kaplan-Meier method).

Suppose that λ is constant in the interval $(t, t + \Delta t)$ and that d_t deaths have been observed among n_t subjects under observation at time t. Then the estimate of the instantaneous rate is $\hat{\lambda} = \dfrac{d_t}{m_t}$ where m_t is the number of person-years of survival of the n_t subjects in the interval (see (1.24)). If we assume that d_t deceased individuals and r_t subjects with censored observations had been living on average for half of the interval, the estimate of λ is

$$\hat{\lambda} = \frac{d_t}{\Delta t \left(n_t - \dfrac{r_t}{2} - \dfrac{d_t}{2} \right)} = \frac{d_t}{\Delta t \left(N_t - \dfrac{d_t}{2} \right)} \tag{1.29}$$

where

$$N_t = n_t - \frac{r_t}{2} \tag{1.30}$$

Therefore, we make the calculation as if N_t subjects were at risk at the beginning of the interval and that d_t deaths were observed among them. The probability of death is then

$$\hat{q}_t = \frac{d_t}{N_t} = \frac{2\hat{\lambda}\Delta t}{2 + \hat{\lambda}\Delta t} \tag{1.31}$$

The above formula (1.31) which links rate and probability has been used in the context of the construction of the life table (see page 26). The assumption that $\lambda(t) = \lambda$ remains constant in the interval should in fact imply

$$\hat{q}_t = 1 - e^{-\hat{\lambda}\Delta t} \tag{1.32}$$

The expressions (1.31) and (1.32) differ only by a term of the order of $(\Delta t)^2$, which is usually negligible.

In the actuarial method, it is the number N_t (*effective number at risk*), which is used as the denominator to calculate the probability of death. Therefore, the survival probability is calculated at the end of each interval by the formula

$$S(t + \Delta t) = S(t) \left(1 - \frac{d_t}{n_t - \dfrac{r_t}{2}} \right) = S(t) \frac{N_t - d_t}{N_t} \tag{1.33}$$

and, furthermore, by using the approximation

$$S(u) = S(t)\left(1 - \hat{\lambda}\, \frac{u-t}{\Delta t} \right)$$

in each interval, the function is linear between t and t + Δt.

The Kaplan-Meier method is much simpler as no assumption is made about λ; the dates of death are now the only information available to estimate the survival probability and it cannot be excluded that λ is zero in the interval between two deaths. Accordingly, survival probability is estimated as constant between two deaths. In other words, if all the dates of death are distinct and if t_i and t_{i+1} are the dates of two successive deaths, survival probability just after t_{i+1} is

$$S(t_{i+1}) = S(t_i)\left(1 - \frac{1}{n_{i+1}} \right) \tag{1.34}$$

where $n_{i+1} = n_i - 1 - r_i$ is the number of subjects remaining under observation just before t_{i+1} if r_i observations are censored between t_i and t_{i+1} (inclusive); function S is now constant between t_i and t_{i+1} and changes its value at the time of each death. Furthermore, it can be shown that S is the maximum likelihood estimate of theoretical survival. In practice, if several deaths occur on the same date, we use the formula

$$S(t_{i+1}) = S(t_i)\left(1 - \frac{d_{i+1}}{n_{i+1}} \right) \tag{1.35}$$

where d_{i+1} is the number of deaths observed on date t_{i+1}, and $n_{i+1} = n_i - d_i - r_i$. When censoring and death occur at the same time, it is considered that death occurs first; in other words, the censored observations at time t_{i+1} are counted in the denominator n_{i+1}.

Note that, in the actuarial method, the exact dates of death or loss to follow-up are not necessarily needed in the calculation; in fact, it is sufficient to know the subjects' status at the limits of the intervals. In the Kaplan-Meier method, the date of each death needs to be known but not the dates when subjects are censored, as only the number of censored observations between two deaths plays a role in the calculation.

Theoretically, the actuarial method could be improved if the exact dates of death and censoring were known; this information would enable the exact computation of the person-years of observation m_j in each interval $[t_j, t_{j+1}]$ to be carried out. If the death rate is constant in each interval and if Δt_j is the length of the interval $[t_j, t_{j+1}]$, survival would be estimated by the function

$$S(t) = e^{-\left[\sum_{j<i} \frac{d_j}{m_j}\Delta t_j + \frac{d_i}{m_i}(t-t_i) \right]} \qquad t_i < t < t_{i+1} \tag{1.36}$$

The argument of the exponential is the estimate of the cumulative rate, which we defined above (see page 13); each d_j/m_j is the estimate of the instantaneous rate in the interval $[t_j, t_{j+1}]$.

If d_j is the number of deaths from a given cause, all the methods estimate the net probability of survival from this cause, to the extent that risks which are related to other causes are independent. In practice, the possibility of estimating this probability presents several problems which will be discussed in Chapter 4; in particular, in the situation which arises when we are interested in deaths due to the disease under study among individuals diagnosed with the disease. The related concept of competing risk will be discussed on page 34 after we have introduced the necessary tools to construct a life table for a given population and discussed a few classical models for survival distributions (see page 29).

The life table

The *life table* is an example of calculating survival in a closed group. It describes, for each sex, the survival of a fictitious cohort of new-borns from one birthday to the next up until the complete extinction of the group, under the hypothesis that it is subject to the force of mortality of the population for which the table is constructed. As only one risk is operating, the group is closed, that is, subjects cannot leave the group for other reasons (such as departures or loss to follow-up); likewise, the group is closed to new entries (new arrivals) and the total number of subjects at each birthday is consequently the same as the number of surviving subjects at the preceding birthday minus the deaths which have occurred between the two birthdays.

The construction of the table is based on mortality rates by age; the rates are calculated from counts of deaths and census results, which explains why most of the tables refer to a period around the census date. The annual mortality rate is in fact often calculated over several calendar years in order to avoid large random fluctuations.

The table is built from a fictitious cohort whose initial total membership is arbitrarily fixed at 100 000 or 10 000 individuals (the radix of the table); it gives the number of surviving individuals at each birthday until a terminal age w at which, by convention, all members of the cohort have died (i.e., the number of cohort survivors at age w + 1 is zero).

The following terms, referred to as biometric functions, describe the principal information which is tabulated on a life table (see Appendix 1)

• x (column 1) indicates the beginning of the age interval, that is, birth and then successive birthdays. For most tables, x is used for males and y for females.

• $\hat{q}_x$ (column 2) is the proportion of individuals who die during the interval out of those who were living at the beginning of this interval. This proportion is the estimate of the probability of dying in the interval; it is obtained from vital statistics as described in (1.42). In the Swiss table given in Appendix 1, $\hat{q}_{25} = 0.001532$ is the proportion of those who died between their 25th and 26th birthdays.

- The quantity $\hat{p}_x = 1 - \hat{q}_x$ is the estimate of the conditional probability of survival between x and x + 1 given that the subject was alive at age x (column 3).
- $\hat{\lambda}_x$ (column 4) is the estimate of the mortality rate (see page 12).
- ℓ_x (column 5) is the number of survivors at the xth birthday, when the mortality at each age is defined by the series q_x. The series ℓ_x is called the *survivor function*. For example, the cohort of 100 000 births still includes $\ell_{25} = 97\,155$ survivors at the 25th birthday; the probability of survival which corresponds to this age is equal to 0.97155. As the group is closed, the probability of survival between x and x + h is given by the ratio of the number of survivors at these two birthdays:

$$\hat{p}_{x,h} = \frac{\ell_{x+h}}{\ell_x} \tag{1.37}$$

- L_x (which is not shown in the Table in Appendix 1) denotes the total number of years lived by the members of the cohort between x and x + 1 (the person-years), taking account of the fraction of years lived by those who died between the two birthdays. If the ages at death are spread uniformly over the interval, it may be written

$$L_x = \ell_x - \frac{1}{2} d_x = \frac{(\ell_x + \ell_{x+1})}{2} \tag{1.38}$$

showing that L_x is equal to the average number of individuals of age x.

- d_x (column 6) is the number of deaths which occurred in the cohort between age x and age x + 1.
- $\overset{o}{e}_x$ (column 7) is the life expectancy (or average number of remaining years of life) at the beginning of each age interval, that is, at each birthday x. (The ^{o} symbol above e indicates that deaths occurring at age x did not take place on the day of the xth birthday but, on average, between birthdays). Life expectancy is calculated by adding the remaining years of life of the ℓ_x survivors up to the terminal age of the table (age w) and by dividing this total by ℓ_x:

$$\overset{o}{e}_x = \frac{L_x + L_{x+1} + L_{x+2} + \ldots + L_w}{\ell_x} \tag{1.39}$$

From formula (1.38), we obtain

$$\overset{o}{e}_x = \frac{1}{\ell_x} \sum_{t=x}^{w} \frac{\ell_t + \ell_{t+1}}{2} = \frac{1}{\ell_x} \sum_{t=x}^{w} \ell_t - \frac{1}{2} = e_x - \frac{1}{2} \tag{1.40}$$

where e_x is obtained directly from the survivor function ℓ_x.

From the table in Appendix 1, the life expectancy on the day of the 25th birthday is

$$\overset{o}{e}_{25} = 49.28 \text{ years}$$

From the preceding definitions, the estimate of the mortality rate at age x is

$$\hat{\lambda}_x = \frac{d_x}{L_x} = \frac{2d_x}{\ell_x + \ell_{x+1}} = \frac{2\hat{q}_x}{2 - \hat{q}_x} \qquad (1.41)$$

The equation is classically used to pass from the annual observed mortality rate to the annual probability of death on which the table is based. However, some authors prefer to calculate the annual probability of death directly without first estimating λ_x. This latter parameter is in fact obtained from $\hat{q}_x$ using (1.41).[2] In this approach, the estimate of $\hat{q}_x$ is obtained by dividing the number of deaths at age x observed in a given birth cohort by the number of persons at risk at the beginning of year t.

$$\hat{q}_x = \frac{d'_t + d''_{t+1}}{n_x(t + 1) + d'_t} \qquad (1.42)$$

Figure 1.5 presents the various elements required to calculate the annual probability of death on a Lexis diagram where d'_t is the number of deaths which have taken place in year t, and d''_{t+1} is the number of deaths which have taken place in year t + 1 in a cohort whose members have their xth birthday in year t; $n_x(t + 1)$ is the number of persons of age x in the population alive on 1 January of year t + 1.

In published tables, probabilities of death are usually smoothed, by using various analytical and graphical procedures, in order to attenuate the effect of random fluctuation [12].

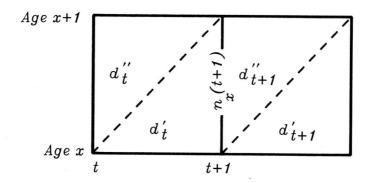

Figure 1.5   Representation of the data needed for the calculation of the annual probability of death on a Lexis diagram

---

[2] In the life table provided in Appendix 1, this formula gives a result which is correct only up to the first two decimal places as the published results have been smoothed.

National or regional tables made by statistical bureaux consider mortality over a short period of time (current life table), that is, as it is observed at a given time (or over one short period) across a range of ages. Mortality at various ages is estimated from different birth cohorts and the table which is constructed in this way thus refers to a fictitious force of mortality made up of the mortality experience of several successive birth cohorts. Cohort life tables can sometimes be constructed retrospectively; they describe the actual mortality experience for successive ages of a given birth cohort by combining the mortality information from several censuses. In the calculation of expected survival of a cohort which is followed for a relatively long time, the change of mortality of the general population must be taken into consideration. It is then advisable to apply the proper mortality rate to the different cohorts instead of using the cross-sectional force of mortality.

Classical models for survival distribution

It was seen on page that a survival distribution may be completely specified by the instantaneous mortality rate. There are several families of distributions which have played an important role in medical applications and whose definition depends on a parametric expression of $\lambda(t)$. Two of these families lead to a simple expression for the survival distribution $S(t)$:

- The Weibull distribution, for which

$$\lambda(t \; ; \; \alpha, \theta) = \theta\alpha \, (\theta t)^{\alpha - 1}$$

$$S(t \; ; \; \alpha, \theta) = e^{-(\theta t)^{\alpha}} \tag{1.43}$$

- The log-logistic distribution for which

$$\lambda(t \; ; \; \alpha, \theta) = \frac{\theta\alpha(\theta t)^{\alpha - 1}}{1 + (\theta t)^{\alpha}}$$

$$S(t \; ; \; \alpha, \theta) = \frac{1}{1 + (\theta t)^{\alpha}} \tag{1.44}$$

It is simple to estimate the parameters θ and α that define respectively the scale and the shape of the survival distribution by using the maximum likelihood method. The log-likelihood may be written

$$L(\alpha, \theta) = \sum_{i=1}^{n} \text{Log} \, [S(t_i \; ; \; \alpha, \theta)] + \sum_{i=1}^{n} \delta_i \, \text{Log} \, [\, \lambda(t_i \; ; \; \alpha, \theta)] \tag{1.45}$$

Note that the exponential distribution discussed on page 16 is a particular case of the Weibull distribution with $\alpha = 1$. In fact, $\lambda(t;1,\theta) = \theta$ and $S(t) = e^{-\theta t}$. The Weibull hazard rate may also be used to describe cancer incidence rate and could in particular be used in the framework of the multistage theory of carcinogenesis. In this context, α would be the number of stages needed for a cell to become malignant. The Weibull distribution is in fact the paradigmatic survival distribution and the starting point for the definition of more complex models which include prognostic factors $z = (z_1,... z_p)$.

First, by writing $\mu = -Log(\theta)$ and $\sigma = 1/\alpha$, it can be shown that the logarithm of survival duration $Y = Log(T)$ is $\mu + \sigma W$, where W has the same distribution as the minimum of a sample of continuous variables (extreme value distribution [13]). An analogous property holds for the log-logistic distribution, with W having in this case a distribution defined by the logistic probability density $e^W/(1 + e^W)^2$. A natural extension is to model the expectation μ of $Log(T)$ with a linear function of the prognostic factors z ($\mu = \beta z$). This model supposes that the factors z act on survival by multiplying (or dividing) the mean duration of survival by a constant ($e^{\beta z}$).

A second approach more commonly used in medical applications starts from the observation that the hazard rates defined by the Weibull family are proportional. Writing $\mu = \theta^\alpha$, the hazard rate of the Weibull distribution becomes

$$\lambda(t) = \mu\alpha t^{\alpha-1}.$$

Considering that each prognostic factor acts on the instantaneous rate by multiplying (or dividing) it by a constant ($\mu = e^{\beta z}$), we obtain an example of a proportional rates model $\lambda(t) = \alpha t^{\alpha-1} e^{\beta z}$. The most general model of this class is the Cox model [14] defined by the relation

$$\lambda(t , z) = \lambda_0(t) \, e^{\beta z} \qquad (1.46)$$

where $\lambda_0(t)$ is left unspecified.

Estimation of the parameter vector β in the model (1.46) is made difficult by the presence in its equation of the arbitrary function $\lambda_0(t)$. The likelihood of the observations given by formula (1.22) depends explicitly on λ_0 and is impossible to maximize without parameterizing $\lambda_0(t)$. However, as one of the goals of the Cox method is to specifically avoid such a parametric distribution, this approach would not be satisfactory. Full mathematical development of the likelihood function under the Cox model is beyond the scope of this text. It is however useful to understand the principles underlying its development in simple situations. In the framework of this model, only the ranks of the observed survival times are informative for the estimation of β: as the rate $\lambda_0(t)$ is *a priori* an arbitrary function, it could be zero between two deaths. Another set of values of survival times with the same rank order should provide the same estimate of β. More precisely, it is simple to check that a change in time scale defined by a monotonic function $\tau = u^{-1}(t)$ would give survival time τ_i with a distribution specified by the same model. The background hazard rate would simply be replaced by $\lambda_0[u(\tau)u'(\tau)]$. As a result, the estimate of β will be the vector of numerical values which maximize the probability that the ranks of the survival time are as observed.

Consider first two complete observations t_1 and t_2 for which **z** equals **u** and **v** respectively. The probability that the death of the subject having covariate value **u** comes first is

$$Pr\,(t_1 < t_2) = \frac{e^{\beta u}}{e^{\beta u} + e^{\beta v}} \qquad (1.47)$$

This intuitive result can be checked from the joint probability distribution of t_1, t_2. This principle may be generalized easily to m complete observations. If $u_i \ldots u_m$ are the values of **z** for the $m - i + 1$ subjects still alive just before the ith death, the probability that the death of the subject with covariate value u_i comes first is given by

$$\frac{e^{\beta u_i}}{e^{\beta u_i} + \ldots + e^{\beta u_m}}$$

The extension of this approach to n observations among which $n - m$ are censored leads to the likelihood

$$V(\beta) = Pr[(t_1 < \ldots < t_m) \text{ and } (t_i < \text{censored observations in } t_i, t_{i+1}\,;\, 1 \le i \le m)]$$

that is

$$V(\beta) = \prod_{i=1}^{m} \frac{e^{\beta u_i}}{\sum_{j \in R_i} e^{\beta u_j}} \qquad (1.48)$$

where
- i indexes the m dates of death t_i ranked in increasing order;
- u_i is the covariate value of the subject who died at time t_i; and
- R_i is the set of subjects still at risk at time t_i of the ith death.

The log-likelihood is

$$L(\beta) = Log\,[V(\beta)] = \sum_{i=1}^{m} \left\{ \beta u_i - Log\left[\sum_{j \in R_i} e^{\beta u_j} \right] \right\} \qquad (1.49)$$

The estimate of β is the value $\hat{\beta}$ which maximizes $L(\beta)$, obtained by equating to zero its derivatives with respect to the coordinates β_k of β:

$$C_k(\beta) = \frac{\partial L(\beta)}{\partial \beta_k} = \sum_{i=1}^{m} [u_{ki} - \bar{u}_{ki}\,(\beta)] \qquad (1.50)$$

where

$$\bar{u}_{ki}\,(\beta) = \frac{\sum_{j \in R_i} u_{kj}\, e^{\beta u_j}}{\sum_{j \in R_i} e^{\beta u_j}} \qquad (1.51)$$

is the average of the covariate values of the subjects still at risk just before time t_i weighted by their respective relative rates. C_k is known as the *score function* and is used to construct the *score test* described below.

The observed information matrix having as elements the negative of the second derivatives of the log-likelihood $L(\beta)$ (see page 17)

$$I_{k\ell}(\beta) = -\frac{\partial^2 L(\beta)}{\partial \beta_k \partial \beta_\ell} = \sum_{i=1}^{m} \iota_{k\ell i}(\beta) \tag{1.52}$$

where

$$\iota_{k\ell i}(\beta) = \frac{\sum\limits_{j \in R_i} u_{ki} u_{\ell i} e^{\beta u_j}}{\sum\limits_{j \in R_i} e^{\beta u_j}} - \bar{u}_{ki}(\beta) \, \bar{u}_{\ell i}(\beta) \tag{1.53}$$

will be used to carry out the maximization using the Newton-Raphson method. This algorithm constructs a sequence of β values which lead by successive iterations to the value $\hat{\beta}$ where $C(\beta) = 0$:

$$\beta_0 = 0 \; ; \quad \beta_n = \beta_{n-1} + I^{-1}(\beta_{n-1}) \, C(\beta_{n-1})$$

This method is used by most computer programs, which estimate the Cox model. The inverse of the observed information matrix $I^{-1}(\hat{\beta})$ provides an estimate of the covariance matrix of the maximum likelihood estimates of the parameter vector β.

The application of these principles leads to unmanageable formulae when the number of deaths d_i occurring at time t_i exceeds more than a few. The likelihood may then be approximated [15] by

$$V(\beta) = \prod_{i=1}^{m} \frac{e^{\beta s_i}}{\left(\sum\limits_{j \in R_i} e^{\beta u_j} \right)^{d_i}} \tag{1.54}$$

where :

$$s_i = \sum_{j=1}^{d_i} u_j \tag{1.55}$$

is the sum of the covariate values of the d_i subjects dying at date t_i. Expressions (1.49) (1.50) and (1.52) then become

$$L(\beta) = \sum_{i=1}^{m} \left[\beta s_i - d_i \, Log \left(\sum_{j \in R_i} e^{\beta u_j} \right) \right] \tag{1.56}$$

$$C_k(\boldsymbol{\beta}) = \sum_{i=1}^{m} [s_{ki} - d_i \, \bar{u}_{ki}(\boldsymbol{\beta})] \tag{1.57}$$

$$I_{k\ell}(\boldsymbol{\beta}) = \sum_{i=1}^{m} d_i \, \iota_{k\ell i}(\boldsymbol{\beta}) \tag{1.58}$$

It is worth noting that the above approximation may be obtained directly from the assumption that the hazard function is constant within intervals, as is the case with the actuarial method. The estimation of the nuisance parameters λ_i, $1 \le i \le m$ and their substitution in the likelihood lead to (1.54) [16].

Several tests for comparison of survival distributions may then be obtained from the likelihood or from the score function [17]. The practical aspects of these methods are described in detail in Chapter 4. Here, we simply note that the test of the hypothesis $\boldsymbol{\beta} = 0$ by the *likelihood ratio test* is based on the statistic

$$T_1 = 2[L(\hat{\boldsymbol{\beta}}) - L(0)] \tag{1.59}$$

which has a χ^2 distribution with r degrees of freedom, dimension of $\boldsymbol{\beta}$, under the null hypothesis $\boldsymbol{\beta} = 0$. The *score test* is based on the evaluation of the score function at $\boldsymbol{\beta} = 0$ which should be close to zero under the null hypothesis since, at the true value of $\boldsymbol{\beta}$, the derivative of L should be close to zero, its value at the maximum likelihood estimate. After standardization by its variance, the score statistic is written

$$T_2 = \mathbf{C}(0)' \, \boldsymbol{\Gamma}^{-1} \, \mathbf{C}(0) \tag{1.60}$$

and also has a χ^2 distribution with r degrees of freedom under the null hypothesis. The *Wald test* is based on the evaluation of $\hat{\boldsymbol{\beta}}$ itself which should be close to zero under the null hypothesis. After standardization by its variance, we obtain the statistic

$$T_3 = \hat{\boldsymbol{\beta}} \, \mathbf{I} \, \hat{\boldsymbol{\beta}}' \tag{1.61}$$

which also has the χ^2 distribution with r degrees of freedom under the null hypothesis.

Similar tests exist when the null hypothesis does not completely specify the value of $\boldsymbol{\beta}$. In this context the null hypothesis is usually defined by one or several constraints on the coordinates of $\boldsymbol{\beta}$ (e.g., $\beta_i = 0$). T_1 and T_2 are then calculated by replacing zero in (1.59) and (1.60) by the maximum likelihood estimate of $\boldsymbol{\beta}$ under the null hypothesis. When the null hypothesis specifies that some coordinates of $\boldsymbol{\beta}$ are zero, this approach is equivalent to setting the other coordinates to their maximum likelihood estimates under the null hypothesis. In this case, the test T_3 is restricted to the coordinates being tested. The number of degrees of freedom of these three tests is equal to the number of coordinates of $\boldsymbol{\beta}$ which specify the null hypothesis. Applications of this methodology are presented in Chapter 4, page 268.

In the preceding discussion, we have concentrated on the properties of the proportional hazards model which enable group comparisons to be carried out. In other words, the problem of estimating β has been seen as more important by considering λ_0 as a nuisance function. In practice, it is often necessary to provide an estimate of the survival distribution for some given value of the covariate z. The same principle as used previously for the Kaplan-Meier procedure (1.34) may be used here, taking into account the fact that the subjects are not at the same risk of death at the time when one of them dies. For a subject with covariate z_j, this risk is characterized by the relative rate of mortality $\hat{\theta}_j = e^{\hat{\beta} z_j}$ where $\hat{\beta}$ is the maximum likelihood estimate of β. Thus, in estimating $\lambda_0(t_i)$, each subject at risk at that time will account for θ_j units instead of one. Therefore the cumulative rate and survival distribution will be given by:

$$\hat{\Lambda}_0(t) = \sum_{t_i \le t} \frac{d_i}{\sum_{j \in R_i} e^{\hat{\beta} z_j}} \tag{1.62}$$

$$\hat{S}_0(t) = \prod_{t_i \le t} \left(1 - \frac{d_i}{\sum_{j \in R_i} e^{\hat{\beta} z_j}} \right) \tag{1.63}$$

The estimate of the survival distribution for a given value of z is then obtained from the fact that the hazard rates are proportional. Therefore

$$\hat{S}(t, z) = \hat{S}_0(t)^{e^{\hat{\beta} z}} \tag{1.64}$$

Interactive risks

Competing risks

We can see from the preceding sections that it is relatively simple to estimate the distribution of survival times while taking account of information provided by incomplete or censored observations. The method which has been discussed depends on the assumption of independence between risk of death and the mechanism which leads to censored observations. In Chapter 4, we will discuss situations in which this assumption can be questioned, most notably when not all the members of the cohort are followed up in the same way. However, the assumption is usually quite reasonable. In fact, the survival time which corresponds to a withdrawal is clearly defined. It could be observed by prolonging the study; it would then be possible to check statistically that censored observations are not associated with either longer or shorter survival times, or equivalently, that survival does not change with time of diagnosis.

The problem presents itself in different terms when our aim is no longer to measure overall mortality but to establish the impact of a specific cause of death, usually corresponding to the diagnosis by which the cohort is defined. Therefore, we should consider that the individuals under observation are subject to other risks of death besides the one which forms the basis of the study. Since the realization of one of the risks excludes the possibility of the realization of the others, the risks are then said to be *competing*. It is tempting to consider deaths due to other causes as censored observations; survival related to the cause under study could then be estimated by simply using the method described earlier. Discussion of the practical problems raised by this approach will be left until Chapter 4; in this section we will treat succinctly the theoretical aspects of competing risks and problems raised by the definition and especially by the evaluation of the independence of risks.

The crude probability of death from a given cause is the probability of death from this cause in the presence of other risks.

The net probability is the probability of death from the given cause when all other risks of death have been eliminated.

The partial crude probability is defined as the probability of death from a given cause when the potential effects of another cause (or group of causes) are eliminated.

The third concept is obviously crucial to competing risk theory. Its recognition probably goes back to the controversy over the efficiency of the smallpox vaccination; in 1760, Bernouilli [18], d'Alembert [19] and other authors were each attempting to evaluate the consequences of eliminating the risk of death from smallpox on the composition and life expectancy of the population. Today, it is relatively straightforward to construct life tables based on probabilities of death after a cause has been eliminated, in order to estimate the cause's impact on life expectancy [20]. For example, it has been calculated that, if mortality from cancer (all sites combined) was totally eliminated, the consequent lengthening of the expectation of life would be about two years. However, these statistics only tell part of the truth: the improvement in survival for patients who suffer from the disease is much more significant both qualitatively and quantitatively. Our goal is to define the survival probability as a measure of the consequence of a specific disease. This concept corresponds better to the net probability, that is, the survival probability from cancer in the absence of mortality from other causes.

The data which are generally available for the study of mortality by cause can be summarized by the three variables T, Δ and z, where T is survival time, Δ the indicator of the cause and z the vector of covariables which influence the risk of death. Δ varies between 1 and m + 1 when m causes of death are studied and the number m + 1 indicates withdrawals other than those due to death. If the withdrawals are independent of death, the same argument that was used on page 19 shows that the contribution of observation t_i, z_i of subject i to the likelihood may be written

- $\lambda_j(t_i, z_i)$ $S(t_i, z_i)$ if death resulted from the jth cause,
- $S(t_i, z_i)$ if the observation is censored at t_i,

where

$$S(t_i, z_i) = e^{-\sum_{i=1}^{m} \Lambda_j(t_i, z_i)}$$

formulae in which λ_j and Λ_j are the instantaneous and cumulative rates of death for the jth cause. The likelihood is thus a product of m terms of the form

$$\prod_{j=1}^{m} \left[\prod_{i=1}^{n} \lambda_j(t_i, z_i)^{\delta_j} e^{-\Lambda_j(t_i, z_i)} \right]$$

where $\delta_j = 1$ if death results from the jth cause ($\Delta = j$) and $\delta_j = 0$ otherwise ($\Delta \neq j$); each of these terms represents the likelihood which would be obtained in the study of the jth cause of death if all deaths from other causes could be considered to be independent censored observations.

From this discussion it is clear that the methods previously described for estimating λ and assessing the effect of covariates z on mortality are appropriate in the presence of competing risks. It is also clear that they are describing a particular risk of mortality within a complex of risk interactions, rather than the risk that would prevail if one or several causes of mortality were eliminated. It was previously stated that it is generally valid to assume that the instantaneous rate of death observed in the presence of censored observations is that which would prevail if the censored observations were eliminated (or completed). However, this assumption may well be questionable when a specific cause of death is being studied in the presence of other risks of death. Indeed, it is very likely that the removal of one cause of death would have noticeable consequences for the risk of death from one or several other causes. We should remember that some individuals can be subject to increased risk of death from several diseases, either because the diseases have similar etiology or because they are linked to the same innate susceptibility. When one of these diseases tends to occur earlier in life or to be associated with a shorter survival probability, it will more often be the cause of death. Any action taken to eliminate one disease or to reduce its associated mortality will tend, therefore, to modify the instantaneous mortality rate of associated competing diseases. For example, it has been suggested that coal miners who survived pneumoconiosis were subject to a reduced risk of lung cancer, as a result of the selection of the most resistant. If this assumption is true, an improvement in the treatment for pneumoconiosis resulting in better survival could lead to an increase in the lung cancer mortality rate. On the other hand, a measure aimed at reducing exposure to coal dusts might result in a decrease in the two risks under consideration.

This example shows that the probabilities of death that are calculated in a given context of risk interaction need not correspond to the instantaneous rates which would prevail if other causes of death were eliminated; it also shows that the direction of the interaction between risks can be modified by the intervention used on one of the risks.

In practice, the existence of a statistical link between competing risks is difficult to identify, and the strength of a link is hard to measure. Independence of risks cannot be verified simply from survival data, since, by definition, the occurrence of death from cause j excludes the possibility of death from all other causes. In fact, data of the type (T, Δ, z) do not contain the information necessary to assess risk interaction. Moreover, it has been shown that, for a given set of such observations, a compatible model of independent risks can always be constructed [21-23]. Some empirical models have been proposed to assess the interaction between risks of death using additional information such as concomitant causes of death [24]. It is however possible that the concomitant causes of death have a direct link with the disease primarily responsible for death or are a consequence of its diagnosis or treatment. In such a situation, information on concomitant causes is of little use in assessing risk dependence and may even lead to a biased evaluation. So far, these models have not proved to be usable. By definition, there is absolutely no information which could allow the correct estimation of the joint distribution of potential survival times for multiple causes. Consequently, the formal specification of this joint distribution cannot be verified and is therefore of little practical value.

For lack of a better alternative, we therefore restrict our discussion to the net probabilities of mortality (and consequently the net survival) with respect to a given environment of risks, while remaining aware of the limitations in their interpretation (see Chapter 4). These difficulties probably explain why life tables routinely published by official statistical services only rarely present net probabilities, and generally restrict themselves to crude probabilities by cause or group of causes.

Relationship between incidence, mortality, survival and prevalence

The most widely available information describing the risk of cancer as a function of space and time are age- and sex-specific mortality statistics. In many countries, these data have been recorded systematically over long time periods for most cancer sites. In some countries, they may even be available for small geographical areas such as census or administrative districts. However, mortality data are frequently of uneven quality and inadequate for the descriptive study of site-specific cancer occurrence.

Information on cancer incidence is provided by the number of new cases of cancer occurring each year, and is generally available from cancer registries. This information is much more reliable than mortality statistics but, except for Nordic countries, it is limited in space and time. Cancer registries may also have information on survival of cancer patients when they have established routine procedures of follow-up (see Chapter 4). Thus, in a region where cancer incidence is recorded, it is possible to estimate the empirical relation which links incidence, mortality and survival and then use this observed relation to estimate cancer incidence in regions where cancer registries do not exist [25-28]. The goal of the present section is to give some insight into the theoretical relationships which link incidence, mortality and survival and to assess the feasibility of estimating one of them from the other two.

This discussion will also introduce the concept of *prevalence*, the number (or proportion) of subjects with a specific condition in a population at a given time. This measure of disease frequency depends on incidence and duration of disease, that is, on survival probability, in the case of a 'non reversible' disease such as cancer, for which an incident case is considered prevalent up to death, even if treatment is effective. In contrast to incidence, which is a concept with a natural link to age and therefore logically described in the context of birth cohorts, prevalence is related to the time period of observation. Incidence is better assessed in a *longitudinal* study, whereas prevalence is measured on a cross-sectional basis. For this reason, the relations between incidence, survival and prevalence are simple only in *stationary* populations in which longitudinal and cross-sectional measures are identical. In this section, the meaning of the term 'stationary' will be explained and the usage of the relationship 'prevalence is the product of incidence and the duration of the disease' will be discussed.

Although it is rarely estimated in cancer registries, prevalence is important to public health planning. When incidence data are not systematically recorded (as for HIV and diabetes), it is often from prevalence surveys that incidence will be estimated.

In order to understand the relationships between these concepts, a fictitious cohort of size ℓ_0 born in year $t = u_0$ and subject to cancer incidence rate λ_y is described in Table 1.4. We assume that the number of years L_y lived without cancer by each individual of the cohort is known for each age y.

In the absence of migration, the number of cancer deaths at age x occurring in year $t = u_0 + x$ among incident cases in the cohort is given by the formula

$$d_x(t) = \sum_{y=0}^{x} L_y \lambda_y \left[S_y \left(x - \frac{1}{2} \right) - S_y \left(x + \frac{1}{2} \right) \right] \tag{1.65}$$

where $S_y(x)$ is the probability that a subject diagnosed at age y survives to age x; $S_y \left(x - \frac{1}{2} \right) - S_y \left(x + \frac{1}{2} \right)$ is then the probability that death occurs at age x. Similarly the cases of age x prevalent in the population during year $t = u_0 + x$ come from the cohort born in year u_0. Their number is given by the formula

$$n_x(t) = \sum_{y=0}^{x} L_y \lambda_y S_y(x) \tag{1.66}$$

which shows that they are calculated from the cases in the cohort diagnosed before age x and still surviving at age x.

Table 1.4   Incident cases, deaths and prevalent cases

Age	Time period					
	$t = u_0$	$t = u_0 + 1$	....	$t = u_0 + y$	....	$t = u_0 + x$
0	$L_0\ \lambda_0$					
1	....	$L_1\ \lambda_1$				
.						
.						
.						
y	....	....	....	$L_y\ \lambda_y$	....	$k_y(t),\ d_y(t),\ n_y(t)$
.						
.						
.						
x	....	....	....	....	....	$k_x(t) = L_x\lambda_x,\ d_x(t),\ n_x(t)$

If ℓ_0 is equal to 100 000, the figures are obtained per 100 000 births in year u_0. The numbers of deaths and cases (incident or prevalent) actually observed are obtained by multiplying the figures in Table 1.4 by the actual number of births $B(u_0)$ in year u_0.

The figures in column $u_0 + x$ of Table 1.4 are generated by successive birth cohorts and depend on factors which change with time, either period– or cohort-wise. Most often, survival probability changes with period, whereas age-specific incidence depends substantially on birth cohort. Each line in column $u_0 + x$ must therefore be calculated from the parameters L_y, λ_y and $S_y(x)$ by taking their evolution over time into account.

The prevalence at age x or *age-specific prevalence* is the proportion $p_x(t) = \dfrac{n_x(t)}{\ell_x(t)}$ where $\ell_x(t)$ is the number of survivors at time t among the individuals of the cohort born in u_0. This figure depends only on the risk environment experienced by this cohort up to age x while the overall prevalence depends on the experience of several successive cohorts:

$$p(t) = \frac{\sum_{x=0}^{g} n_x(t)}{\sum_{x=0}^{g} \ell_x(t)} \qquad (1.67)$$

where each term in the above sums is generated by different birth cohorts for each of the g age groups.

A deeper understanding of the relationship linking the survival, incidence and prevalence requires more detailed modelling which involves explicit mathematical definitions. Let

- $\lambda(t,x)$ be the incidence rate at age x and time t for the disease under study,

- $\mu(t,x)$ be the mortality rate at age x from causes other than the disease, for individuals without the disease,

- $v_y(t,x)$ be the mortality rate at age x of patients diagnosed with the disease at age y and time t,

- $\beta(u)$ be the average annual number of births, considered to be a Poisson process and depending on year u.

It is then possible to write formulae similar to (1.65) and (1.66) as well as formulae for the number of individuals with and without a particular health condition living in the population at time t.

The probability of being alive and free of cancer at age x and time t for an individual born in year u = t − x can be written

$$H(t,x) = e\left\{ - \int_0^x [\mu(u+y,y) + \lambda(u+y,y)]\, dy \right\} \tag{1.68}$$

This expression shows that to be alive and without cancer, an individual must escape both the force of cancer incidence and the force of mortality in the interval between birth and age x. Therefore, the number of individuals of age x without cancer at time t is on average

$$h(t,x) = \beta(t-x)\, H(t,x) \tag{1.69}$$

In the same way, the probability that an individual with cancer is alive at age x and time t may be written

$$\pi(t, x) = \int_0^x H(u+y,y)\, \lambda(u+y,y)\, S_y(u+y,x)\, dy \tag{1.70}$$

where :

$$S_y(u+y,x) = e^{-\int_y^x v_y(u+y,z)\, dz} \tag{1.71}$$

is the probability of surviving up to age x when diagnosed at time u+y and age y. The number of individuals of age x who have been diagnosed with the disease in the population is therefore at time t

$$n(t, x) = \beta(t-x)\, \pi(t, x) \tag{1.72}$$

The prevalence p(t), the proportion of individuals with the disease living in the population at time t, is then obtained in a simple way from the ratio of the number of individuals diagnosed with the disease to the number without the disease (prevalence odds). This ratio can be written from (1.69) and (1.72):

$$\frac{p(t)}{1 - p(t)} = \frac{\int_0^\infty \beta(t - x)\, \pi\,(t, x)\, dx}{\int_0^\infty \beta(t - x)\, H(t, x)\, dx} \tag{1.73}$$

In a stationary population where λ, μ and β are all independent of t, the above formulae lead to simple relationships. It is however important to realize how restrictive the stationary hypothesis is; it implies that the birth rate, the cancer incidence rate, the cancer survival probability and mortality rate from other causes all remain constant with time. We will nevertheless give the main results which are obtained under the stationary hypothesis, since most epidemiological textbooks define prevalence in this situation.

In a stationary population, the various rates do not depend on time so that formulae (1.68) and (1.70) simplify to

$$H(x) = e\left\{-\int_0^x [\mu(y) + \lambda(y)]\, dy\right\} \tag{1.74}$$

$$\pi(x) = \int_0^x H(y)\, \lambda(y)\, S_y(x)\, dy \tag{1.75}$$

The integrals of these functions which no longer depend on t are respectively

$$\int_0^\infty H(x)\, dx = E_0(X) \tag{1.76}$$

which is the mean duration of life for individuals who remain without the given disease over their lifetime, since H(x) is their survival distribution. By exchanging the order of integration

$$\int_0^\infty \pi\,(x)\, dx = \int_0^\infty [H(y)\, \lambda(y) \int_y^\infty S_y(x)\, dx]dy \tag{1.77}$$

which is, except for division by $R = \int_0^\infty H(y)\, \lambda(y)\, dy$, the mean duration of disease for those who have contracted it. In other words

$$\int_0^\infty \pi\,(x)\, dx = R\; E_1(X - Y) = R\; E_1(V) \tag{1.78}$$

is the product of the crude risk of disease [see (1.41)] and the mean survival of the patients which, in the case of a 'non-reversible' disease (see above), is the duration of the disease.

Since β is constant, formula (1.73) simplifies to become the ratio of (1.78) and (1.76), that is

$$\frac{p}{1 - p} = \frac{R\, E_1(V)}{E_0(X)} \tag{1.79}$$

Furthermore, the ratio of $R/E_0(X)$ may be written as a function of H and λ, using their respective definitions:

$$\frac{R}{E_0(X)} = \frac{\int_0^\infty H(x)\, \lambda(x)\, dx}{\int_0^\infty H(x)\, dx} = \bar{\lambda} \tag{1.80}$$

This last result leads to the classical statement that 'prevalence is the product of incidence and the duration of the disease' since we can write from (1.79) and (1.80)

$$\frac{p}{1-p} = \bar{\lambda}\, E_1(V) \tag{1.81}$$

The above approach to the concept of prevalence is taken from a paper by Keiding [38]. We will also describe the method of Verdecchia and Capocaccia [39], who showed that under certain conditions the information needed to carry out the various calculations is contained in the net probability distributions of age at the occurrence of cancer and at death from cancer.

Let X, Y and V be respectively the age at death from the disease of interest, the age at diagnosis and the survival time up to death from cancer. We may then write

$$X = Y + V$$

Consequently, the age at death from cancer has the probability density

$$d(x) = \int_0^x i(y)\, s_y(x - y)\, dy \tag{1.82}$$

where i and s_y are the probability densities of Y and V. As explained previously, this function is known only from the corresponding incidence rates because of censoring. (1.82) must therefore be written

$$d(x) = \int_0^x \lambda(y)\, e^{\left\{ -\int_0^y [\lambda(u) + \mu(u)]\, du \right\}} v_y(x - y)\, e^{\left\{ -\int_y^x [v_y(u-y) + \mu_y^*(u)]\, du \right\}} dy \tag{1.83}$$

where

• $v_y(v)$ is the mortality rate from the disease v years after diagnosis for a patient diagnosed at age y; and

• $\mu_y^*(u)$ is the mortality rate from causes other than the disease at age u for a patient diagnosed at age y.

Denoting by $\mu_y^e(x)$ the difference $\mu_y^*(x) - \mu(x)$ which represents the excess death from other causes for a patient diagnosed at age y, we can write

$$d(x) = \int_0^x \lambda(y)\, e^{-\Lambda(y)}\, v_y(x - y)\, e^{\left\{ -\int_y^x [v_y(u-y) + \mu_y^e(u)]\, du \right\}} dy\, e^{-\int_0^x [\mu(y)\, dy]} \tag{1.84}$$

The rate $v_y^*(u - y) = v_y(u - y) + \mu_y^e(u)$ is the mortality rate experienced by patients after diagnosis taking into account the excess (or the reduction) of the hazard of death from other causes. This rate is connected to the relative survival rate (see Chapter 4, page 231), whereas v_y corresponds to net survival. If most deaths of cancer patients are in fact certified as due to cancer, we can replace v_y by v_y^* in (1.84) and obtain

$$\delta(x) \, e^{-D(x)} = \int_0^x \lambda(y) \, e^{-\Lambda (y)} \, v_y^*(x - y) \, e^{[- N_y^* (x- y)]} \, dy \qquad (1.85)$$

where δ is the mortality rate for the given cancer and D, Λ and N* denote the cumulative rates associated respectively with δ, λ and v*. Formula (1.85) results from the fact that $d(x) = \delta(x) \, e^{-M(x)}$ since $M(x) = D(x) + \int_0^x \mu(y) \, dy$ is the cumulative mortality rate from all causes.

The relationship initially given for the crude probability density in (1.82) therefore remains true for net density in (1.85) if net and relative survivals are identical. However, this relationship is only simple when survival probability does not depend on age at diagnosis or depends on it according to a simple model. In this situation, the relationship between mortality, incidence and survival distribution can be written as a convolution and corresponding mathematical tools are available to carry out its analysis.

The probability $\pi(x)$ of having cancer and still being alive at age x may be calculated in the same way. Thus

$$\pi(x) = \int_0^x \lambda(y) \, e^{-\Lambda (y)} \, e^{[-N^*_y(x-y)]} \, dy \, e^{-\int_0^x \mu(y) \, dy} \qquad (1.86)$$

The number of cancer cases of age x in the corresponding birth cohort is $n(x) = B \, \pi(x)$ where B is the number of births in this cohort. Furthermore, the number of survivors without cancer of age x is $h(x) = B \, H(x)$, where $H(x)$ is obtained from (1.74). Therefore the age-specific prevalence is given by

$$\frac{p(x)}{1 - p(x)} = \frac{n(x)}{h(x)} = \frac{\pi_c(x)}{1 - R_i(x)} \qquad (1.87)$$

where $\pi_c(x)$ is the first integral of the right-hand side of formula (1.86) and $R_i(x)$ is the net risk of disease before age x.

Denoting the net probability densities of age at death, age at diagnosis and survival time by d, i and s_y, the following two equations can be written:

$$d(x) = \int_0^x i(y) \, s_y(x - y) \, dy \qquad (1.88)$$

$$\pi_c(x) = \int_0^x i(y) \, S_y(x - y) \, dy \qquad (1.89)$$

The derivative with respect to x of $\pi_c(x)$ is by definition

$$\pi'_c(x) = \lim_{\Delta x \to 0} \frac{1}{\Delta x} [\pi_c (x + \Delta x) - \pi_c (x)]$$

$$= \lim_{\Delta x \to 0} \int_0^x i(y) \frac{S_y(x + \Delta x - y) - S_y(x - y)}{\Delta x} dy + \frac{1}{\Delta x} \int_x^{x + \Delta x} i(y) S_y(x + \Delta x - y) dy$$

which may be written, using the rules of calculus and the fact that the derivative of S_y is $-s_y$:

$$\pi'_c(x) = - \int_0^x i(y) s_y(x - y) dy + i(x)$$

$$= - d(x) + i(x)$$

and therefore

$$\pi_c(x) = \int_0^x i(y) dy - \int_0^x d(y) dy \qquad (1.90)$$

which expresses the fact that the numerator of the prevalence odds in (1.87) is the difference between the net risk of having cancer before age x and the net risk of dying from this cancer before age x. Thus the age-specific prevalence of cancer may be obtained from:

$$\frac{p(x)}{1 - p(x)} = \frac{R_i(x) - R_d(x)}{1 - R_i(x)} \qquad (1.91)$$

where $R_d(x)$ denotes the net risk of dying from the given cancer.

This result is obtained under some fairly general assumptions about the inter-actions between the risk of dying from the given cancer and the risk of dying from other causes. When the cancer risk is not stationary, the formula 1.91 must be used in conjunction with the modelling of the time trend in incidence and mortality by birth cohort (see page 189)

Preston has provided a useful and intuitive approach to calculate prevalence when the population is not stationary [40].

Bibliographical notes

Mathematical arguments used in basic epidemiological texts, and in particular those which form the theoretical basis of descriptive epidemiology, are often ap-proximate, and for a good reason: a satisfactory mathematical approach, based on the statistical analysis of stochastic processes, quickly leads to advanced mathe-matics [29] in even the simplest situations. Moreover, this level of sophistication is rarely required to meet the real problems of descriptive epidemiology, which are more often of a different kind. The approach we have taken in this first chapter is similar to that used in demography [30], where data of this type were first analysed rigorously. The modern trend in mathematical statistics is to treat the analysis of censored data using the concepts of stochastic processes, which provide very general results on the convergence and the speed of convergence of the estimates. It is not surprising that, in medical research, most effort in this direction has been in the context of clinical trials, because these often have relatively few subjects and the validity of the statistical conclusions is a paramount requirement. Readers interested in this approach can find the necessary concepts in Hill et al. [31], particularly the appendix. Anderson [32] has published a fairly complete and non-technical introduction to this method. To the extent that the fundamental principles of descriptive epidemiology do not differ from those of cohort studies, several sections of chapters 2, 3 and 4 in the book by Breslow and Day [11] make profitable reading, and give a more complete bibliography of the various formalizations.

Chapter 9 in Pressat [30] provides a complete presentation of the concepts involved in the life table. The estimation of the life table is discussed in depth by Chiang [20] in chapter 9. Classical survival models are described in detail in Kalbfleisch and Prentice [33] [see pages 21-30] and in Cox and Oakes [34] [see pages 13-28]. Since Cox [14] was first published, the proportional hazards model has had so many applications, that even an abridged list would be difficult to provide. References [35,36 and 37] provide a clear discussion of its application in epidemiology.

The theory of competing risks is discussed in Chiang [20], chapter 2; a monograph has also been written on this subject [41]. Makeham [42] is generally recognized as having originated the concept of multiple decremental forces, from which the essentially similar idea of latent survival time was largely derived. In this approach, the observed survival of a subject is the smallest of the [unobserved] latent survival times, with each of these times corresponding to the causes of death under study. This approach is described in the monograph by David and Moeschberger [41], and discussed in reference [23]. The problem of estimating mortality when the competing risks cannot be assumed to be independent is reviewed in an article by Duchene [43].

The concept of prevalence and its calculation has been discussed by many authors. The texts by MacMahon and Pugh [44], and Kleinbaum and co-workers [45] can be consulted, and an article by Freeman and Hutchison [46] gives a detailed overview. Reference [38] also provides a full bibliography on the subject.

REFERENCES

[1] Day NE, Muñoz N. Oesophagus. In D Schottenfeld, JF Fraumeni (eds) : *Cancer Epidemiology and Prevention,* (2nd Edition). Philadelphia, WB Saunders, in press

[2] *IARC Monographs on the Evaluation of the Carcinogenic Risk of Chemicals to Humans,* Vol. 38, *Tobacco Smoking.* Lyon, IARC, 1986

[3] DOLL R, PETO R. The causes of cancer. *J Epidemiol Commun Health* 1981, **66**

[4] BRESLOW NE, ENSTROM JE. Geographic correlations between cancer mortality rates and alcohol – Tobacco consumption in the United States. *J Nat Cancer Inst* 1974, **53** : 631-39

[5] JENSEN OM. *Cancer morbidity and causes of death among Danish brewery workers.* 1980, Lyon, International Agency for Research on Cancer

[6] ARMSTRONG BK, DOLL R. Environmental factors and cancer incidence and mortality in different countries with special reference to dietary practices. *Int J Cancer* 1975, **15** : 617-31

[7] WILLETT WC, STAMPFER MJ, COLDITZ GA et al. Dietary fat and risk of breast cancer. *N Engl J Med* 1987, **316** : 22-8

[8] BEESE DH, Ed. *Tobacco consumption in various countries.* London, Tobacco Research Council, 1972, research paper 6, 3rd edition

[9] WATERHOUSE J, MUIR C, SHANMUGARATNAM K, POWELL J. *Cancer incidence in five continents,* Vol. IV (IARC Scientific Publications No 42), Lyon, IARC, 1982

[10] LYON JL, GARDNER JW, WEST DW. Cancer in Utah : Risk by religion and place of residence. *J Nat Cancer Inst* 1980. **65** : 1063-71

[11] BRESLOW NE, DAY NE. *Statistical methods in cancer research. Vol II : The Design and analysis of cohort studies.* (IARC Scientific Publications No. 82), Lyon, IARC, 1987

[12] DUCHÊNE J. *Un essai de modélisation de la répartition des décès selon l'âge et la cause dans les pays industrialisés.* Louvain-la-Neuve, Cabay, 1980

[13] JOHNSON NL, KOTZ S. *Distribution in statistics. Continuous univariate distribution.* New York, Wiley, 1970, chapter 21

[14] COX DR. Regression models and life tables. *J Roy Stat Soc B* 1972, **34** : 187-220

[15] PETO R. Contribution to the discussion of paper by DR Cox. *J Roy Stat Soc B* 1972, **34** : 205-7

[16] BRESLOW NE. Covariance analysis of censored survival data. *Biometrics* 1974, **30** : 89-99

[17] RAO CR. *Linear statistical inference and its applications.* New York, Wiley, 1973, pp. 417-8

[18] BERNOULLI D. Essai d'une nouvelle analyse de la mortalité causée par la petite vérole et des avantages de l'inoculation pour la prévenir. *Mémoire de l'Académie Royale des Sciences,* 1760, pp. 1-45

[19] D'ALEMBERT. Sur l'application du calcul des probabilités à l'inoculation de la petite vérole. Opuscules II, 1761, pp. 26-95

[20] CHIANG CL. *Introduction to stochastic process in biostatistics.* New York, Wiley, 1968

[21] COX DR. The analysis of exponentially distributed life times with two types of failures. *J Roy Stat Soc B* 1959, **21** : 411-21

[22] TSIATIS A. A non-identifiability aspect of the problem of competing risks. *Proc Nat Acad Sci USA* 1975, **72** : 20-2

[23] PRENTICE RL, KALBFLEISCH JD, PETERSON AV, FLOURNOY N, FAREWELL TT, BRESLOW NE. The analysis of failure times in the presence of competing risks. *Biometrics* 1978, **34** : 541-54

[24] WONG O. A competing risk model based on the life table. Procedures in epidemiological studies. *Int J Epidemiol* 1977, **6** : 153-60

[25] DOLL R. The geographical distribution of cancer. *Br J Cancer* 1969, **23** : 1-8

[26] BENHAMOU E, LAPLANCHE A, WARTELLE M, FAIVRE J, GIGNOUX M, MÉNÉGOZ F, ROBILLARD J, SCHAFFER P, SCHRAUB S, FLAMANT R. *Incidence des cancers en France, 1978-1982.* Paris, Les Éditions INSERM, 1990

[27] JENSEN OM, ESTÈVE J, MØLLER H, RENARD H. Cancer in the European Community and its member states. *Eur J Cancer* 1990, **26** : 1167-1256

[28] VERDECCHIA A, CAPOCACCIA R, EGIDI V, GOLINI A. A method for estimation of chronic disease, morbidity and trends from mortality data. *Stat Med* 1989, **8** : 201-16

[29] BRILLINGER DR. The natural variability of vital rates and associated statistics. *Biometrics* 1986, **42** : 693-734

[30] PRESSAT R. *L'analyse démographique.* Paris, Presses Universitaires de France, 1973

[31] HILL C, COM-NOUGUÉ C, KRAMAR A et al. *Analyse statistique des données de survie.* INSERM/Médecine-Sciences Flammarion, 1990, Paris

[32] ANDERSEN PK. Counting process for life history data : A review. *Scand J Stat* 1985, **12** : 97-158

[33] KALBFLEISCH JD, PRENTICE RL. *The statistical analysis of failure time data.* New York, Wiley, 1980

[34] COX DR, OAKES D. *Analysis of survival data.* London, Chapman and Hall, 1984

[35] BRESLOW NE. The proportional hazards model : Applications in epidemiology. *Commun Stat,* (Ser A) 1978, **7** : 315-32

[36] BERRY G. The analysis of mortality by the subject years method. *Biometrics* 1983, **39** : 173-84

[37] BRESLOW NE, LUBIN JH, MAREK P, LANGHOLZ B. Multiplicative models and cohort analysis. *J Am Stat Assoc* 1983, **78** : 1-12

[38] KEIDING N. Age-specific incidence and prevalence : a statistical perspective. *J R Statist Soc* A 1991, **154** : 371-412

[39] VERDECCHIA A, CAPOCACCIA R. Discussion of the paper by Keiding. *J R Statist Soc A* 1991, **154** : 405-6

[40] PRESTON SH,. Relations among standard epidemiologic measures in a population. *Am J Epidemiol* 1987, **126** : 336-45

[41] DAVID HA, Moeschberger MC. *The theory of competing risks.* London, Charles Griffin, 1978

[42] MAKEHAM WM. On an application of the theory of the composition of decremental forces. *J Hist Actuaries* 1874, **18** : 317-22

[43] DUCHÊNE J. Dépendances entre processus morbides et mesures de la mortalité par cause de décès. *In* Chaire Quételet : 82 : *Morbidité et mortalité aux âges adultes dans les pays développés.* Louvain-la-Neuve, Cabay-Jezierski, 1983

[44] MACMAHON B, PUGH TF. *Epidemiology : principles and methods.* Boston, Little-Brown, 1970

[45] KLEINBAUM DG, KUPPER LL, MORGENSTERN H. *Epidemiologic research : Principles and quantitative methods.* Belmont, Life-time Learning, 1982

[46] FREEMAN J, HUTCHISON GB. Prevalence, incidence and duration. *Am J Epidemiol* 1980, 112 : 707-23

Chapter 2

Techniques for the analysis of cancer risk

Measurement of the risk of cancer

Age- and sex-specific rates

The annual incidence rate for a specific tumour, for a group and for a given time period is equal to the ratio between the number of new cases of the tumour observed in the group over the given time and the number of *person-years* accumulated by the members of the group in the same time interval.

The calculation of an incidence rate is more meaningful when the group is homogeneous and when there is a constant risk during the time period. Moreover, it is only under these conditions that the observed incidence rate can be considered as an estimate of the underlying instantaneous rate which plays a key role in the definition of the risk of cancer (see Chapter 1, page 11). The homogeneity condition justifies the calculation of rates separately by age and sex, known as *specific incidence rates* because they refer to subgroups of the population and not to the population as a whole.

In the following, we first describe methods for calculating specific incidence rates, and then examine techniques of estimating their precision since, like all indexes calculated from observed data, the incidence rate is subject to random variation. Finally, we describe some typical incidence curves.

The calculation of a specific rate

The only problems involved in the determination of the numerator are the completeness of registration and respect for whatever guidelines have been adopted to define new cases. We will return to this point later in detail with the study of time trends, which are particularly vulnerable to changes in the definition adopted (see Chapter 3, page 176).

The determination of the denominator depends on available demographic statistics. In theory, the calculation of the exact number of person-years of observation requires individual data, but statistical offices provide at best reports including cross-sectional characteristics of the population at periodic intervals, obtained from censuses or other population estimates. Thus, the denominator can be estimated only by making assumptions about the evolution of the population between two of these points, that is, about the way in which individuals traverse the age × time rectangle of the Lexis diagram (see Figure 1.1). Let us suppose, for example, that we wish to estimate the annual incidence of breast cancer for women aged 45 to 49 years in Zaragoza (Spain) between the beginning of 1973 and the end of 1977. Theoretically, we should add up the number of years lived in this age group by each woman of the population of Zaragoza during the period 1973-1977: thus, a woman who turned 45 years of age on 1 January 1977 will contribute one year to the person-years, in the same way as a woman who turned 49 on 1 January 1973 will contribute one year. In reality, it is known only that 27 699 women were between 45 and 49 years of age in 1975, the year of the census. It is supposed that there are as many women each year joining the age group as there are leaving it and that the number counted at the mid-point is consequently an estimate of the average number throughout the interval. Therefore, the estimate of the number of person-years accumulated between 1973 and 1977 is obtained by multiplying the number at the mid-point by five (27 699 × 5). Then, as the Cancer Registry recorded 109 cases of breast cancer for women between 45 and 49 years of age in the interval under consideration, the specific rate of breast cancer in this age group is

$$109/(27\ 699 \times 5) = 78.7 \text{ cases per } 100\,000 \text{ women per year.}$$

In most situations, this method for approximating the denominator is acceptable. However, the example below shows that the method can sometimes lead to aberrant results.

In Calvados, France, the resident population in the age group 60 to 64 years at the first of January evolved as follows from 1977 to 1982:

Number in age group 60 to 64 years at 1 January	
1977	20 790
1978	18 592
1979	16 886
1980	15 643
1981	18 757
1982	22 106

To calculate the incidence rate in the interval between 1 January 1977, and 31 December 1981, using the previously described method, we would take as the denominator five times the average population for the year 1979, that is

$$5 \times \frac{(16\,886 + 15\,643)}{2} = 81\,323 \text{ person-years}$$

However, a careful examination of the annual figures reveals fluctuations due to the effects of the decline in the birth rate during the first world war. Therefore, the calculation of incidence rate should take the figures for each year of the interval

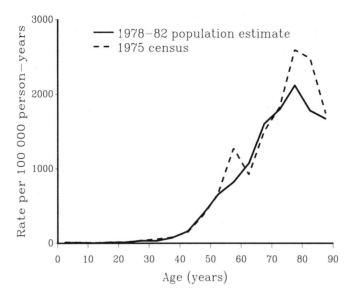

Figure 2.1   Influence of the denominator estimates on the age-specific incidence curve. All cancer sites, Calvados (France), males, incident cases 1978-1982
Source : Robillard [1]

into consideration; supposing that, on average, the number of individuals at risk in the group under study can be estimated each year by the arithmetic average of the number of individuals in the age group at the beginning and the end of the year, then we have

$$20\,790/2 + 18\,592 + 16\,886 + 15\,643 + 18\,757 + 22\,106/2,$$

that is, a total of 91 326 person-years [1].

In this example, the previous approximation under-estimated the calculation of person-years accumulated in the interval by 11%. The solution which takes as denominator a demographic estimate that does not correspond to the mid-point of the interval being considered can lead to even more serious inaccuracies. Figure 2.1 shows, again in Calvados, biases in the age-specific incidence curve when the number of cases observed for the interval 1978-82 (males) is related to data from the 1975 census. Even if variations from one year to the next are rarely as marked as those in our example, successive annual estimates should be used in the calculations when they are available.

The accuracy of the estimate of a rate

Regardless of the bias that a wrong evaluation of the denominator causes, we should question the accuracy of the estimate of the rate being calculated.

For reasons that were discussed earlier (see Chapter 1, page 20), the denominator can be considered as a non-random quantity; thus, the accuracy of a rate only depends on the variability of the number of cases observed (K). We can therefore suppose that K is a variable that follows a Poisson distribution whose expectation and variance are equal to the theoretical rate (λ) that we are attempting to estimate, multiplied by the number of person-years (m) accumulated within the period of the study:

$$K \rightsquigarrow P(\lambda m)$$

$$E(K) = \lambda m$$

$$Var(K) = \lambda m$$

Therefore, the variance of the rate estimator (K/m) is

$$Var\left(\frac{K}{m}\right) = \frac{Var\,(K)}{m^2} = \frac{\lambda}{m}$$

Its estimate is obtained by replacing λ by k/m in the above formula, k being the observed value of K; it is given by

$$V\hat{a}r\left(\frac{K}{m}\right) = \frac{k}{m^2} = \frac{\hat{\lambda}^2}{k}$$

an expression which has already been obtained in Chapter 1, page 20. It is then possible to construct a confidence interval of level $1 - \alpha$ for λ. When k is large, we can consider that the distribution of K/m is normal with mean λ and standard deviation $\frac{\sqrt{k}}{m}$, therefore

$$Prob\left[\left|\frac{\frac{K}{m} - \lambda}{\frac{\sqrt{k}}{m}}\right| < Z_{\alpha/2}\right] = \alpha$$

hence the confidence interval:

$$\left[\frac{k}{m} - Z_{\alpha/2}\frac{\sqrt{k}}{m}\;;\;\frac{k}{m} + Z_{\alpha/2}\frac{\sqrt{k}}{m}\right]$$

The usual value of α is 0.05 and $Z_{\alpha/2} = 1.96$. As an example, if nine cases have been observed in a population of 10 000 persons followed up during three years, the incidence rate is 30 per 100 000; its variance is $9/(30\,000)^2$, and its standard error is 10/100 000. Therefore, the confidence interval may be written:

$$30/100\,000 \pm (1.96 \times 10/100\,000) = [10.40/100\,000\;;\;49.6/100\,000]$$

It is also possible to use directly a confidence interval for the expectation of K as calculated from the Poisson distribution (see page 64). Table 2.3 below gives the values [4.12 ; 17.08], which leads to a confidence interval for the rate equal to [13.70/100 000 ; 56.93/100 000]. This exact interval is fairly different from the above conventional interval. It is therefore recommended to use the Poisson distribution when the number of cases observed is less than 50.

In practice, it is usual to assess the accuracy of the rate on a relative scale. The relative error in the estimation of a rate is given by the coefficient of variation of the estimated rate, which is defined as the ratio between its standard error and its mean:

$$CV = \frac{\sqrt{\lambda/m}}{\lambda} = \frac{1}{\sqrt{\lambda m}}$$

The expected value of K being λm, $1/\sqrt{k}$ provides a simple estimator of the accuracy of the rate measured on a relative scale. In the previous example, the relative error in the calculated rate is $1/\sqrt{9} = 33\%$. If we had observed four cases, the relative error would have been $1/\sqrt{4} = 50\%$. These examples reveal the substantial inaccuracies which can affect measures of rare cancers.

The coefficient of variation that we defined above has a natural interpretation when it is appropriate to consider the rates after logarithmic transformation (see next page). In fact, in this case, variability is measured by the standard error of the logarithm of the specific rate which can be calculated in the usual way:

$$Var\left[Log\left(\frac{K}{m}\right)\right] = Var\left[Log(K) - Log(m)\right] = Var\left[Log(K)\right]$$

$$\approx \left(\frac{d\,Log\,[E(K)]}{dK}\right)^2 \times Var\,(K) = \left(\frac{1}{\lambda m}\right)^2 \times Var\,(K)$$

$$Var\left[Log\left(\frac{K}{m}\right)\right] \approx \frac{1}{\lambda m} \tag{2.1}$$

Thus, not surprisingly, the standard error of the logarithm of the rate is equal to the coefficient of variation. Using the same principle as before and the data from the previous example, the confidence interval of the logarithm of the rate is

$$Log\,(30/100\,000) \pm (1.96 \times 0.33)$$

which leads, by taking the exponential of the interval end-points to a new confidence interval for the rate itself

$$CI_{95\%} = [15.7\,/\,100\,000\,;\,57.3\,/\,100\,000]$$

It is worth noting that, by improving the required normality, the logarithmic transformation has led to a result which is closer to the exact interval than the conventional interval based on the rate itself.

As the accuracy of the estimate depends only on the number of observed cases, it can theoretically be increased by lengthening the observation time. However, if incidence is not constant over time, the accumulation of cases over several years can only lead to a less meaningful result. In practice, the choice of interval is a compromise between these two requirements. The situation is similar when we consider that a region covered by a registry is too heterogeneous to give only one estimate of the rate. If we decide to divide the area into subgroups which are more homogeneous, the accuracy of the rate estimates in each subregion is lower. Therefore, a compromise between interpretability and accuracy has to be found (see Chapter 3).

The incidence curve

Age-specific rates are usually calculated for seventeen five-year age groups between the age of 0 and 85 years, with an eighteenth group for 85 years and over. As a rule, the rates should be represented on a graph by a step-function with five-yearly increments. However, it is customary to join the points that mark the mid-point of each age group; the line obtained by doing so is called *the incidence curve*. In a population where the age-specific incidence might remain constant over a period of time, such as would occur in the absence of a cohort effect, the curve could be seen as an estimate of the function $\lambda(t)$ which we defined in Chapter 1. However, as incidence does tend to change with time, the shape of the curve is a result of the combined effect of age and observation time: incidence rates for older age-groups describe a relationship between risk and age that does not necessarily correspond to that described by incidence for the youngest individuals living at the same time. In other words, when older people today were young, they did not have the same risk as the young people of today.

As we stated previously, incidence according to age is sometimes shown after logarithmic transformation of age-specific rates. This sort of representation is used firstly for practical reasons. Rates of very different orders of magnitude can be represented on the same graph, allowing a clear visualization of incidence levels for ages where rates are low. It is also worth noting that a constant ratio of age-specific incidence rate between two populations will produce, on a logarithmic scale, two parallel incidence curves.

A logarithmic scale may also be used on the age axis. Thus, a log-log graph is designed to place the observed data in the context of the multi-stage model of carcinogenesis [2,3]. According to this model, incidence is a power function of age and should therefore be represented by a straight line on a log-log scale. However, such a model can only be identified by this procedure in the absence of a cohort effect [4].

The mortality from colorectal cancer in France for the period 1978-1982 is represented in Figure 2.2 by using various scales. In this case it is clear that Figure 2.2(c) provides a remarkably concise description of the increase in risk with age. However, other more complex incidence curves are often seen (Figures 1.2 and 2.5). In particular, the incidence curve for breast cancer shows a characteristic drop in the rate of increase around 50 years of age; Clemmesen has demonstrated the universality of this phenomenon. [5]

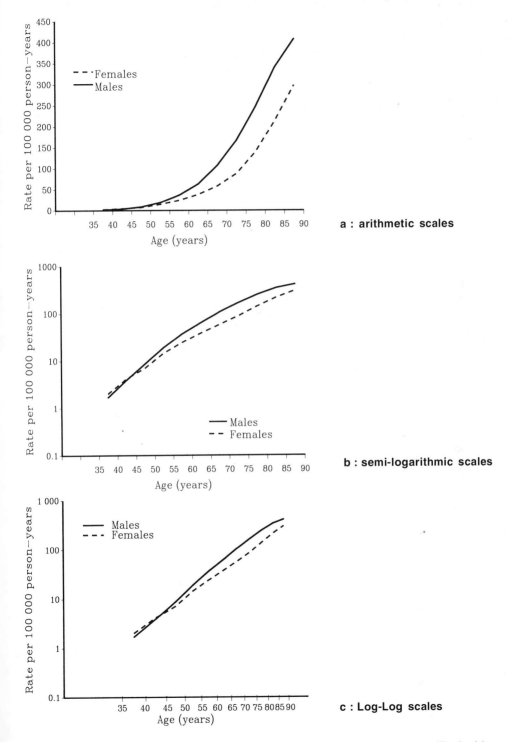

Figure 2.2   Influence of the choice of scale on the shape of age-specific incidence curves. Mortality from colorectal cancer in France, 1978-1982

Standardized rates

One of the principal aims of collecting incidence data is the investigation of etiological factors for the disease being considered. In order to compare observed incidence for different regions or groups or years, we should be in a position to take account of the factors which are already recognized as possible explanations of observed differences in rates. Among these factors, age is the first candidate. The effects of age are large and, in general, the various populations being compared differ in their age structures. The control of the confounding effect of a factor, by methods to be discussed below, implies that we know its distribution in the populations that we wish to compare. This is the reason why the following methods cannot be applied to biasing factors such as the quality of registration or the accuracy of diagnosis. On the other hand, when denominators are not available, the method described on page 95 could be used.

Direct standardization

The principle of this method is to determine the annual rate that would be observed in a *standard*, or theoretical, population of a given age structure, were it subjected to the force of incidence of the population under study. The procedure is based on the calculation of the expected number of cases in each age-group of this *standard population* by applying to the corresponding person-years the estimated rate of the population under study. The total number of expected cases is then divided by the total number of person-years in the theoretical population.

Let:

• g be the number of age groups under consideration, which is usually 18 but can change if we are calculating a truncated rate for a subset of adjacent age-groups, for example, 35-64 years;

• L be the size of a standard population,

• L_x be the number of individuals in the xth age-group of this standard population,

• k_x be the number of cases observed in the xth age-group of the population under study

• m_x be the number of person-years accumulated in the xth age-group of the population under study

• $t_x = k_x/n_x$ be the specific rate of the xth age-group of the population under study.

$L_x t_x$ is thus the number of expected cases that might be observed in one year in the xth age group of the standard population if it were exposed to a level of risk defined by the rate t_x. The *standardized rate* is then:

$$\bar{t} = \frac{1}{L} \sum_{x=1}^{g} L_x t_x \qquad (2.2)$$

It may also be written

$$\bar{t} = \sum_{x=1}^{g} w_x t_x \qquad (2.3)$$

where $w_x = L_x/L$ is the proportion of individuals in the xth age group in the standard population with

$$\sum_{x=1}^{g} w_x = 1$$

This expression shows that the rate $\bar{t}$ is a weighted average of age-specific rates, with the weights being the proportion of individuals in the various age groups of the standard population.

We should note that the calculation presumes that the number of person-years of observation and the number of observed cases in each age-group of the population under study (or at least the age-specific rates) are known. Furthermore, the calculation requires the choice of a standard population. In practice, this choice depends on our objective and it influences the numerical result that we obtain. The principal standard populations that have been suggested are presented in Table 2.1. For routine comparisons, it is preferable to use the world population as a standard. The European population figures are suitable when we are comparing observed incidences in countries where the age structure is similar to that usually observed in developed countries. In the same way, the African population can be used as a standard for developing countries. A *truncated population* is used to restrict the comparison to the adult age groups where the most interesting differences appear. It also has the advantage of eliminating from the standardized rate the contribution of the oldest age groups that are particularly subject to the risk of being under-registered. When we are not dealing with routine comparisons, other standards are sometimes adopted; for example, if we wish to describe the risk in several subsets of a region or a country, it is reasonable to take the total population of the region or the country as the standard population. In the particular case where we are interested in two regions or countries, the sum of their populations is sometimes taken as the standard.

Table 2.2 presents the calculation of the standardized rate of stomach cancer for males in the French region of the Côte-d'Or from 1976 to 1980, using the European population as a standard.

The calculation of a directly standardized rate uses age-specific rates that have been estimated from observations which are subject to a certain amount of random variability. This variability affects the estimate of the standardized rate and can lead to spurious conclusions if the observed difference between standardized rates is in fact mainly due to random variation. In order to evaluate the importance of this kind of variation, the standardized rate (t) should be presented with its standard error or its confidence interval.

Table 2.1 Age structure of commonly used standard populations [6]
(valid for either sex)

Age group	World	African	European	World truncated
0-4	12	10	8	–
5-9	10	10	7	–
10-14	9	10	7	–
15-19	9	10	7	–
20-24	8	10	7	–
25-29	8	10	7	–
30-34	6	10	7	–
35-39	6	10	7	6
40-44	6	5	7	6
45-49	6	5	7	6
50-54	5	3	7	5
55-59	4	2	6	4
60-64	4	2	5	4
65-69	3	1	4	–
70-74	2	1	3	–
75-79	1	0.5	2	–
80-84	0.5	0.3	1	–
85 +	0.5	0.2	1	–
Total	100	100	100	31

As we saw previously when discussing the estimation of λ_x, from K_x observations resulting from m_x person-years in age group x,

$$K_x \rightsquigarrow P(\lambda_x m_x)$$

$$E(K_x) = \text{Var}(K_x) = \lambda_x m_x$$

The variance of the specific rate $t_x = K_x/m_x$ is then obtained using the classical method

$$\text{Var}(t_x) = \frac{\text{Var}(K_x)}{m_x^2} = \frac{\lambda_x}{m_x}$$

Therefore, the variance of the standardized rate is, from formula (2.3)

$$\text{Var}(\bar{t}) = \sum_{x=1}^{g} w_x^2 \, \text{Var}(t_x)$$

$$\text{Var}(\bar{t}) = \sum_{x=1}^{g} w_x^2 \left(\frac{\lambda_x}{m_x} \right) \tag{2.4}$$

λ_x being unknown, $\text{Var}(\bar{t})$ must be estimated by replacing λ_x by its estimate k_x/m_x in the above expression. Then

$$\hat{\text{Var}}(\bar{t}) = \sum_{x=1}^{g} \left(\frac{w_x^2}{m_x^2} \right) k_x$$

If the theoretical standardized rate is denoted by $\mu = \sum_x w_x \lambda_x$ and if s is the estimate of its standard error, then we can consider that $(\bar{t} - \mu)/s$ is approximately a standard normal variable; the confidence interval at level $1 - \alpha$ for μ is then obtained as explained previously:

$$[\bar{t} - Z_{\alpha/2} \sqrt{\hat{\text{Var}}(\bar{t})} \; ; \; \bar{t} + Z_{\alpha/2} \sqrt{\hat{\text{Var}}(\bar{t})} \,]$$

In practice, rates are given per 100 000 person-years ($10^5 \, t_x$); the variance that is calculated is therefore in the form $10^{10} \, \text{Var}(\bar{t})$.

Table 2.2 also gives the data required to calculate the variance of the standardized rate, from which we obtain a standard error of 1.55 and its 95% confidence interval [20.49 ; 26.58].

We should note again that the procedure which enables the confidence interval to be constructed from the standard error of the estimator implies that the distribution of this estimator is reasonably close to normal. This is in fact only true in the present situation if the total number of cases is sufficiently large. It is however difficult to tell what 'sufficiently' means in the present context because the numerator of a standardized rate is no longer a Poisson variate. Its variance depends not only on the total number of observed cases but also on the weighting scheme w and the accuracy of the age-specific rates. This may be seen by writing the formula (2.4) in the following way:

$$\text{Var}(\bar{t}) = \frac{1}{m} \sum_{i=1}^{g} w_x \frac{\kappa_x}{m_x} = \frac{\tau}{m}$$

where $\kappa_x = L_x \lambda_x$ and L_x, the numerator of w_x, is chosen in such a way that:

$$\sum_{i=1}^{g} L_x = \sum_{i=1}^{g} m_x = m$$

This expression shows that the variance may be badly assessed from the total number of expected cases especially if the majority of them (κ_x) originated from an age group where m_x is low (see page 100).

The quotient of two standardized rates calculated from the same standard population is known as the *comparative incidence figure* (CIF). It is a measure of the relative risk of a population compared with another population and is generally expressed as a percentage. The standardized rate in a subgroup of a population that is itself used as the standard, divided by the crude rate in the whole population

Table 2.2 Calculation of a directly standardized rate (stomach cancer in Côte-d'Or, France, males, 1976-1980, European standard)

x	Age	k_x	m_x	$10^5 \, t_x$	w_x	$10^5 \, w_x t_x$	$10^{10} \left(\dfrac{w_x^2 k_x}{m_x^2} \right)$
(1)	(2)	(3)	(4)	(5)	(6)	(7)	(8)
1	0-4	0	91 228	0.00	0.08	0.000	0.0000
2	5-9	0	95 230	0.00	0.07	0.000	0.0000
3	10-14	0	95 869	0.00	0.07	0.000	0.0000
4	15-19	0	98 744	0.00	0.07	0.000	0.0000
5	20-24	0	101 131	0.00	0.07	0.000	0.0000
6	25-29	0	101 103	0.00	0.07	0.000	0.0000
7	30-34	0	83 544	0.00	0.07	0.000	0.0000
8	35-39	1	67 580	1.48	0.07	0.104	0.0107
9	40-44	3	68 577	4.37	0.07	0.306	0.0313
10	45-49	6	68 126	8.81	0.07	0.617	0.0633
11	50-54	10	63 708	15.70	0.07	1.099	0.1207
12	55-59	17	51 007	33.33	0.06	2.000	0.2352
13	60-64	27	37 695	71.63	0.05	3.582	0.4751
14	65-69	34	44 374	76.62	0.04	3.065	0.2763
15	70-74	51	36 768	138.71	0.03	4.161	0.3395
16	75-79	46	24 196	190.11	0.02	3.802	0.3143
17	80 +	42	17 491	240.12	0.02	4.802	0.5491
Total		237	1 146 371		1.00	23.537	2.4155

Columns 1 to 4 and 6 are given and columns 5, 7 and 8 are calculated.
k_x : observed number of cases of stomach cancer in Côte-d'Or from 1976 to 1980 for the xth age group.
m_x : estimate of the number of person-years for males in each age group x, obtained by summing the numbers of the Côte-d'Or population from 1976 to 1980 (INSEE, PRUDENT).
t_x : age-specific rate per 100 000 persons per year.
w_x : structure of the standard population by age.

(which in this case is equal to the standardized rate with respect to itself) is also a CIF.

The value of a CIF is independent of the standard population used only if the ratio of the age-specific incidence rates is constant, in other words, only when the two incidence curves that are being compared are parallel when the log scale is used on the rate axis. This property often holds for incidence curves (see Figure 2.3) and can be checked with a statistical test which evaluates the assumption of the homogeneity of age-specific relative rates (see page 80).

Cumulative rates

The overall incidence observed in a population can also be described by the *cumulative rate* [7] which provides, as we shall see below, an approximation of the risk of developing a disease before age b (or between two ages a and b) in the absence of mortality (see the concept of net risk in Chapter 1, page 34). The cu-

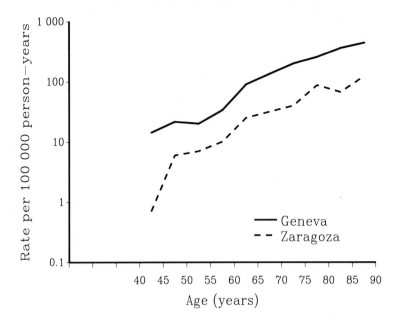

Figure 2.3   Age-specific incidence of colon cancer in Zaragoza (Spain) and Geneva (Switzerland) males, 1973-1977

mulative rate over a whole lifetime is an integral of the function represented by the incidence curve. This rate can be estimated by adding up the age-specific incidence over each year of age. Assuming that the incidence is constant within an age group (x) of five years, we will write

$$t_{0,b} = \sum_{x=1}^{j} 5 \times t_x = 5 \sum_{x=1}^{j} t_x \tag{2.5}$$

to estimate the cumulative rate from zero to the upper limit b of age group j, and

$$t_{a,b} = 5 \sum_{x=i}^{j} t_x \tag{2.6}$$

to estimate the cumulative rate from the lower limit a of age group i to the upper limit b of the age group j.

For example, the cumulative rate of stomach cancer between 35 and 65 years of age can be calculated from the data in Table 2.2 by adding up the numbers in column 5 from line 8 to line 13 and multiplying the result by 5/100 000, i.e.

$$t_{35,65} = 0.0068 = 0.68\%$$

Estimation of the cumulative rate over a whole lifetime presents a problem because the last age group is open and, unlike the other age-groups, does not contain five years. If the last age-group is 80 years and over, we can suppose that the estimate of the rate in this age-group is almost identical to the rate in the age group 80-85 years, and consider that the value we obtain is the cumulative rate up to 85 years. With this convention, the cumulative rate over life of stomach cancer can be estimated by

$$t_{0,85} = 0.0390 = 3.90\%.$$

In practice, it is preferable not to calculate the cumulative rates beyond the upper limit of the last closed age group. In fact, cumulative rates are rarely published above 75 years, the age at which competing causes of death begin to play a major role (see Chapter 1, page 34).

Note that the cumulative rate is proportional to the arithmetic average of the age-specific rates, that is, to a rate that would be standardized to a population in which every age-group contained the same proportion of individuals ('rectangular' population). Note also that the probabilistic interpretation mentioned above assumes that the cross-sectional incidence curve, constructed for a given time period from different cohorts, correctly represents the force of incidence applicable to an individual for whom we wish to evaluate risk; in fact, the risk obtained in this way is that of a 'fictitious' individual who synthesizes the experience of several cohorts.

The standard error and confidence interval of a cumulative rate are obtained in the same way as those for a direct standardized rate; the application of formula (2.4) with $w_x = 5$ gives

$$\text{Var} (t_{a,b}) = 25 \sum_{x=i}^{j} \frac{k_x}{m_x^2} \tag{2.7}$$

for example, the standard error of the cumulative rate of stomach cancer between age 35 and 65 years is

$$\sqrt{\text{Var} (t_{35,65})} = 0,0009$$

from which we derive a confidence interval of [0.51% ; 0.85%].

Indirect standardization

While direct standardization could be called the method of the standard population, the procedure described in this paragraph could be called the method of standard incidence. The principle is based on the comparison between the total number of cases observed in the population under study and the number that could be expected if the population was subject to a given force of incidence (λ_x), the standard incidence.

The number of expected cases in the population under study is

$$E = \sum_{x=1}^{g} m_x \lambda_x \qquad (2.8)$$

where λ_x is the incidence rate of group x in the standard population, and m_x is the number of person-years accumulated by group x in the population under study.

The ratio between the total number of cases observed in the population under study (O) and the expected number (E) is called the *standardized incidence ratio* (SIR). Like the CIF, it is a measure of relative risk of the population under study compared with the standard population. It is usually expressed as a percentage,

$$SIR = \frac{O}{E} \times 100 \qquad (2.9)$$

Therefore, a value of 150 for this index means that 50% more cases were observed in the population under study than if the incidence was that of the standard population.

For reasons already discussed, the variability of the SIR depends only on the numerator, whose distribution can be considered to be Poisson. The estimate of the SIR variability can be obtained accurately from Table 2.3 which gives the 95% confidence interval of the expectation μ of a Poisson variable given an observed number of cases O.

The results in Table 2.3 are obtained by defining the lower and upper limits of the confidence interval μ_0 and μ_1 according to the formulae:

$$P[X \geq O | \mu_0] = \alpha/2 \; ; \; P[X \leq O | \mu_1] = \alpha/2$$

such an interval will contain the true value μ with probability $1 - \alpha$. On the other hand, the Poisson distribution is related to the χ^2 distribution by the relation:

$$Pr[X \geq k | \mu] = Pr[\chi^2_{2k} < 2\mu]$$

in other words, if F_{2k} is the distribution function of χ^2 with 2k degrees of freedom, we can write:

$$\sum_{x=k}^{\infty} e^{-\mu} \frac{\mu^x}{x!} = F_{2k}(2\mu)$$

$$F_{2O}(2\mu_0) = \alpha/2$$

$$F_{2(O+1)}(2\mu_1) = 1 - \alpha/2$$

therefore, if F^{-1} denotes the reciprocal function of F:

$$\mu_0 = \frac{1}{2} F^{-1}_{2O}(\alpha/2)$$

$$\mu_1 = \frac{1}{2} F^{-1}_{2(O+1)}(1 - \alpha/2)$$

**Table 2.3   Exact 95 % confidence interval for the expectation (μ)
of a Poisson distribution according to the number of observed cases (O)**

Observed cases (O)	95 % Confidence interval		Observed cases (O)	95% confidence interval	
	μ_0	μ_1		μ_0	μ_1
0	0.00	3.00	31	21.06	44.00
1	0.03	5.57	32	21.89	45.17
2	0.24	7.22	33	22.72	46.34
3	0.62	8.77	34	23.55	47.51
4	1.09	10.24	35	24.38	48.68
5	1.62	11.67	36	25.21	49.84
6	2.20	13.06	37	26.05	51.00
7	2.81	14.42	38	26.89	52.16
8	3.45	15.76	39	27.73	53.31
9	4.12	17.08	40	28.58	54.47
10	4.80	18.39	41	29.42	55.62
11	5.49	19.68	42	30.27	56.77
12	6.20	20.96	43	31.12	57.92
13	6.92	22.23	44	31.97	59.07
14	7.65	23.49	45	32.82	60.21
15	8.40	24.74	46	33.68	61.36
16	9.15	25.98	47	34.53	62.50
17	9.90	27.22	48	35.39	63.64
18	10.67	28.45	49	36.25	64.78
19	11.44	29.67	50	37.11	65.92
20	12.22	30.89	51	37.97	67.06
21	13.00	32.10	52	38.84	68.19
22	13.79	33.31	53	39.70	69.33
23	14.58	34.51	54	40.57	70.46
24	15.38	35.71	55	41.43	71.59
25	16.18	36.90	56	42.30	72.72
26	16.98	38.10	57	43.17	73.85
27	17.79	39.28	58	44.04	74.98
28	18.61	40.47	59	44.91	76.11
29	19.42	41.65	60	45.78	77.23
30	20.24	42.83	61	46.66	78.36

When the number of observed cases is zero, X is greater than the observed number with probability 1 whatever μ_0 may be. To keep the correct level of confidence $1 - \alpha$, we construct the interval $[0 ; \mu_1]$ such that $P[X = 0|\mu_1] = e^{-\mu_1} = \alpha$. This interval covers the theoretical value μ with probability $1 - \alpha$. For example, when $\alpha = 5\%$, $\mu_1 = -\mathrm{Log}\,(0.05) = 3.00$.

When O is greater than 50, we can assume that Log (O) follows a normal distribution with expectation Log(μ) and variance $1/\mu$. Thus, to obtain a 95% confidence interval we make use of the inequality

$$\frac{|\,\mathrm{Log}\,(O) - \mathrm{Log}\,(\mu)\,|}{1/\sqrt{\mu}} < 1.96$$

which gives after replacing μ with its estimate O

$$O\,e^{\left(-\frac{1.96}{\sqrt{O}}\right)} < \mu < O\,e^{\left(\frac{1.96}{\sqrt{O}}\right)}$$

for example, when O = 50 and E = 45.6, the 95% confidence interval of μ is

$$[\mu_0 \; ; \; \mu_1] = [37.9 \; ; \; 66.0]$$

therefore, the interval of the corresponding SIR is [83.1 ; 144.7]. If instead we use Table 2.3, the confidence intervals are respectively

$$[37.1 \; ; \; 65.9] \text{ and } [81.4 \; ; \; 144.5].$$

Another more reliable approach is based on the approximation of the distribution of $\sqrt{X}$ by a normal distribution with mean $\sqrt{\mu}$ and variance 1/4 [8]; the confidence interval is then

$$[\mu_0 \; ; \; \mu_1] = \left[\left(\frac{Z_{\alpha/2}}{2} - \sqrt{O}\right)^2 \; ; \; \left(\frac{Z_{\alpha/2}}{2} + \sqrt{O+1}\right)^2\right]$$

for O = 50, this method gives [37.1 ; 66.0].

The calculation of the SIR requires only the number of person-years accumulated in each of the different groups x in the population under study and not the number of cases occurring in these groups. It requires the choice of a standard distribution which, in practice, is dictated by the use that we intend to make of the SIR, as will be shown subsequently.

As the SIR is an estimate of relative risk with respect to a reference force of incidence, the product of the SIR and the crude rate in the standard population which provides the standard incidence rates is in fact a form of standardized rate known as the *indirectly standardized rate*.

Table 2.4 provides the data required to calculate the standardized incidence ratio of colon cancer for males in the French city of Dijon between 1976 and 1980, using rates observed in the whole region of the Côte-d'Or as a standard. We obtain

$$SIR = 100 \times \frac{123}{98.7} = 124.6$$

and the 95% confidence interval of the SIR is [104.5 ; 148.9] obtained using the first normal approximation above. We can calculate the indirect standardized rate from the crude rate of 24.3 (see Table 2.4) and we can obtain the indirectly standardized rate

$$\tilde{t} = 1.246 \times 24.3 = 30.3$$

**Table 2.4 Calculation of a standardized incidence ratio (SIR)
for colon cancer in the town of Dijon for the period 1976-1980
with the overall incidence in the French département of Côte-d'Or as a standard**

x	k_x	m_x	$10^5 \lambda_x$	e_x
0-4	0	45 626	0.0	0.00
5-9	0	41 145	0.0	0.00
10-14	0	39 284	0.0	0.00
15-19	0	43 469	0.0	0.00
20-24	0	52 794	1.0	0.53
25-29	0	54 321	1.0	0.54
30-34	0	40 848	0.0	0.00
35-39	2	31 559	5.9	1.86
40-44	2	30 703	4.4	1.35
45-49	3	29 875	14.7	4.39
50-54	10	27 228	22.0	5.99
55-59	17	21 808	47.1	10.27
60-64	7	15 002	45.2	6.78
65-69	17	14 556	81.2	11.82
70-74	33	11 841	206.7	24.47
75-79	20	7 762	214.9	16.68
80 +	12	6 112	228.8	13.98
Total	O = 123	513 933	24.3	E = 98.70

k_x : observed number of cases in age group x in Dijon.
m_x : person-years of observation in age group x in Dijon.
λ_x : observed colon cancer rate in age group x in Côte-d'Or.
e_x : expected number of cases in age group x in Dijon if the incidence rates were λ_x (i.e., that of Côte-d'Or).

Probability of developing a specific form of cancer

The cumulative rate discussed previously is an approximation to the *net cancer risk*, that is, of the probability of developing cancer in the absence of mortality. In fact, we may also be concerned with the *crude probability* of developing a particular form of cancer; in other words, the risk actually incurred by an individual subjected not only to the risk of cancer but also to the risk of death. For a given level of incidence, this probability will be higher when the general mortality is low and vice versa.

The method of calculation of this probability is derived directly from formula 1.4 of Chapter 1. It was shown there that the raw probability of developing cancer is the sum for all ages of the product of the age-specific rate and the probability of survival without cancer up to this age. In practice, we shall estimate the probability of cancer from the life table neglecting the probability of not having cancer at age x which is close to 1 for most cancer sites.

Let:

• t_x be the incidence rate in the age group x;

• L_x be the number of years lived by the survivors of age x during the age interval starting at x if they are subject only to the force of mortality of the general population.

• ℓ_0 be the size of this population at the beginning of the first age interval under consideration (ℓ_0 and the L_x are provided by the life table, see Chapter 1, page 26). Then the probability of developing a given cancer is

$$p = \frac{1}{\ell_0} \sum_{x=1}^{g} L_x t_x = \frac{K}{\ell_0} \tag{2.11}$$

In fact, the summation in formula (2.11) gives the number K of expected cancers between the beginning of the first age interval and the end of the last if L_x is an acceptable approximation of person-years lived in each age group by cancer-free survivors.

When the probability of cancer (all sites) is being calculated, it might be better to construct a life table giving at each age the number of cancer-free survivors. The improvement obtained in this way is, however, somewhat illusory, as we shall see below.

When the current life table (see Chapter 1) is used in this calculation, the predictive value of this parameter should be viewed with caution. The actual mortality that will be experienced by cohorts for which the prediction is carried out may differ substantially from the reference mortality which has been used in the standard life table. This is why it is important to clarify the concept and to refer to it as being the *current probability* of developing cancer.

If we wish to compare probabilities in several regions or from several time periods, we can use the same life table; in this way, we obtain adjusted probabilities that play the same role as standardized rates. Note, however, that the standardization refers to mortality and not age, for which control is implicitly assured by the very definition of the parameter. For comparisons of this kind, it is much more simple to use the cumulative rates defined previously which provides the same type of information. When they are low, they actually provide a good approximation to the net probability R_b of developing a disease before a given age b, also known as the *cumulative risk*.

We shall give below a simple proof of this result that has previously been discussed in Chapter 1. First of all, consider an age group [x, x + Δx] in which the incidence rate is constant, and subdivide this interval into n equal parts; the probability of not developing the cancer under consideration at age x + Δx is the product of the probabilities of remaining healthy throughout each of the successive intervals thus defined. This probability is approximately

$$s_n = \left(1 - \lambda \frac{\Delta x}{n}\right)^n$$

the smaller the interval Δx/n, the more accurate the approximation will be. Now, it is known that the limit of s_n when n tends to infinity is $e^{-\lambda \Delta x}$. In other words, the probability of developing cancer between x and x + Δx is equal to $(1 - e^{-\lambda \Delta x})$.

Secondly, suppose that the age interval [0 – b] can be subdivided into j age groups of length Δx_i in which the rate λ_i is considered to be constant; the probability of not developing cancer before age b is obtained using the same principle as before:

$$1 - R_b = \prod_{i=1}^{j} e^{-\lambda_i \Delta x_i}$$

$$1 - R_b = e^{-\sum_{i=1}^{j} \lambda_i \Delta x_i}$$

If the Δ_x correspond to five-year age groups, the argument of the exponential is, except for the minus sign, the cumulative rate.

In practice, we calculate the estimate $t_{0,b}$ of the cumulative rate as was shown on page 61 and the estimate of the cumulative risk R_b according to the formula:

$$\hat{R}_b = 1 - e^{-t_{0,b}} \qquad (2.12)$$

Up to a cumulative rate of 10%, the two numbers $t_{0,b}$ and R_b are very close: the approximation of the cumulative risk R_b by the cumulative rate $t_{0,b}$ is therefore good for most cancer sites. As an example, the cumulative risk of stomach cancer between 35 and 65 years for the Côte-d'Or is 0.68%, while the life-time cumulative risk for the same region is 3.83% (the corresponding cumulative rates are respectively 0.68% and 3.90%; see Table 2.2).

Table 2.5 presents the three indexes that have been discussed, to evaluate the overall life-time cancer risk from data from New York State between 1969 and 1971 [9,10]. Note that the values of the two indexes defined by probabilities (cumulative risk and current probability) are relatively close to each other before 65

Table 2.5   Cumulative rate, cumulative risk, and current probability of cancer in New York State, USA (1969-1971) [6]

	Males		Females	
	All sites	Lung	All sites	Breast
Cumulative rate (%)				
0-65 years	12.3	3.0	12.8	4.0
0-75 years	28.8	7.0	22.6	6.2
Cumulative risk				
0-65 years	11.6	3.0	12.0	3.9
0-75 years	25.0	6.8	20.2	6.0
0-85 years	42.0	10.6	30.7	8.7
Current probability				
0-65 years	10.0	2.4	11.6	3.6
0 + (^{a})	27.1	5.8	27.8	7.2

(^{a}) In this instance, the probability is calculated up to the terminal age of the table (see page 27).

years, particularly for females. Beyond this age, mortality has played a greater role effectively preventing incidence to manifest itself. In addition, we can see that the approximation of the cumulative risk by the cumulative rate is not very satisfactory when incidence is high, such as occurs when all cancer sites are combined.

As an index of comparison between populations, the cumulative risk has two main advantages over the standardized rate; it avoids the arbitrary choice of the weighting and it expresses the risk on a probability scale which is interpretable immediately.

The number of years of life lost

Descriptive epidemiology is fundamental to etiologic research. In this capacity, it attempts to link characteristics of time and place to cancer development. It is therefore natural that the measurement of incidence or, failing that, the measurement of mortality will be the key instrument of the epidemiologist. But descriptive epidemiology should also provide information that could be useful in the establishment of public health priorities and policies, by addressing the consequences of cancer, the main one from a public health perspective being the amount of human life lost from the disease. This objective is already partially achieved by the determination of survival rates, but they do not provide an overall picture of the impact of cancer on the general population. In order to obtain this picture, we must measure the impact of cancer on the potential duration of life that individuals of the given population should have, on average, in the absence of the disease. The concept of *potential years of life lost* (PYLL) has exactly this objective, since it measures the average reduction of duration of life due to premature death caused by the given disease.

In order to assess the reduction in duration of life, two conceptual approaches have been proposed. The first suggests that the years lost from death due to the cause under study should only be taken into consideration up to an age limit that is arbitrarily fixed to mark the normal end of life; only deaths occurring at ages lower than this limit are then taken into account in the estimation of the reduction of duration of life. The second approach assumes that the reduction in potential life is equal to the number of years which the individual would otherwise have expected to live at the age of death. Thus this approach takes into account the force of general mortality exerted on the population under consideration. The two concepts differ in the same way as do the net and crude probabilities of dying from a certain cause of death, since the parameter is calculated respectively without and with taking other causes into account (see Chapter 1, page 34).

Several upper limits have been proposed in the context of the fixed age limit method. It has also been suggested to adopt a lower limit in order to exclude infant mortality from the definition of premature death. The approach based on life expectancy also has several variants. We will, however, only discuss the most common ones here.

Years of life lost with respect to a fixed age limit

If h is the fixed age limit, then the number of years potentially lost for an individual in age group x dying from a certain cause can be denoted by

$$h - a_x$$

where a_x is the average age of death in age group x, which is, in practice, taken as the centre of the age interval. If d_x denotes the number of deaths in age group x, then the total number of years of life lost in the population may be written

$$PYLL = \sum_{a_x < h} d_x (h - a_x) \qquad (2.13)$$

and, consequently, the number of years of life lost per death on average is

$$\frac{PYLL}{\sum_x d_x}$$

which is simply $h - \bar{a}$, where $\bar{a}$ is the average age of death from the cause under consideration.

Rather than calculating this number of years per number of deaths, some authors prefer to compute years lost per number of person-years M which has produced these deaths. The number $(10^5 \times PYLL)/M$ then measures the number of years of life lost in a year per 100 000 people who have the same age structure and mortality as the population under consideration. This ratio is described as the *rate of years of life lost*. Note that the index $\dfrac{PYLL}{M} = \dfrac{\sum_x d_x}{M} (h - \bar{a})$ is in fact the product of the crude mortality rate and the average number of years lost by the individuals who have died from the given cause.

The rate of life years lost can be standardized for the purpose of comparison between groups. Let m_x be the number of person-years of age x in the given group, and L_x be the number of person-years of age x in the standard population and $L = \sum_x L_x$; the standardized rate of years of life lost may then be written

$$\frac{1}{L} \sum_{a_x < h} L_x \frac{d_x}{m_x} (h - a_x) = \frac{1}{L} \left(\sum_{a_x < h} d'_x \right) (h - \bar{a}') \qquad (2.14)$$

where d'_x and $\bar{a}'$ are, respectively, the age-specific number of deaths and the average age of death which would be observed in a population with the age structure of the standard population, and the mortality rate of the given group.

$$d'_x = L_x \frac{d_x}{m_x}$$

Table 2.6 Calculation of number and standardized (^{a}) rate of potential years of life lost with a fixed limit at age 70
(male, lung cancer, canton of Neuchâtel, Switzerland, 1974-1976)

x	a_x	$70 - a_x$	d_x	m_x	$PYLL_x$	w_x	$10^5 \, PYLL_x$	$\dfrac{w_x}{m_x}$
(1)	(2)	(3)	(4)	(5)	(6)	(7)	(8)	
40-44	42.5	27.5	5	15 270	137.5	0.214	192.7	
45-49	47.5	22.5	4	15 102	90.0	0.214	127.5	
50-54	52.5	17.5	12	14 946	210.0	0.179	251.3	
55-59	57.5	12.5	18	13 044	225.0	0.143	246.7	
60-64	62.5	7.5	31	10 830	232.5	0.143	307.0	
65-69	67.5	2.5	38	9 843	95.0	0.107	103.3	
Total			108		990.0	1.000	1 228.5	

Columns 1, 4, 5, 7 are given and columns 2, 3, 6, 8 are calculated.
(^{a}) World population 40-69 years.

$$\overline{a}' = \frac{\displaystyle\sum_x d'_x \, a_x}{\displaystyle\sum_x d'_x}$$

Formula (2.14) is therefore the product of the standardized mortality rate and the average number of years of life lost in a population that would have the standard age structure and experience the mortality of the given group.

When they are calculated in this way, the rates from different causes have the advantage of being additive. In other words, the sum of the rates corresponding to several given causes is equal to the rate which is calculated from the sum of deaths due to these combined causes.

As an example, Table 2.6 presents the calculation of the years of life lost from lung cancer for Neuchâtel, Switzerland; only deaths occurring after 40 years are taken into consideration and the age limit is 70 years. Years of life lost are also expressed as rates, standardized to the European population. This example shows the weight that is given to deaths, however few in number, occurring long before the age limit.

Years of life lost with respect to life expectancy

In this situation, potential life is the number of years which would theoretically be left to live at the time of death, according to the life table.

If we let $\overset{o}{e}_x$ (see Chapter 1, page 27) be the life expectancy at the mid-point a_x of age group x, then, as previously explained, the years of life lost from a given cause are the sum of the potential duration of life of all those who have died from this cause

$$PYLL' = \sum_{x=1}^{g} d_x \overset{o}{e}_x \tag{2.15}$$

For comparisons between populations, rates and standardized rates can of course be calculated, although the justification for doing so is not obvious when the life expectancy differs among the populations being compared. Table 2.7 shows the calculation of the rates and standardized rates from data for lung cancer in Neuchâtel, taking values of life expectancy from the life table for the whole of Switzerland (see Appendix 1).

The rate obtained (2395 years per 100 000) is twice that given by the fixed limit method. The difference arises partly from the fact that deaths are taken into account at whatever age they occur, including those well after the fixed age limit. However, it also results from the fact that, for all ages less than 70 years, the life expectancy is greater than that which would be obtained with a life potential limited to 70 years. A higher fixed limit could possibly have led to the opposite conclusion.

We have stated that life expectancy implicitly took into account competing risks due to other causes that could manifest their effects at any age, including the years before the arbitrarily fixed age-limit. From this perspective, it would be more appropriate to recalculate the life expectancy at each age from a life table that excludes the deaths for which the years of life lost are calculated. This approach has some connection with the concept of additional years of life due to elimination of a cause

Table 2.7 Calculation of number and standardized rate of potential years of life lost compared to life expectancy ([a]) at age of death (male, lung cancer, canton of Neuchâtel, Switzerland – 1974-1976)

Age (x)	$\overset{o}{e}_x$	d_x	m_x	$PYLL'_x$	w_x	$10^5\ PYLL_x\ \dfrac{w_x}{m_x}$
(1)	(2)	(3)	(4)	(5)	(6)	(7)
40-44	32.77	5	15 270	163.9	0.188	201.8
45-49	28.24	4	15 102	113.0	0.188	140.7
50-54	23.89	12	14 946	286.7	0.156	299.2
55-59	19.85	18	13 044	357.3	0.125	342.4
60-64	16.12	31	10 830	499.7	0.125	576.8
65-69	12.78	38	9 843	485.6	0.094	463.7
70-74	9.84	29	7 656	285.4	0.063	234.9
75-79	7.35	22	5 787	161.7	0.031	86.6
80-84	5.38	13	2 721	69.9	0.015	38.5
85 +	4.59	2	1 323	9.2	0.015	10.4
Total				2 432.4	1.000	2 395.0

([a]) Swiss life table, 1978-1983. Office fédéral de la Statistique, Berne, 1985; see Annex 1.

of death (see Chapter 1, page 35). In practice, this subtlety is only necessary for the causes of death that themselves play an appreciable role in the life table, and besides, it has the disadvantage of making the procedure lose its additive property: the estimate of the years of life lost from a combination of causes could then be less than the sum of the individual estimates [11].

Methods for comparison

When we wish to compare incidence in several populations, the first step is to examine standardized rates. However, as explained in the previous section, these rates are affected by random variability. It is therefore important to know if an observed difference between two incidence curves described in this way is real or only due to chance. Knowing the confidence intervals of the rates being compared is not always sufficient to make a judgement about the difference: there exist situations in which incidence curves are significantly different even when the confidence intervals of the rates overlap.

The statistical significance of an observed difference between two rates can be roughly estimated by a method that requires only the total number of cases in both populations in addition to the two rates under study. Because it is not precise, this method, described in the next paragraph, should be reserved for use in situations in which age-specific data are unavailable. We discuss therefore in a following section the methods that are appropriate when age-specific data are available (see page 77).

Finding a statistically significant difference generally leads us to attempt to define the nature of the difference. Although age-specific rates are obtained from cross-sectional data, it is not unusual for them to differ in a constant ratio between the two populations (the proportionality assumption). When such a model (known as the *multiplicative model*) is acceptable, it is reasonable to estimate the constant factor, that is simply the *relative rate* of one population compared with another (see page 79) When it is not acceptable, the incidence ratio varies with age; this situation is known as *interaction* between group and age. On page 81, we present a general test to decide wether the assumption of proportionality is acceptable and in a following paragraph a test against the more specific assumption of increasing or decreasing trend of the incidence ratio with age; the test against the existence of a linear trend, which is the model most frequently considered, is discussed. Lastly, we give an example on page 83 to show the practical use in a complex situation of the tests that have been discussed.

In the second part of this section we deal with the problems that arise from the comparison of incidence in several populations or in different subgroups of the same population. A series of pairwise comparison of rates can actually produce contradictory results, as well as being inappropriate: by multiplying the number of comparisons that have been made, we increase the risk of concluding wrongly that a difference is significant. We first consider an approximate method which involves the comparison of the incidence of all the subgroups of a population with a standard incidence, which is usually that of the whole population. Then the correct test for deciding wether several forces of incidence can be considered identical is introduced on page 87. In a final paragraph of this section we briefly introduce the analysis of incidence using the log-linear model which allow this type of problem to be approached in a more systematic fashion (see page 90).

Comparison of incidence of a disease in two groups

The approximate method

We can obtain a rough idea of the significance of the difference between two standardized rates when we only have these rates and the total number of individuals in the populations in which the incidence was measured.

If we were comparing crude rates, it would be sufficient to know their variances (page 51). Let t_1 and t_2 be the rates to be compared and m_1 and m_2 the person-years of observation. Since the variance of a difference of independent variables is equal to the sum of their variances, we may write

$$\text{Var}\,(t_1 - t_2) = \left(\frac{1}{m_1} + \frac{1}{m_2}\right)\lambda = \frac{2}{h}\,\lambda \qquad (2.16)$$

where λ is the theoretical common rate in the two populations and h the harmonic mean of m_1 and m_2. Then if we replace λ by its estimate under the null hypothesis

$$\hat{\lambda} = (m_1 t_1 + m_2 t_2)\,/\,(m_1 + m_2)$$

we can write

$$\text{Var}\,(t_1 - t_2) = \frac{m_1 t_1 + m_2 t_2}{m_1 m_2} \qquad (2.17)$$

Thus, the variable

$$Z = \frac{t_1 - t_2}{\sqrt{\dfrac{m_1 t_1 + m_2 t_2}{m_1 m_2}}}$$

has a standard normal distribution and we shall reject the hypothesis of equality of the rate in the two populations at the $\alpha = 5\%$ significance level when $|Z|$ is greater than 1.96.

When the rates to be compared t_1 and t_2 are standardized, the variance of the denominator calculated in this way is only an approximation to the variance of the difference of the two rates. Writing t_1 and t_2 as an explicit function of the age-specific rates t_{1x} and t_{2x}, the expression (2.17) becomes

$$V_a (t_1 - t_2) = \sum_x w_x \frac{m_1 t_{1x} + m_2 t_{2x}}{m_1 m_2}$$

$$= \frac{2}{h} \sum_x w_x \bar{t}_x \qquad (2.18)$$

where $\bar{t}_x$ is the mean of t_{1x} and t_{2x} weighted by m_1 and m_2, the size of the groups to be compared.

The average of the $\bar{t}_x$ in (2.18) gives only a partial description of the variability of $t_1 - t_2$. Its exact variance is slightly different and is obtained from the variance of the differences of the specific rates; using formula (2.16) in each age group and replacing λ by its estimate, we get

$$V_e (t_1 - t_2) = \sum_x w_x^2 \left(\frac{2}{h_x} \hat{\lambda}_x \right) = \sum_x w_x^2 \frac{k_{1x} + k_{2x}}{m_{1x} m_{2x}} \qquad (2.19)$$

where $\hat{\lambda}_x$ is the estimate of the common rate λ_x and h_x the harmonic mean of m_{1x} and m_{2x}. Writing $w_x = L_x / h$, we get

$$V_e (t_1 - t_2) = \frac{2}{h} \sum_x w_x \frac{L_x \hat{\lambda}_x}{h_x} = \frac{2}{h} \sum_x w_x t_x^*$$

a formula which suggests that the values V_a and V_e may be close together if the structure of the standard population is not too different from that corresponding to the harmonic mean of the populations being compared.

As an example, consider the rates of stomach cancer for males in Zaragoza and Geneva, standardized to the world population restricted to the age range 35 to 74 years (see Table 2.8 and Figure 2.4). We obtain respectively $t_1 = 56.82/100\ 000$ and $t_2 = 43.52/100\ 000$. The approximate variance of the difference between the rates is thus (see (2.17))

$$V_a (t_1 - t_2) = \frac{(5 \times 167\ 022 \times 56.82) + (5 \times 71\ 298 \times 43.52)}{5 \times 71\ 298 \times 5 \times 167\ 022} \times 10^{-5} = 2.12 \times 10^{-9}$$

$$Z_a = \frac{|56.82 - 43.52| \times 10^{-5}}{\sqrt{2.12 \times 10^{-9}}} = 2.89$$

whereas the exact variance calculated using formula (2.18) above is

$$V_e (t_1 - t_2) = 2.11 \times 10^{-9}$$

$$Z_e = \frac{|56.82 - 43.52| \times 10^{-5}}{\sqrt{2.11 \times 10^{-9}}} = 2.89$$

Table 2.8   Cases of stomach cancer in males and population size by age group in Zaragoza, Spain, and Geneva, Switzerland.
Incident cases 1973-77 [6]

x	Age	Incident cases		Population size 1975	
		Zaragoza k_{1x}	Geneva k_{2x}	Zaragoza $m_{1x}/5$	Geneva $m_{2x}/5$
1	35-39	8	10	22 801	13 506
2	40-44	8	6	27 291	12 480
3	45-49	36	7	26 762	11 012
4	50-54	54	18	25 899	9 887
5	55-59	53	17	19 853	7 010
6	60-64	96	25	17 431	6 845
7	65-69	115	35	15 024	6 066
8	70-74	145	37	11 961	4 492
Total		515	155	167 022	71 298

k_{1x} : Observed cases in age group x in Zaragoza between 1973 and 1977.
m_{1x} : number of person-years of observation in age group x in Zaragoza between 1973 and 1977.
k_{2x} and m_{2x} : similar definition for Geneva.

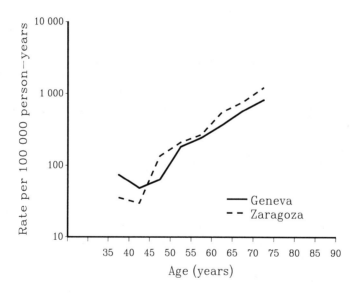

Figure 2.4   Age-specific incidence of stomach cancer in Zaragoza (Spain) and Geneva (Switzerland) males, 1973-1977

In this case, we see that the two values calculated from the variance are almost identical. The comparison of the two standardized rates by this method leads us to conclude that the incidence rate of stomach cancer observed in Zaragoza (56.82/100 000) is significantly greater than that observed in Geneva (43.52/100 000). It could, however, happen that $\bar{t}_x$ and t_x^* have different mean values.

Therefore the approximate method is not recommended when the data permit the correct calculation to be carried out.

Mantel-Haenszel test

Standardized rates have a descriptive function and the method of comparison previously proposed above is essentially aimed at avoiding gross errors in interpretation. When a comparative study of incidence is envisaged, the comparison problem should be approached in another way that requires knowing the age-specific rates and the number of person-years from which they were calculated.

Cochran [12] has shown how the performance of the χ^2 test could be improved by explicitly taking into account alternatives to the null hypothesis that we are trying to test. He proposed a method for the combination of 2 × 2 tables that was adapted by Mantel and Haenszel [13] in the context of case-control studies. It can also be applied with little change for the comparisons of incidence. The numerous applications of the Mantel-Haenszel method justify the amount of attention that we will give to its presentation.

Often incidence curves are approximately parallel when they are represented on a logarithmic scale. This overall shift in the curve corresponds to the fact that the ratio of the age-specific rates in the two populations being compared is more or less constant. The Mantel-Haenszel test basically involves testing the alternative assumption of proportionality of age-specific rates against the null hypothesis of equal rates.

The method involves summing the observed differences in each age group; if the differences tend to be of the same sign, as is supposed under the alternative hypothesis, their cumulative value will not be compatible with the null hypothesis of equality of age-specific rates. Small differences can thus be identified more easily whereas, if they were considered individually or incorporated into a sum of squared differences, no conclusions could be drawn.

Suppose that the hypothesis of equal rates is true. Then, apart from random variation, the total number of observed cases in each age-group is divided between the two populations in proportion to the number of person-years accumulated in each one. Summing these expected numbers over all age groups will provide the overall expected difference between the two populations which must be compared to the overall observed difference. Since the total number of expected cases is made equal to the total number of observed cases, it is sufficient, in practice, to calculate the difference between the total number of cases observed and the total number of cases expected under the hypothesis of equal rates in just one of the populations. We illustrate this method using data presented in Tables 2.8 and 2.9.

If we use data for the second population, that is, in Geneva (Table 2.8), the number of cases expected in age group x is

$$e_{2x} = K_x \frac{m_{2x}}{M_x} \tag{2.20}$$

where $M_x = m_{1x} + m_{2x}$ and $K_x = k_{1x} + k_{2x}$. The test is then based on the overall difference between observed and expected cases in the second population, that is, if g
age groups are used:

$$T = \sum_{x=1}^{g} (k_{2x} - e_{2x}) = O_2 - E_2$$

It is then evident from this latter formula that the statistic T is designed to
detect systematic differences of the same sign between the observed and expected
numbers in the different age-groups. In order to find out if the value of the statistic
is significantly different from zero, we need to know its variability under the null
hypothesis. Under this hypothesis, the total information available on the common
rate λ_x in age group x is contained in the variable K_x. Therefore, K_x being fixed at
its observed value, the statistical distribution of the number of cases in the age
group x of the second population is independent of λ_x; it may be described as the
result of K_x independent choices between the two populations with probability m_{2x}/M_x
that the second population is chosen. In other words, k_{2x} has a binomial distribution
with mean e_{2x} and variance

$$\text{Var}(k_{2x}) = K_x \frac{m_{2x}}{M_x} \frac{m_{1x}}{M_x} \tag{2.21}$$

and consequently, the variance of the statistic T is

$$\text{Var}(T) = \sum_{x=1}^{g} \text{Var}(k_{2x} - e_{2x}) = \sum_{x=1}^{g} K_x \frac{m_{2x} \times m_{1x}}{M_x^2}$$

$Z = T/\sqrt{\text{Var}(T)}$ approximately follows a standard normal distribution; thus, if we observe an absolute value of Z greater than 1.96, we can reject the null hypothesis
of equality of rates at the 0.05 level (two-sided test).

This statistic has low power if the alternative hypothesis is not the one specified
above; for example, an incidence that is clearly higher at young ages and clearly
lower in older age groups might give a result which is not statistically significant,
even though the null hypothesis is not true. The test is actually much less effective
the further one moves away from the assumption of proportionality of rates. We
examine its use in particular situations, notably when curves cross over, on page 83.

Table 2.9 gives the various steps of the calculation of the Mantel-Haenszel
test, using the data presented in Table 2.8.

The value of the statistic Z is therefore:

$$Z = \frac{155 - 188.7}{\sqrt{135.3}} = -2.90$$

The differences observed cannot therefore be attributed to random variation
and we can conclude that the incidence of stomach cancer is higher in Zaragoza

Table 2.9 Comparison of incidence rates in two populations; Mantel-Haenszel test. Data from Table 2.8

x	$M_x/5$ (1)	K_x (2)	k_{2x} (3)	e_{2x} (4)	$Var(k_{2x})$ (5)
1	36 307	18	10	6.7	4.2
2	39 771	14	6	4.4	3.0
3	37 774	43	7	12.5	8.9
4	35 786	72	18	19.9	14.4
5	26 863	70	17	18.3	13.5
6	24 276	121	25	34.1	24.5
7	21 090	150	35	43.1	30.7
8	16 453	182	37	49.7	36.1
Total	238 320	670	$O_2 = 155$	$E_2 = 188.7$	135.3

than in Geneva. Note that in this case the value of |Z| only differs slightly from that obtained by the approximate method (see page 75).

Overall measure of incidence ratio

When the multiplicative model is acceptable, the rate ratio of the two populations is independent of age:

$$\frac{\lambda_{2x}}{\lambda_{1x}} = \rho$$

It is therefore natural to try to estimate ρ. Mantel and Haenszel have proposed a weighted average of the ratio of the age-specific rates which proved to be very efficient:

$$\hat{\rho} = \frac{\sum\limits_{x=1}^{g} \dfrac{k_{2x} m_{1x}}{M_x}}{\sum\limits_{x=1}^{g} \dfrac{k_{1x} m_{2x}}{M_x}} \tag{2.22}$$

From data in Table 2.8 and from intermediate calculations presented in the first two columns of Table 2.10, we obtain

$$\hat{\rho} = \frac{110.73}{144.46} = 0.766$$

which means that the risk of stomach cancer is 1.3 times $(1/\hat{\rho})$ greater in Zaragoza than in Geneva. We can easily calculate a confidence level for ρ, although it would mainly be of theoretical interest in the context of most descriptive analysis.

Table 2.10 Calculation of the relative risk of stomach cancer in Geneva, Switzerland, with Zaragoza, Spain, as baseline. Data from Tables 2.8 and 2.9

x	$\dfrac{k_{2x}\,m_{1x}}{M_x}$ (1)	$\dfrac{k_{1x}\,m_{2x}}{M_x}$ (2)	$\dfrac{m_{1x} + \hat{\rho}\,m_{2x}}{5}$ (3)	$\dfrac{K_x\,m_{1x}\,m_{2x}}{M_x\,(m_{1x} + \hat{\rho}\,m_{2x})}$ (4)
1	6.28	2.98	33 146.60	4.61
2	4.12	2.51	36 850.68	3.25
3	4.96	10.49	35 197.19	9.53
4	13.03	14.92	33 472.44	15.39
5	12.56	13.83	25 222.66	14.38
6	17.95	27.07	22 674.27	26.23
7	24.93	33.08	19 670.56	32.95
8	26.90	39.59	15 401.87	38.59
Total	110.73	144.47	221 636.27	144.93

In fact, the variance of $\text{Log}(\hat{\rho})$ is approximately [14-16]:

$$V = \frac{\displaystyle\sum_{x=1}^{g} \text{Var}\,(k_{2x})}{\hat{\rho}\left(\displaystyle\sum_{x=1}^{g} \dfrac{K_x m_{1x} m_{2x}}{M_x(m_{1x} + m_{2x}\hat{\rho})}\right)^2} \tag{2.23}$$

which, using the data in Table 2.9 (column 5) and 2.10, gives

$$V = \frac{135.3}{0.766\,(144.93)^2} = \frac{135.3}{16\,094.95} = 0.0084$$

from which we obtain the standard error $\sqrt{V} = 0.0917$.

Considering that $\text{Log}(\hat{\rho})$ has a normal distribution with mean $\text{Log}(\rho)$ and variance V, a confidence interval $[\rho_1 ; \rho_2]$ at the $(1 - \alpha)$ level can then be derived as

$$\left[\hat{\rho}\,e^{-Z_{\alpha/2}\sqrt{V}} \;;\; \hat{\rho}\,e^{+Z_{\alpha/2}\sqrt{V}}\right]$$

which gives, for $\alpha = 0.05$, the lower and upper confidence bounds, respectively:

$$\left[\hat{\rho}\,e^{-1.96\sqrt{V}} \;;\; \hat{\rho}\,e^{1.96\sqrt{V}}\right]$$

in the above example

$$\rho_1 = 0.766 \times 0.835 = 0.64$$

and

$$\rho_2 = 0.766 \times 1.1969 = 0.92$$

Test of a multiplicative model

The assumption of proportionality also can be tested using the same principle as before. Under the hypothesis of a constant relative risk regardless of the age group, the means of the Poisson distributions in the two populations for age group x are respectively $\lambda_x m_{1x}$ and $\rho \lambda_x m_{2x}$, where λ_x is the age-specific rate in the first population and ρ is the rate ratio. The K_x cases observed will tend to be distributed among the two populations in proportion to these values, so that, using the same principle as in the previous paragraph,

$$k_{2x} \rightsquigarrow \text{Binom}(K_x, p_x)$$

where

$$p_x = \frac{\rho \lambda_x m_{2x}}{\lambda_x m_{1x} + \rho \lambda_x m_{2x}} = \frac{\rho m_{2x}}{m_{1x} + \rho m_{2x}} \qquad (2.24)$$

Therefore, under the assumption of proportionality, the expectation and variance of the number of cases in age group x of population 2 are now dependent on ρ and are respectively:

$$e_{2x}(\rho) = K_x p_x$$

$$\text{Var}(k_{2x}; \rho) = K_x p_x (1 - p_x)$$

and will be estimated by replacing ρ in (2.24) by $\hat{\rho}$ given by (2.22).

If the hypothesis of a constant risk ratio is not true, we will observe substantial differences between the observed and the expected numbers of cases in some age groups; overall, these differences will be detected by the sum of standardized squared differences d_x^2 in each age group,

$$X^2 = \sum_x d_x^2 = \sum_x \left[\frac{[k_{2x} - e_{2x}(\hat{\rho})]^2}{\text{Var}(k_{2x}; \hat{\rho})} \right] \qquad (2.25)$$

Table 2.11 Calculation for interaction tests. Data from Tables 2.8, 2.9 and 2.10

x (1)	k_{2x} (2)	$e_{2x}(\hat{\rho})$ (3)	$\text{Var}(k_{2x}; \hat{\rho})$ (4)	d_x^2 (5)	$(1) \times (2-3)$ (6)	$(1) \times (4)$ (7)	$(1) \times (7)$ (8)
1	10	5.62	3.87	4.96	4.38	3.87	3.87
2	6	3.63	2.69	2.09	4.74	5.38	10.76
3	7	10.31	7.84	1.40	− 9.93	23.52	70.56
4	18	16.29	12.60	0.23	6.84	50.40	201.60
5	17	14.90	11.73	0.38	10.50	58.65	293.25
6	25	27.98	21.51	0.41	−17.88	129.06	774.36
7	35	35.43	27.06	0.01	− 3.01	189.42	1 325.94
8	37	40.66	31.58	0.42	−29.28	252.64	2 021.12
Total	155	154.82	118.88	9.90	−33.64	712.94	4 701.46

which is approximately distributed as a χ^2 with g-1 degrees of freedom. This test is also known as the *homogeneity test*.

In the above example, its value can be calculated from Table 2.11 (column 5):

$$\sum_x d_x^2 = 9.90$$

as this value is lower than the critical value 14.07 at the significance level $\alpha = 0.05$ for a χ^2 with seven degrees of freedom, we cannot reject the null hypothesis of proportionality.

Trend test

The test with $(g - 1)$ degrees of freedom described above is not very sensitive to small departures from proportionality; nevertheless, even small differences can be interpretable if they increase or decrease systematically with age. If such a situation is expected, it is preferable to use a trend test (with one degree of freedom) which is aimed more specifically at this alternative hypothesis. The relevant statistic is given by the weighted sum of the differences between observed and expected numbers

$$T = \sum_{x=1}^{g} u_x [k_{2x} - e_{2x} (\hat{\rho})]$$

where u_x varies with age according to a specified structure; for example, it could be assigned the age group's number if one was allowing for a linear divergence of the two curves with age.

We can show that

$$Var\,(T) = \sum_{x=1}^{g} u_x^2 \, Var\,(k_{2x}\,;\hat{\rho}\,) - \frac{\left[\sum_{x=1}^{g} u_x \, Var\,(k_{2x}\,;\hat{\rho}\,)\right]^2}{\sum_{x=1}^{g} Var\,(k_{2x}\,;\hat{\rho}\,)} \qquad (2.26)$$

$Z = T/\sqrt{Var(T)}$ is a standard normal variable that we will use to test for the alternative hypothesis specified by the series of coefficients u_x; this test is also known as the Armitage test [17]. Details of the calculations are presented in Table 2.11 (columns 6 to 8); from these data we obtain

$$Z = \frac{-33.64}{\sqrt{4\,701.5 - \dfrac{(712.9)^2}{118.9}}} = -1.63$$

The hypothesis of proportionality can therefore not be rejected even when the alternative hypothesis is more narrowly specified. However, the value of Z is relatively high; this can be understood well enough by examining Figure 2.4 where we can see that, because incidence is initially higher in Geneva, there is a slight departure from the null hypothesis of proportionality.

Example : Hodgkin's lymphoma

The methods that we introduced above might seem unnecessarily sophisticated for estimating differences as obvious as those which appear between Zaragoza and Geneva with regard to stomach cancer. Their usefulness does not appear in routine contexts, but is apparent in borderline or complex situations. For example, a more precise method is needed to interpret population differences when incidence in different periods of life is described by different models. The above approach may then be extremely useful. To illustrate this idea, consider the comparison of incidence of Hodgkin's disease for males in Connecticut and the province of Zaragoza for the time period 1973 to 1977 [7] (see also Figure 2.5).

If we use the method described on page 76, we obtain a value Z = 0.56 for the Mantel-Haenszel test, which tempts us to conclude that there is no difference in incidence between the two populations. Note also that the standardized rates (respectively 3.8 and 4.0 per 100 000 in Zaragoza and Connecticut) yield the same interpretation. On the other hand, one should be warned by the high value (53.65 with seventeen degrees of freedom) obtained with the homogeneity test, suggesting that the incidence curves very likely cross; this phenomenon, which can be clearly

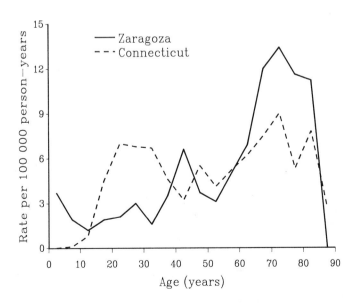

Figure 2.5   Age-specific incidence of Hodgkin's disease in Zaragoza (Spain) and Connecticut (USA) males, 1973-1977

seen on the graph in Figure 2.5 is not *a priori* surprising since we know that Hodgkin's disease has at least two forms with different etiologies. It is then natural that we should look separately at differences in younger age groups and in older age groups.

If we use the Mantel-Haenszel test on the age groups from one to 24 years, we obtain 85 observed cases as opposed to 83.22 expected in Connecticut and a value of $\hat{\rho} = 1.13$ with $Z = 0.45$. Although the test is not significant, given the appearance of the two incidence curves, it is still advisable to continue the analysis using the methods presented page   and ; the homogeneity test gives a value of 38.85 with four degrees of freedom (p < 0.001), and the linear trend test gives 5.65 for one degree of freedom. This last value means that the difference between observed and expected numbers increased significantly with age. The observed and expected values under the hypothesis of parallel curves with $\hat{\rho} = 1.13$ are shown in Table 2.12 and, from close examination, it can be clearly seen why the hypothesis of proportionality is not justifiable. Actually, the disease is significantly more frequent in children in Zaragoza ($Z = -5.40$ with the Mantel-Haenszel test performed on the first two age groups); a reversal of risk takes place at adolescence. In Connecticut, the risk is significantly higher for young adults: if we restrict our analysis to age groups 20-34 years, the disease is three times more frequent in Connecticut (($\hat{\rho} = 3.06$, $Z = 3.41$). On the other hand, differences between the two countries are no longer observed after 35 years: the homogeneity test gives values of $Z = -1.05$ and $\chi^2_{10} = 6.59$. These diverse results force us to suspect that Hodgkin's disease might involve a group of three pathological entities with different etiologies and not two as was previously assumed [18]. The observed difference could also originate in different definitions of the disease in the two countries.

The example demonstrates that the procedures introduced in this section can be valuable tools to help avoid erroneous interpretations when random variation are substantial and when the pattern of incidence deviates markedly from the simple shapes observed for epithelial tumours. They must nevertheless be applied with caution and their use be motivated by biological hypotheses defined *a priori*.

Table 2.12 Hodgkin's disease in Connecticut (USA) and Zaragoza (Spain). Male, 1973-1977 [7]

| Age | Connecticut | | | Zaragoza |
	Observed cases	Expected cases for $\hat{\rho} = 1.13$	Rate	Rate
1-4	0	4.74	0.00	3.67
5-9	1	3.38	0.13	1.89
10-14	6	6.65	0.85	1.23
15-19	32	29.20	4.51	1.88
20-24	46	41.07	7.02	2.10

Comparison of incidence among several populations

Often in descriptive epidemiology we have to interpret differences in incidence among a series of populations, or subgroups of the same population. This is a standard procedure when routinely published data are studied. Therefore, the analysis has no longer the goal of studying specific differences between a few given groups. Its objective is instead to find all differences which may exist. We present below the standard methods that can evaluate whether each incidence rate in a series of groups or populations is significantly different from an overall expected value. The problem with these methods, like all those which involve multiple comparisons, is that they are bound to identify some differences produced by random fluctuations as being significant. It is therefore preferable to use a test that provides an overall assessment of the homogeneity of incidence. This is introduced on page 87. We shall also discuss in Chapter 3 (see page 134) other methods which are appropriate in this context.

Comparison with an overall expected value

If the total number of cases is available in a subpopulation whose age structure is known, then it is possible to check if this observation is compatible with a given incidence rate, such as the incidence rate of the whole population. It is straightforward to use this incidence rate to calculate the number of expected cases in each age group, their total E, the SIR and its confidence interval in the subpopulation. We will take it that the SIR is different from 100 when its confidence interval does not include 100 (see page 64). When the total number O of observed cases is sufficiently large, the normal approximation to the Poisson distribution can be used. In other words, we consider that O is a normal variable with expectation E and variance E; accordingly, we can calculate the quantity: $X^2 = \dfrac{(O - E)^2}{E}$ which follows a χ^2 distribution with one degree of freedom.

Because of its simplicity, this method is often used systematically to find out if the incidence rate in selected subpopulations deviates significantly from the total population incidence rate, as though this incidence were known *a priori* and not calculated from the observations themselves.

To illustrate the method, let us consider the regional subdivisions of the French département of Côte-d'Or that is covered by the Burgundy Registry of digestive tract tumours. The number of cases of colon cancer observed in each five-year age group, from 1976 to 1980, as well as the number of person-years accumulated in each age-group for the same period are summarized in Table 2.13. The total number of observed cases in each region, and the calculations of expected value under the hypothesis that the rates in the whole département of Côte-d'Or apply to each region of the département, are given in Table 2.14.

Table 2.13 Colon cancer cases and person-years ([a]) in Côte-d'Or, France, Male, incident cases 1976-1980

	Dijon		Côte Viticole		Châtillonnais		Plaine de la Saône		Auxois		Morvan		Côte-d'Or (Total)	
x	k_x	m_x	k_x	m_x	k_x	m_x	k_x	m_x	k_x	m_x	k_x	m_x	k_x	m_x
0-4	0	45 626	0	9 273	0	7 309	0	19 970	0	8 094	0	905	0	91 177
5-9	0	41 145	0	9 653	0	9 683	0	24 135	0	9 500	0	1 171	0	95 287
10-14	0	39 284	0	10 255	0	10 758	0	23 297	0	10 483	0	1 819	0	95 896
15-19	0	43 469	0	11 054	0	10 360	0	21 195	0	10 870	0	1 770	0	98 718
20-24	0	52 794	0	10 073	0	8 402	0	19 034	1	9 539	0	1 186	1	101 028
25-29	0	54 321	0	10 499	0	7 984	1	19 009	0	7 936	0	1 345	1	101 094
30-34	0	40 848	0	8 588	0	7 482	0	19 040	0	6 633	0	979	0	83 570
35-39	2	31 559	1	6 459	0	6 707	0	16 017	0	6 012	1	779	4	67 533
40-44	2	30 703	0	6 860	0	7 273	0	15 762	1	6 775	0	1 120	3	68 493
45-49	3	29 875	1	7 181	0	6 869	3	15 242	3	7 377	0	1 481	10	68 025
50-54	10	27 228	2	6 955	0	7 313	1	13 265	1	7 489	0	1 422	14	63 672
55-59	17	21 808	0	5 636	1	5 211	5	10 951	1	6 066	0	1 275	24	50 947
60-64	7	15 002	2	4 041	0	4 638	5	8 249	3	4 729	0	975	17	37 634
65-69	17	14 556	4	5 203	3	6 322	7	10 287	4	6 350	1	1 595	36	44 313
70-74	33	11 841	4	4 310	7	5 129	18	8 397	13	5 764	1	1 336	76	36 777
75-79	20	7 762	3	2 425	10	3 375	11	5 625	6	4 187	2	825	52	24 199
80 +	12	6 112	10	1 894	4	2 167	11	3 913	3	2 795	0	604	40	17 485
Total	123	513 933	27	120 359	25	116 982	62	253 388	36	120 599	5	20 587	278	2 245 848

([a]) Person-years of observation were calculated by summing the mid-year populations from 1976 to 1980.

Table 2.14 Calculation of the SIRs in the different regions of Côte-d'Or (France) with the overall incidence in the département as standard, males, colon cancer, 1976-1980

Region	Observed number	Expected number	SIR	95% confidence interval ([a])
Dijon	123	98.7	124.6	[103.6 ; 148.7]
Côte viticole	27	30.6	88.2	[58.1 ; 128.4]
Châtillonnais	25	36.0	69.4	[44.9 ; 102.5]
Plaine de Saône	62	62.8	98.7	[75.7 ; 126.6]
Auxois	36	41.0	87.8	[61.5 ; 121.6]
Morvan	5	8.9	56.2	[18.2 ; 131.1]

([a]) Exact method (Poisson distribution).

As the confidence interval of the SIR for Dijon excludes 100, we conclude that the incidence of colon cancer is higher here than in the whole département. We could also have tested the observed difference by calculating χ^2 with one degree of freedom; its observed value $(123 - 98.7)^2/98.7 = 5.98$ leads to the same conclusion. However, observations in the other cantons of Côte-d'Or are compatible with the overall incidence in this département.

Note that an analysis of the SIR without an indication of its precision would not be sufficient to provide the correct conclusion about the variation of incidence in the region. For example, the value of 56.2, that appears to indicate that Morvan is a low-risk area, is actually only due to the low value of the expected number which, in turn, implies large random variation in the observed number. In this case, the probability of obtaining five or fewer cases simply by chance, when the expected number is E = 8.9, is actually 13%, therefore too high to reject the null hypothesis of equality of the incidence rate in Morvan and in the whole département.

Although interpretation of the values obtained for the different SIRs is much more convincing when their confidence intervals are taken into account, the method is still approximate. In fact, the incidence for the whole of the Côte-d'Or that is used as a standard is calculated from observations made in the different subgroups; the SIR obtained for each of the subgroups is by definition systematically closer to unity than it would be if the standard incidence had been defined *a priori*. To avoid this problem, which is more significant when the subpopulation consists of a larger proportion of the total, some authors have proposed taking as a standard the incidence in the population complementary to the subpopulation for which the SIR is calculated. In other words, to use the incidence in all of the other populations as the standard incidence. As the variability of the rates in the complementary population is not taken into account, this approach is unfortunately not much more satisfying. The first approach is conservative, as it too often tends to favour the null hypothesis, while the second method is too liberal as it often wrongly rejects the null hypothesis.

Homogeneity test for incidence

The appropriate method is actually quite similar in conception to that previously described for the situation of two populations (see page 77). Its principle has been mainly applied to survival analyses (log rank test, see Chapter 4, page 247) and case-control studies, but its application to descriptive incidence or mortality data is also straightforward.

If the theoretical incidence is the same in all groups, the total number of observed cases K_x in each age group x would be divided among the different groups in proportion to the person-years accumulated in each of them. It can then be shown that the distribution of observed cases follows a multinomial distribution. To be defined completely, the distribution should be specified by the expected number in each group and by the variance-covariance matrix which quantifies not only the variability but also the correlation of the observed numbers in these groups.

Letting

- I be the number of subgroups to be compared ($1 \leq i \leq I$),

- k_{ix} be the number of observed cases in the xth age interval of the ith subgroup,

- m_{ix} be the number of person-years accumulated in the xth age interval of the ith subgroup,

- $K_x = \sum\limits_{i=1}^{I} k_{ix}$ and $M_x = \sum\limits_{i=1}^{I} m_{ix}$ the total number of cases and person-years in age-group x,

the mean and the variance of the observed number of cases in each age interval of each subgroup may be written ($1 \le i \le I$ and $1 \le x \le g$):

$$e_{ix} = \frac{K_x m_{ix}}{M_x} \qquad (2.27)$$

and

$$\text{Var}\,(k_{ix}) = \frac{K_x m_{ix}\,(M_x - m_{ix})}{M_x^2} \qquad (2.28)$$

Furthermore, the covariance between observations in two subgroups is

$$\text{Cov}\,(k_{ix}\,,\,k_{jx}) = \frac{-\,K_x m_{ix} m_{jx}}{M_x^2} \qquad (2.29)$$

As was done in the situation of two populations, we sum the quantities e_{ix} over all age groups to obtain the expected numbers E_i in subpopulation i. The variance and covariance of the observed numbers calculated under the assumption of equality of incidence are also summed over the age groups in order to obtain the variance-covariance matrix of the total number of cases in the subpopulations. The expected numbers are obviously the same as those given in Table 2.14, which were also defined by the overall incidence rate in the département of the Côte-d'Or:

$$E_i = \sum_x \frac{K_x m_{ix}}{M_x}$$

Table 2.15 gives the variance-covariance matrix V of the observed numbers O_i; it shows on the one hand that the variances are lower than the expected numbers. In other words, they are lower than the variance under the Poisson distribution; on the other hand, the table shows that all the covariances are negative, a predictable result since the total observed number in age group x is fixed at its observed value K_x (see (2.29)). If the observed numbers had themselves been allocated in the various populations according to a multinomial distribution, we would have the classic χ^2 test obtained from the normal approximation to the multinomial. Thus, we would calculate the test statistic

$$T_1 = \sum\limits_{i=1}^{I} \frac{(O_i - E_i)^2}{E_i} \qquad (2.30)$$

Table 2.15   Variance-covariance of the observed numbers of colon cancer cases in Côte-d'Or, France, under the hypothesis of risk homogeneity ([a]) within the département. Data from Table 2.13

Dijon	63.03				
Côte viticole	− 10.85	27.24			
Châtillonnais	− 12.59	− 3.97	31.27		
Plaine de la Saône	− 22.22	− 6.92	− 8.15	48.6	
Auxois	− 14.30	− 4.52	− 5.38	− 9.29	34.83
Morvan	− 3.09	− 0.99	− 1.17	− 2.02	−1.34	8.61

([a]) The variance of observed numbers is on the diagonal. The covariance of one region with the regions preceding it in the first column is under the diagonal. For example, in Auxois, the variance is 34.83; the covariance of observed numbers in Auxois and Morvan is −1.34.

which, in the present example, is 12.10, a value that is greater than 11.07, the 5% critical value of χ^2 with five degrees of freedom. This leads us to reject the hypothesis of homogeneity of the incidence rates in the six cantons of Côte-d'Or.

However, as the total number of cases K_x is fixed, the O_i are distributed as the sum of multinomial variables and T_1 is on average smaller than χ^2 with I−1 degrees of freedom. The appropriate calculation is based on another quadratic function T_2 of the $(O_i − E_i)$ where these differences are weighted inversely to their variances. Calculation of this statistic therefore requires the inverse of the variance-covariance matrix of the differences $O_i − E_i$; the elements w_{ij} of this inverted matrix provide the necessary weights. The statistic can thus be written:

$$T_2 = \sum_{i=1}^{I-1} w_{ii} (O_i − E_i)^2 + 2 \sum_{i<j} w_{ij} (O_i − E_i) (O_j − E_j) \qquad (2.31)$$

Note that the restriction of the sum to the first I−1 populations is related to the same principle involved in the Mantel-Haenszel test where only one group is used for calculating the test statistic. Because the sum of O_i is fixed, the last region does not contribute any further information to the test. The matrix inversion can be computed with readily available software. In the present example, the weights are provided by the inverse of the matrix in Table 2.15 and the statistic T_2 has a value of 12.25 which follows a χ^2 distribution with five degrees of freedom and, like T_1, leads us to reject the homogeneity hypothesis. In this situation, the calculation of T_1 would have been sufficient.

In practice, we often need to find the basis for this demonstrated heterogeneity, particularly to determine whether one or a few regions are responsible for the statistical significance of the test. The appropriate tool to answer the question is similar to a trend test with one degree of freedom; $\sum_i u_i O_i$ is compared with its expectation $\sum_i u_i E_i$ where the coefficients u_i which equal + 1, −1 or zero are chosen such that the statistic will enhance the contrast between the regions which are suspected to be different for *a priori* reasons. We thus calculate the statistic

$$T_3 = \frac{\left[\sum_i u_i (O_i - E_i)\right]^2}{\sum_i u_i^2 E_i - \sum_x \frac{\left(\sum_i u_i e_{ix}\right)^2}{K_x}} \tag{2.32}$$

where the denominator, which is **U'VU** in matrix notation, is the variance of $\sum_i u_i O_i$.

For example, for comparing Morvan ($i = 6$) with the rest of Côte-d'Or, we set $u_6 = 1$ and $u_i = -1$ if i is different from 6. We obtain $T_3 = 1.77$, a value which is not significant. The use of the same principle to compare the city of Dijon with the rest of the département gives $T_3 = 9.4$, a highly significant value for χ^2 with one degree of freedom (p = 0.002). For Châtillonnais, we obtain a borderline value, that is, $\chi_1^2 = 3.86$. Although formally significant, a value of this kind should be treated with caution because the multiplicity of the tests carried out increases the chance of wrongly rejecting the hypothesis of equality. Strictly speaking, the test has one degree of freedom only if the comparisons result from hypotheses defined *a priori*. For example, if the subgroups could be characterized according to a sociodemographic variable, such as the average income, a test with a single degree of freedom could be carried out by choosing for the u_i the rank of the regions after ordering them according to the value of this variable. In the same manner, if we wanted to compare northern and southern areas of a region, we could perform the test choosing $u_i = 1$ for the north and $u_i = -1$ for the south.

A further hypothesis which could be considered in the context of this example is whether the rural regions (all except Dijon) are homogeneous with respect to the incidence of colon cancer. The above approach would lead to a χ^2 with four degrees of freedom with the value 3.26 for the test of homogeneity of incidence in rural areas. The conclusion of the analysis is therefore that the incidence is different in the rural and urban regions of the département (see below).

Use of the log-linear model

The analysis of descriptive incidence data can also be conducted with modelling techniques that allow for greater flexibility in interpretation. As a rule, the idea is to look for a model which provides the estimate of the parameters of interest in particular the relative rate and to select the simplest among those that are statistically compatible with the observations. This approach is particularly easy with access to modern computer software.

The linear regression, a widely used statistical tool, consists of modelling the expectation of a normal variable, using a linear function of the covariates that influence its value (see Chapter 3, page 158). it has been proposed to generalize this technique to other probability distributions, including the binomial distribution and the Poisson distribution. It can be shown that, in order to obtain the optimal statistical properties, it is more effective to model a function of expectation rather than expectation itself; thus, for a binomial distribution, the logit of the probability is modelled, and for the Poisson distribution it is the logarithm of the mean which is modelled as a linear function of the relevant covariables.

The observations in the context of this manual are most often Poisson variables, whose expectation depends on the unknown incidence rate and person-years of observation according to the formula

$$E(K_{ix}) = m_{ix}\lambda_{ix}$$

that is

$$Log[E(K_{ix})] = Log(m_{ix}) + Log(\lambda_{ix})$$

The aim of this section is to show how $Log(\lambda_{ix})$ can be modelled linearly to provide most of the results which have been previously presented. The hypothesis of proportional incidence rates that has been introduced on several occasions may be written

$$\lambda_{2x} = \rho\lambda_{1x}$$

thus

$$Log(\lambda_{2x}) = Log(\lambda_{1x}) + Log(\rho) \tag{2.33}$$

Formula (2.33) is therefore a particular *log-linear model* which describes the incidence rate in group 1 (λ_{1x}) and the relative rate ρ of group 2 with respect to group 1. It can easily be generalized to more than two groups in the following form:

$$Log(\lambda_{ix}) = Log\lambda_{(1x)} + Log(\rho_i) \quad 2 \le i \le I \tag{2.34}$$

where ρ_i is the relative rate of group i with respect to group 1. In practice, $\beta_x = Log(\lambda_{1x})$ and $\theta_i = Log(\rho_i)$ are estimated by the maximum likelihood method, then $\hat{\lambda}_{1x}$ and $\hat{\rho}_i$ are derived by exponentiation. In the present situation involving two factors, age and subgroups $\hat{\lambda}_{1x}$ and $\hat{\rho}_i$ are in fact given by close formulae

$$\hat{\rho}_i = \frac{O_i}{\sum\limits_{x=1}^{g} m_{ix}\hat{\lambda}_{1x}} = \frac{O_i}{E_i} \tag{2.35}$$

$$\hat{\lambda}_{1x} = \frac{\sum\limits_{i} k_{ix}}{m_{1x} + \sum\limits_{i>1} \hat{\rho}_i m_{ix}} \tag{2.36}$$

where O_i is the total number of observed cases in group i and E_i is the expected number, taking $\hat{\lambda}_{1x}$ as a standard. It can be seen that this method provides a statistic related to the SIR; it serves the same purpose of locating the subpopulation on the risk scale. It is known as the internal method of standardization [19,20]. The special role given to the first subgroup is obviously the result of an arbitrary choice. An appropriate computer programme is required to estimate the parameters by the maximum likelihood method; the calculations reported below have been carried out using the program GLIM [21] and are described in detail in Appendix 2.

When the rates of stomach cancer in Geneva and Zaragoza are compared, the value of the parameter $\hat{\rho}$ is found to be 0.77 which means that there is about 30% more stomach cancer in Zaragoza. This value can be compared with results obtained from other methods previously presented in this chapter:

- SIR, using the marginal incidence rate as standard is

$$\frac{155}{188.73} \div \frac{515}{481.26} = 0.77$$

- $\hat{\rho}$ according to Mantel-Haenszel formula: 0.77
- Ratio of cumulative rates: 2.38/3.20 = 0.74
- Ratio of rates standardized to world population:

$$CIF = 43.52/56.82 = 0.77$$

When the two incidence curves are parallel, as in this example (see Figure 2.4), these various estimates are close together. It is however recommended to use the internal standardization, i.e., the log-linear model, which has optimal statistical properties in this context or to use the Mantel-Haenszel estimate which has been shown to be particularly robust.

The validity of the model (2.34) may be judged by comparing observed values k_{ix} and values $\hat{k}_{ix}$ calculated from the model itself. The ordinary goodness of fit statistic $T = \sum_{i,x} \frac{(k_{ix} - \hat{k}_{ix})^2}{\hat{k}_{ix}}$ may be used for this purpose. The measure of goodness of fit may also be based on the ratio between the likelihood of the accepted model and the likelihood of a model that would describe the observations exactly; this latter is known as a saturated model. This statistic

$$D = -2 \, Log[V(model) / V(saturated \ model)]$$

is referred to as the deviance. In the context of the classical linear model with normal error, it coincides with the above χ^2 for goodness of fit T. In the present situation, both T and the deviance D have a chi-squared distribution whose number of degrees of freedom is the number of observations h less the number of estimated parameters ν

$$T, D \rightsquigarrow \chi^2_{h-\nu}$$

When testing the goodness of fit of the proportional hazards model to the data from Geneva and Zaragoza, we obtain D = 9.392. The corresponding number of degrees of freedom is 7: 16 observations minus 9 fitted parameters (eight age groups + the relative risk). This value suggests an acceptable fit (p = 0.23): the difference between the values estimated by the model and the observed values is of an order of magnitude compatible with the random fluctuations allowed for by the Poisson distribution.

An hypothesis about the value of a parameter, for example, ρ = 1, can be tested by evaluating the significance of the increase in deviance which results from giving the tested value to the parameter of interest. When the increase is too large the proposed value is rejected. Thus, the comparison of deviance between the two models: (1): $\lambda_{2x} = \rho\lambda_{1x}$ and (2): $\lambda_{2x} = \lambda_{1x}$ is equivalent to the test of the hypothesis ρ = 1. In practice, the more general model is fitted (model 1) and the increase in deviance evaluated by fitting the restricted model (model 2). The calculations for the above examples are listed in Appendix 2.

When fitting model 2 to the present data, the deviance changes from 9.392 to 18.14. The difference of 8.75, value of a χ^2 variable with one degree of freedom, is highly significant and leads to reject the hypothesis of equality of the incidence rates (ρ = 1).

The variance and covariance of the parameter estimates are also derived from the likelihood (see Chapter 1, page 17). The variable

$$Z = \frac{\text{Log}\,(\hat{\rho}) - \text{Log}\,(\rho)}{\sqrt{\text{Var}\,(\text{Log}\,(\hat{\rho}))}}$$

is approximately a standard normal variate. We can then construct a $100\,(1 - \alpha)\,\%$ confidence interval:

$$\text{Log}\,(\hat{\rho}) \pm Z_{\alpha/2}\,\sqrt{\text{Var}\,(\text{Log}\,(\hat{\rho}))}$$

The value of Log($\hat{\rho}$) and its standard error are provided by the computer program GLIM (see Appendix 2) and are respectively for the current example Log($\hat{\rho}$) = − 0.2651 and Var(Log($\hat{\rho}$)) = 0.00841. Therefore, if the theoretical value of ρ were equal to one,

$$Z = \frac{-0.2651}{0.09168} = -2.89$$

a value which is too large for a standard normal deviate. We therefore conclude that ρ is significantly lower than 1 and its value is estimated at 0.77. This second way of testing the hypothesis ρ = 1 is known as the Wald test which here is the same as checking whether this confidence interval includes one.

The confidence interval of Log(ρ) calculated as shown above is [−0.448 ; −0.0854] from which we can derive the confidence interval of ρ by exponentiation [0.64 ; 0.92] which is identical in the present case to that obtained earlier from the Mantel-Haens-zel estimate (see page 80).

As a second example, we return to previous data on colon cancer incidence in Côte-d'Or (Table 2.13). We shall describe the incidence data observed among men older than 20 years by a proportional hazards model:

$$\lambda_{ix} = \rho_i \, \lambda_{1x} \quad 2 \leq i \leq 6$$

that is, since $E(K_{ix}) = \lambda_{ix} m_{ix}$:

$$\text{Log}\,[E(K_{ix})] = \text{Log}\,(m_{ix}) + \text{Log}\,(\lambda_{1x}) + \text{Log}\,(\rho_i)$$

This is an 18 parameter model (13 parameters for age and 5 for the relative rates); we have 78 observations available to carry out their estimation.

The fit of the model (see Appendix 2) leads to a deviance of 68.20 for 60 degrees of freedom; the goodness of fit is satisfactory (p = 0.219) showing that the proportional hazards model is acceptable. The relative rate of the 5 cantons with respect to Dijon (taken as a reference) are respectively 0.70 (côte Viticole), 0.55 (Châtillonnais), 0.79 (Plaine de la Saône), 0.70 (Auxois) and 0.45 (Morvan). How-ever, only the risk for Châtillonnais is significantly less than 1.

The confidence intervals of these parameters, which are obtained as explained above in the context of the comparison of two populations, confirm our previous conclusion. Only the relative rate for Chatillonnais is significantly less than one (see Appendix 2). This result implies logically that the rates of colon cancer are not homogeneous; it is however preferred to test formally this hypothesis by fitting the previous model under the constraint:

$$\rho_i = 1 \quad 2 \leq i \leq 6$$

We find a deviance of 80.78 for this new model; the increase $80.78 - 68.20 = 12.58$ is significant when compared to the critical value of χ^2 with $65 - 60 = 5$ degrees of freedom (p = 0.03). This confirms the heterogeneity of the rates.

The modelling approach is particularly well suited for carrying out the test of homogeneity of the rural regions made previously (see page 90). The hypothesis is then written:

$$\rho_i = \rho_j = \rho* \quad \rho* \neq 1 \quad 2 \leq i, j \leq 6$$

The fit of this model increases the deviance of 3.46 which is just below its expectation (the χ^2 in this example has $64 - 60 = 4$ degrees of freedom). The esti-mate of $\rho*$, relative rate of rural cantons is obtained from the fit and it is equal to 0.69 (95% CI = [0.54 ; 0.88]).

We therefore conclude that Dijon has the greater risk of colon cancer and that there is no evidence of rate heterogeneity in the rural regions of Côte-d'Or.

The modelling done for the factor region may also have been done for the factor age; it is clear that 13 parameters are not needed for describing the age effect which could be smoothed by a polynomial function (the age effect estimates for younger age groups have in fact a very low precision). The resulting model would be more parsimonous and would have the same ability for doing the above geo-graphical comparison (see Appendix 2).

The mathematical complexity of this approach is largely compensated for by its interpretative power. The clear terms of the hypotheses, the statistical evaluation of the results, the flexibility of use and the cohesiveness of the approach are qualities that make its systematic introduction into descriptive epidemiology worthy of serious consideration.

Extension and limitations of the present methodology

Risk analyses in the absence of denominators

As we have seen in previous sections, the descriptive analysis of cancer risk requires the estimation of person-years of observation. For descriptive studies in-volving large areas, national bureaux of statistics are usually able to provide the necessary information. In most countries, however, the data are generally not broken down by variables of epidemiological interest, such as occupation and country of birth. In contrast, these variables are usually available for incident cases or deaths. This section will show how it is possible to take advantage of this information to carry out the analysis of risk despite the lack of corresponding denominators.

The methods which have been proposed are based on an analysis either of the distribution of cases by site (e.g., correspondence analysis) or, where the interest is mainly in cancer of a particular site, of the proportion of this cancer occurring among all other sites. These are known as relative frequency or proportional inci-dence (or mortality) methods. The discussion will be restricted to the situation where interest is centred on a specific cancer site.

The relative frequency of a specific cancer in a population is defined as the ratio between the number of cases of the cancer and the total number of cancer cases in the population during the same period. The comparison of relative frequen-cies of a given cancer between two populations is at best an indirect measure of the absolute risk difference. This comparison will be more reliable when the cancer site of interest accounts for a small proportion of all cancer cases. For example, buccal cavity and pharyngeal cancers represent only 2.1% of all cancers in men in the United Kingdom, whereas in France they represent 8.6%. The corresponding crude rates in the two countries are respectively 9.2 and 42.4 per 100 000 person-years. In this situation, the information provided by the absolute and relative indices is identical: this cancer is four times more frequent in France than in the United Kingdom.

As a rule, however, risk estimates obtained from studies of relative frequency are less precise. The methods proposed below provide only a partial remedy for their intrinsic weakness. We will discuss briefly methods of standardization of relative frequencies and the modelling of proportional incidence in the following sections.

Standardized indices of relative frequency

The relationship between cancer incidence or mortality and age is generally site-specific. Consequently, it will generally not be the same for the site of interest and for all cancers. For example, the proportion of buccal cavity and pharyngeal cancers in France is 13.9% between 45 and 64 years and only 5.5% after 65 years [23]. The ratio of the age-specific incidence rate of the cancer under consideration and all cancers combined (λ_x / μ_x) will therefore depend on age; standardization is necessary to account for confounding by age when comparisons are carried out.

Two standardized indices have been proposed: ASCAR [24], which was initially developed for studies in developing countries, and the proportional incidence ratio (PIR). These indices are the equivalents, for relative frequencies, of the direct and indirect methods of standardization discussed previously.

ASCAR is the average of the age-specific relative frequencies, weighted by a standard distribution of age at which cancer occurs. If k_x is the number of cases of age x for the cancer of interest, K_x the total number of cancer cases and w_x the proportion of cancer of age x in the standard population ($\sum_x w_x = 1$), then

$$ASCAR = \sum_x w_x \frac{k_x}{K_x}$$

The PIR is the ratio between the total observed number of cancer cases at a given site and the number expected if the cases occurred according to a standard relative frequency p_x which was a function of age:

$$PIR = \frac{\sum\limits_x k_x}{\sum\limits_x K_x p_x}$$

The total number of cancer cases K_x in age group x being fixed at its observed value, the number k_x of cancer cases at a given site is distributed as a binomial variable. It is possible to make statistical inferences based on ASCAR and PIR using this distribution. This approach is however of limited interest since neither ASCAR nor PIR estimates population parameters which are interpretable in terms of risk or relative risk. The following approach overcomes this difficulty to some extent.

Modelling incidence data in the absence of the denominator

Suppose that we are studying the risk of a specific cancer C in two populations P_0 and P_1 in which cancer incidence rates are respectively λ_0 and λ_1 for cancer C and μ_0 and μ_1 for all cancers (Table 2.16). Let $v_1 = \mu_1 - \lambda_1$ and $v_0 = \mu_0 - \lambda_0$ be the incidence rate for all cancers other than C (denoted A), and ρ and θ be respectively the relative rates of cancers C and A, that is, $\lambda_1 = \rho\lambda_0$ and $v_1 = \theta v_0$. If a cancer occurs in population P_1, the probability that it is the specific cancer C is:

$$p_1 = \frac{\lambda_1}{\mu_1} = \frac{\rho\lambda_0}{\rho\lambda_0 + \theta v_0} \qquad (2.37)$$

and therefore

$$\frac{p_1}{1 - p_1} = \frac{\rho}{\theta} \times \frac{\lambda_0}{v_0} = \frac{\rho}{\theta} \frac{p_0}{1 - p_0} \qquad (2.38)$$

The odds of cancer C occurring in population P_1 are ρ/θ times the odds of its occurring in population P_0. This odds ratio is equal to the relative risk only if $\theta = 1$, that is, if the incidence rate of other cancers A is the same in the two populations. The observed odds ratio $k_1\ell_0 / k_0\ell_1$, which is an estimate of ρ/θ, is therefore somewhat difficult to interpret. When cancer C is rare and other cancers have approximately the same incidence in the populations being compared, the method is perfectly adequate.

When a confounding variable is considered, tables similar to Table 2.16 are constructed for each category of this variable and the Mantel-Haenszel method is used to provide an estimate of ρ/θ [25], for example if the number of cases are distributed by age group (x):

$$\left(\frac{\rho}{\theta}\right) = \sum_x \frac{k_{1x}\ell_{0x}}{K_x} \div \sum_x \frac{k_{0x}\ell_{1x}}{K_x} \qquad (2.39)$$

In practice, the logistic model is preferable, since formula (2.38) is equivalent to

$$\text{Logit}(p_1) = \text{Logit}(p_0) + \text{Log}\left(\frac{\rho}{\theta}\right)$$

More generally, if we adapt the model for confounding variables and study the risk in more than two groups, the probability of cancer C occurring in group j at age x is:

$$p_{jx} = \frac{p_j \lambda_{0x}}{p_j \lambda_{0x} + \theta_j v_{0x}}$$

Table 2.16 Distribution of cancer cases in age group x

	Number of cases		
	Population P_1	Population P_0	Total
Cancer under study (C)	k_{1x}	k_{0x}	$k_{.x}$
Other cancers (A)	ℓ_{1x}	ℓ_{0x}	$\ell_{.x}$
Total	K_{1x}	K_{0x}	$K_{.x}$

which leads to the logistic model

$$\text{Logit}(p_{jx}) = \alpha_x + \beta_j$$

where

$$\alpha_x = \text{Logit}(p_{0x}) \quad \beta_j = \text{Log}\left(\frac{p_j}{\theta_j}\right)$$

The parameters of the logistic model may be estimated from data k_{jx} for cancer C and ℓ_{jx} for other cancers A over exposure categories j.

This methodology is exactly that of a case-control study in which cases are patients with cancer C and controls are all other cancer patients. Given the similarity, this approach will not be developed further. A detailed discussion can be found in Chapter 6 of Breslow and Day [25]. An example of the use of this method is found in Chapter 3, page 168 where it is applied to a study of migrants. The proportional mortality method has also been extensively used in the estimation of occupational risk [26].

Choosing between various risk measures

Describing a complex situation by a single value is inevitably a difficult exercise and the interpretation of such a numerical summary should be made with great care. Standardization is a step towards a better understanding of the phenomena under study, but it is certainly not the universal method used to solve problems of comparison of incidence. Epidemiologists should be aware of the limitations of this method and should not ignore the fact that, in extreme situations, these statistics can behave pathologically.

We have introduced three principal index classes in this Chapter: i) indices of risk that are based on probability, such as cumulative risk; ii) average rates based on standard populations that give more or less importance to different subgroups of the population under study, such as direct standardized rates; and iii) relative measures of incidence, such as the standardized incidence ratio (SIR), whose objective is to measure the risk of disease relative to a standard incidence that can be interpreted in other respects. In this section, we examine the respective advantages and disadvantages of these indices, and, in particular, the interpretability, the absence of bias and the precision of the indices, three essential requirements of statistics intended to summarize disease incidence in a population.

Cumulative risk places the population under consideration on an immediately interpretable scale of risk. Moreover, it has the advantage of being consistent, since truncated risk is less than total risk. However, a truncated standardized rate obviously does not have this property; its value is inevitably arbitrary since it provides only a rough estimate of the annual number of cases that might be observed in a fictitious population. So, in Côte-d'Or, an individual has 38 chances out of 1000 of developing stomach cancer before 85 years of age, if he does not die before this age and he has 6.8 chances out of 1000 of developing it between the ages of 35 and 65 years. Among 100 000 persons in the same population and given the present level of risk, there would be 14.0 stomach cancers per year if the age structure was that of the world population, and 18.9 stomach cancers if the population comprised only individuals aged from 35 to 65 with the same age structure as the world population. Cumulative risk can be interpreted in a practical way by anyone who has an understanding of the concept of risk. Conversely, standardized rates appear as more abstract indices whose interpretation demands some epidemiological training and a familiarity with their orders of magnitude.

Furthermore, the situation is considerably complicated by the existence of a multitude of standards. For example, using the European standard, the same comparative rates discussed in the previous paragraph become 23.5 and 19.8, illustrating how important the choice of a standard population is in the interpretation of the number of cases observed. We should remember that a standardized rate is an average of values that varies with age in a ratio of 1:1000 for most cancers under study and it is not surprising that the weights used play a large role in the determination of the rate. In the situation where the differences of specific rates being compared do not all have the same sign, it can be shown that any desired result can be obtained by manipulating the standard population. Remember too that all the indices are summaries of the incidence curve at a given point in time and synthesize estimates of rates from various cohorts, which might have been exposed to different risk factors or to different levels of the same risk factor. One should be extremely cautious when using the indices to analyse temporal trends in cancer risk, or to examine the covariation with the level of a factor (see Chapter 1, page 8, and Chapter 3).

All these direct measures of incidence are also sensitive to random variation, and the combination of a substantial weight w_x and a very imprecise specific rate can cause surprising results (see Table 2.16 below). This is a problem to which routinely produced indices are particularly sensitive because they are not necessarily subjected to close examination before publication.

Relative measures of incidence are generally used when we want to compare subgroups of a population with its overall incidence that is considered to be free of random fluctuations. The standardized incidence ratio (SIR) is by its construction such a measure, and the comparative incidence figure (CIF) can also be used for this purpose. If the ratio of incidence rates does not depend on age, these relative measures are estimates of this ratio, and the SIR is constructed for this particular situation. Conversely, when this hypothesis does not hold, the SIR can behave pathologically.

If t_x denotes the incidence rate observed in the age group x and λ_x denotes the standard incidence, the SIR may be written

$$SIR = \sum_{x=1}^{g} u_x \frac{t_x}{\lambda_x}$$

where u_x is a weighting factor proportional to $m_x \lambda_x$, the inverse of the variance of t_x / λ_x. It is therefore a minimum variance estimator of the relative rate. Note here that this estimate can provide an absolute measure of risk if it is multiplied by the crude rate in the standard population.

With the same notation, let h_x and L_x denote the observed number of cases and the number of person-years in the standard population $\left(\lambda_x = \dfrac{h_x}{L_x} \right)$, and $H = \sum_x h_x$. The CIF may then be written

$$CIF = \frac{\displaystyle\sum_{x=1}^{g} w_x t_x}{\displaystyle\sum_{x=1}^{g} w_x \lambda_x} = \frac{\displaystyle\sum_{x=1}^{g} L_x t_x}{H} = \frac{1}{H} \sum_{x=1}^{g} h_x \frac{t_x}{\lambda_x}$$

If t_x / λ_x was *strictly* constant, the CIF would be equal to it; however, as t_x is subject to random variation, the CIF is a relative rate estimate which can be quite inaccurate, since, when it is expressed as a weighted average of the relative rates t_x / λ_x,

$$CIF = \sum_{x=1}^{g} u_x \frac{t_x}{\lambda_x}$$

the weight u_x are proportional to h_x the number of expected cases in the standard population. Once again we have the problem that has already been mentioned of heavily weighting very imprecise estimates. These difficulties are illustrated in the following example.

Suppose we study a young, healthy population such as that described in Table 2.17:

Table 2.17   Example of data distribution leading to a directly standardized rate of low precision

Age	Study population			Standard population	
	k_x	m_x	$10^3 \, t_x$	w_x	$10^3 \lambda_x$
15-24	196	98 000	2.00	0.24	3
25-34	2	1 000	2.00	0.20	3
35-44	2	600	3.30	0.19	7
45-54	3	300	10.00	0.19	22
55-64	2	100	20.00	0.18	62
Total	205	100 000	–	1.00	–
Crude rate	–	–	2.05	–	18

the direct standardized rate is then

$\bar{t} = (0.24 \times 2) + (0.20 \times 2) + (0.19 \times 3.3) + (0.19 \times 10) + (0.18 \times 20) = 7.01$ per 1000

consequently,

$$CIF = 100 \times \frac{7.01}{18} = 38.9\%$$

Furthermore, the expected number of cases if the population is subject to the incidence rate λ_x is:

$$E = \sum_{x=1}^{g} m_x \lambda_x = (98 \times 3) + (1 \times 3) + (0.6 \times 7) + (0.3 \times 22) + (0.1 \times 62) = 314$$

therefore, the SIR can be calculated as

$$SIR = 100 \times \frac{205}{314} = 65\%$$

We can see that the last age group (in which the incidence estimate is very imprecise) contributes 3.6 cases to the direct standardized rate, that is, more than all other age groups combined. If no cases were observed in this age-group, the CIF would be 19%; if, on the other hand, four cases were observed, the CIF would be 59%. In fact, both these possibilities are equally and reasonably likely. In contrast, under such hypotheses, the SIR would only vary from 65% to 66%.

However, it would be a mistake to believe that the SIR has only good qualities and the direct rate only faults. In reality, as we have said on a number of occasions, the strengths of the SIR depend on the hypothesis of proportionality of rates. As an illustration, consider the example in Table 2.18, where two populations with grossly different age distributions are compared.

The age-specific incidence is the same in both populations (5 and 20 per 1000) and the direct rates will therefore be the same for both populations, regardless of the standard population used. The standard rates calculated by the indirect method will also be the same if the marginal incidence rate is used as the standard incidence. However, because of the inversion of the distribution of person-years, they

**Table 2.18 Example of data distribution
leading to meaningless standardized incidence ratios**

Age	Population 1		Population 2		Total	
	k_{1x}	m_{1x}	k_{2x}	m_{2x}	$k_{.x}$	$m_{.x}$
1	5	1 000	25	5 000	30	6 000
2	100	5 000	20	1 000	120	6 000
Total	105	6 000	45	6 000	150	12 000

can be very different for standard rates that are not proportional to the common observed rates; for example, when $\lambda_1 = 10$ and $\lambda_2 = 15$,

$$SIR\,(1) = 100 \times \frac{105}{10 + 75} = 124$$

and

$$SIR\,(2) = 100 \times \frac{45}{50 + 15} = 69$$

The difference in person-years distribution has led to an excess of expected cases in the first population and a deficit in the second. The direction of the difference will in fact depend on how the chosen standard differs from the common incidence rate. In other words, two standardized incidence ratios cannot be compared if the populations under study do not have incidence rates proportional to those of the standard population. If, however, the hypothesis of proportionality is valid as is often the case in cancer epidemiology, it is perfectly legitimate to compare two SIRs, and an appropriate test even exists for assessing their equality.

To test whether the same exposure leads to the same effect in two populations with different background incidence λ_{1x}, λ_{2x}, It is justifiable to test whether the relative rates of exposed subgroups (the SIRs) are the same in the two populations.

Let K_1 and K_2 be the observed numbers of cases in the exposed subgroups of the two populations; then K_1 follows a Poisson distribution of parameter $\rho_1 E_1$ where $E_1 = \sum_x m_{1x}\lambda_{1x}$ and, similarly, K_2 follows a Poisson distribution of parameter $\rho_2 E_2$ where $E_2 = \sum_x m_{2x} \lambda_{2x}$. Consequently, the test of equality of the SIRs ρ_1 and ρ_2 is standard and is based on similar arguments to those developed on page 81 of this chapter: the total number of observed cases $K_1 + K_2$ being fixed, K_1 has a binomial distribution with parameter $K_1 + K_2$ and $\dfrac{E_1}{E_1 + \theta E_2}$ where $\theta = \rho_2/\rho_1$. The hypothesis of equality of the SIRs can then be tested as the hypothesis $\theta = 1$ which is itself equivalent to a test of the parameter of the binomial distribution.

Extreme examples should not make us doubt the efficiency of standardization methods. In fact, in 80% of situations that we encounter, the SIR and the CIF are very close [22]. Nevertheless, we should remember that these indices are only summaries of a more complex situation and that they have their limitations. Sometimes it is advisable to analyse incidence data by age and if necessary by cohort in order to obtain appropriate results, and in this situation the more specific procedures introduced on page 82 and in Chapter 3 should be used.

A thorough understanding of the concepts that we have discussed should help to avoid the main pitfalls encountered in the statistical analysis of descriptive epidemiological data. It is essential that methods are kept in their proper perspective when they are used: no statistical recipe book can ever replace a good intuitive understanding obtained from practical experience.

Bibliographical notes

As we have already noted, epidemiology, and specifically, descriptive epidemiology, has borrowed a great deal from demography. Direct and indirect standardized rates, the key tools of the epidemiologist, were devised by demographers. Readers interested in referring to the source of these techniques can consult two classical works on demography which remain current in their field: those of Pressat, in French, and Benjamin, in English [28].

Breslow and Day's monograph (Volume 1) on the analysis of case-control studies provides a fundamental description, at both a theoretical and practical level, of the calculation of risk and its interpretation [25]. Volume 2 by the same authors deals with cohort studies which, as we have noted in Chapter 1, show the basic concepts and techniques of descriptive epidemiology [29].

Two articles by these authors usefully complete this bibliographical summary. The first [16] is a discussion of the statistical tests presented in this chapter, particularly, the Mantel-Haenszel and related tests. The second [30] discusses the properties of the standardized incidence ratio and its advantages and disadvantages compared to the CIF, the principles of the heterogeneity test for comparing incidence in several populations, and the use of log-linear models for this type of analysis. Once again, although the methods are presented in the context of cohort studies, they are directly applicable to descriptive studies.

In his book on rates and proportions, Fleiss [31] devotes about twenty pages to standardization, with a special focus on the case where there are several variables for which adjustment is required. In fact, most epidemiological texts consider the calculation of direct and indirect standardized rates [32]. Some discuss the problem of variability of standardized rates, but few clearly explain the conditions necessary for the application of these methods. The recent publication from the International Agency for Research on Cancer on the techniques of cancer registration devotes a chapter to basic statistical methods in this area, and discusses routine techniques for comparison when denominators are unavailable (ASCAR and PIR) [33]. An older WHO manual on mortality analysis is out-dated with respect to comparative methods, but provides a useful description of the calculation of demographic indices and an empirical approach to the analysis of all-cause mortality, when such data are available [34].

McCullagh and Nelder's monograph provides a deeper analysis of the theory of log-linear models [35] while Aitkin and coworkers' introductory work is more oriented towards practical application [36]. Finally, Healy provides an introduction to the software GLIM [37], in more detail than the brief description in Appendix 2 of this book.

REFERENCES

[1] ROBILLARD JM. Estimation post-censitaire d'une population par projection : application dans le cas d'un registre des cancers du Calvados, 1978. *Rev Epidémiol Santé Publ* 1983, **31** : 337-340

[2] ARMITAGE P, DOLL R. Stochastic models for carcinogenesis. *In* : Proceedings of the 4th Berkeley Symposium on mathematical statistics and probability : biology and problems of health. Berkeley, University of California Press, 1961, pp. 19-38

[3] PETO R. Epidemiology, multistage models and short-term mutagenicity tests. In : HH Hiatt, JD Watson, JA Winsten (eds): *Origins of human cancer*. Cold Spring Harbor, NY, Cold Spring Harbor Laboratory, 1977, pp. 1403-1428

[4] COOK PJ, DOLL R, FELLINGHAM SA. A mathematical model for the age distribution of cancer in man. *Int J Cancer* 1969, **4** : 93-112

[5] CLEMMESEN J. *Statistical studies in the aetiology of malignant neoplasms : I. Review and results*. Kobenhavn, Munksgaard, 1965, pp. 249-340

[6] WATERHOUSE JAH, MUIR C, CORREA P, POWELL J. (eds). *Cancer incidence in five continents*, Vol. III (IARC Scientific Publications, No. 15), Lyon, IARC, 1976

[7] WATERHOUSE J, MUIR C, SHANMUGARATNAM K, POWELL J (eds). *Cancer incidence in five continents*, Vol. IV. (IARC Scientific Publications, No. 42), Lyon, IARC, 1982

[8] RAO CR. *Linear statistical inference and its applications*. New York, John Wiley, 1965, pp. 426-427

[9] ZDEB MS. The probability of developing cancer. *Am J Epidemiol* 1977, **106** : 6-16

[10] MUIR C, WATERHOUSE J, MACK T, POWELL J, WHELAN S (eds). *Cancer incidence in five continents*, Vol. V. (IARC Scientific Publications, No. 88), Lyon, IARC, 1987

[11] ROMEDER M, McWHINNIE JR. Potential years of life lost between ages 1 and 70 : an indicator of premature mortality for health planning. *Int J Epidemiol* 1977, **6** : 143-151

[12] COCHRAN WG. Some methods for strengthening the common χ^2 tests. *Biometrics* 1954, **10** : 417-449

[13] MANTEL N, HAENSZEL W. Statistical aspects of the analysis of data from retrospective studies of disease. *J Natl Cancer Inst* 1959, **22** : 719-748

[14] HAUCK WW. The large sample variance of the Mantel-Haenszel estimator of a common odds ratio. *Biometrics* 1979, **35** : 817-819

[15] BRESLOW NE, LIANG KY. The variance of the Mantel-Haenszel estimator. *Biometrics* 1982, **38** : 943-952

[16] BRESLOW NE. Elementary methods of cohort analysis. *Int J Epidemiol* 1984, **13** : 112-115

[17] ARMITAGE P. Tests for linear trends in proportions and frequencies. *Biometrics* 1955, **11** : 375-386

[18] ALEXANDER FE, McKINNEY PA, WILLIAMS J, RICKETTS TJ, CARTWRIGHT RA. Epidemiological evidence for the « Two-disease hypothesis » in Hodgkin's disease. *Int J Epidemiol* 1991, **20** : 354-361

[19] MANTEL N, STARK CR. Computation of indirect adjusted rates in the presence of confounding. *Biometrics* 1968, **24** :997-1005

[20] BRESLOW NE, DAY NE. Indirect standardization and multiplicative models for rates, with reference to the age adjustement of cancer incidence and relative frequency data. *J Chron Dis* 1975, **28** :289-303

[21] BAKER RJ, NELDER JA. *The GLIM system : release 3.77.* Oxford, Numerical Algorithms Group, 1985

[22] Occupational mortality 1970-72 : England and Wales. Series DS n° 1. London, Her Majesty's Stationery Office, 1978, 244 p.

[23] JENSEN OM, ESTÈVE J, MOLLER H, RENARD H. Cancer in the European Community and its Member States. *Eur J Cancer* 1990, **26** : 1167-1256

[24] TUYNS AJ. Studies on cancer relative frequencies (ratio studies) : a method for computing an age-standardized cancer ratio. *Int J Cancer* 1968, **3** : 397-403

[25] BRESLOW NE, DAY NE. *Statistical methods in cancer research : (Vol. 1) : The analysis of case-control studies.* (IARC Scientific Publications, No. 32), Lyon, IARC, 1980

[26] SHANMUGARATNAM K, LEE HP, DAY NE. *Cancer incidence in Singapore, 1968-1977.* (IARC Scientific Publications, No. 47), Lyon, IARC, 1983

[27] PRESSAT R. *L'analyse démographique, concepts, méthodes, résultats (2nd edition).* Paris, Presses Universitaires de France, 1969

[28] BENJAMIN B. *Demographic analysis.* London, George Allen and Unwin, 1968

[29] BRESLOW NE, DAY NE. *Statistical methods in cancer research. Vol. 2. The design and analysis of cohort studies* (IARC Scientific Publications No. 82), Lyon, IARC, 1987

[30] BRESLOW NE, DAY NE. The standardized mortality ratio. *In :* PK Sen (ed) : *Biostatistics in biomedical, public health and environmental sciences.* Amsterdam, Elsevier North Holland, 1985

[31] FLEISS JL. *Statistical methods for rates and proportions.* New York, Wiley, 1981 (2nd ed)

[32] RUMEAU-ROUQUETTE C, BRÉART G, PADIEU R. *Méthodes en épidémiologie.* Paris, Flammarion, 1985

[33] JENSEN OM, PARKIN DM, MACLENNAN R, MUIR CS, SKEET RG. *Cancer registration : principles and methods.* (IARC Scientific Publications No. 95), Lyon, IARC, 1991

[34] World Health Organisation. *Manual of mortality analysis.* Geneva, WHO Div. of Health Statistics, Dissemination of statistical information, 1977

[35] McCULLAGH P, NELDER JA. *Generalized linear models.* Chapman and Hall, London 1983

[36] AITKIN M, ANDERSON D, FRANCIS B, HINDE J. *Statistical modelling in GLIM.* Oxford Science Publications (OUP), Oxford, 1989

[37] HEALY MJR. *GLIM : An introduction.* Oxford Science Publications (OUP), Oxford, 1989

Chapter 3

Space-time variations and group correlations

Geographical analysis

The objectives of cartography

Like all phenomena which vary across regions, spatial differences in cancer occurrence can be represented on a map. A remarkable degree of sophistication has been achieved in this area. Geographers are convinced that a map can provide, through the simple play of colours, both an overall impression of major differences between regions (such as the juxtaposition of plains and mountains on a geophysical map) as well as a partial or detailed view of the characteristics of a given region.

The design of a map is not only based on aesthetic concerns. In contrast to a table of regional results, a map provides supplementary information on the contiguity and the proximity of regions. The fact that neighbouring regions might be similar with regard to the phenomenon under study can be an essential element in interpretation.

The cartographic illustration of mortality by cause is not a new idea. It has for some time formed the basis for political discussions on inequalities between regions and been a tool for health planners, for example, in the regional planning of health services. There has been a revival of interest in this approach over the past few years mainly as a result of the development of specific computing techniques. In the field of cancer, the development of cartography is relatively recent, with some notable exceptions such as Figure 3.1, showing crude cancer mortality in Switzerland for the period 1911-1914 [1].

Over the past few years, a number of cancer atlases have been produced, generally from mortality data. Examination of these atlases reveals many differences in the methods used, suggesting that their objectives differed somewhat. Some are designed to show only broad spatial patterns (for example, through a limited number of regions or colours), others indicate a systematic attempt to show, by magnification, highly localized differences through the use of a rich array of colours or a fine division of geographical units. Despite these differences, it seems obvious that the main objective of cancer atlases is to provide basic information for etiological research. Their implicit goal is therefore to allow the image of geographical variation in the rate of a given cancer to be superposed on other maps, real or imaginary,

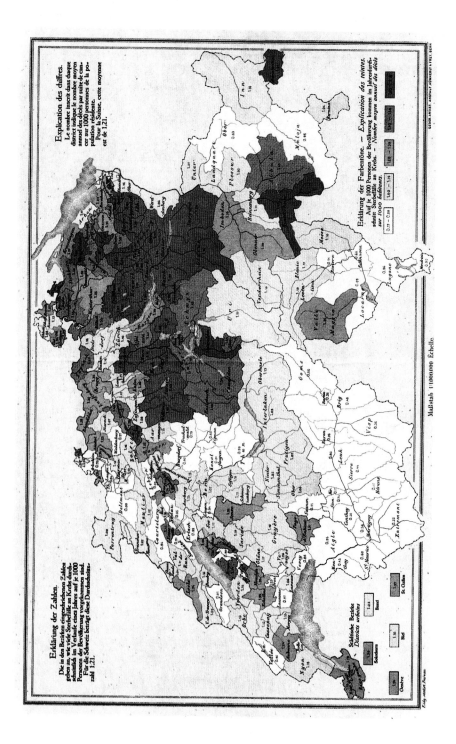

Figure 3.1   Cancer mortality (crude rates) in Switzerland in 1901-1910
Source : Swiss Bureau of Statistics [1]

of one or more environmental characteristics or individual behaviour potentially im-plicated in the variation of cancer risk. It is not certain that such superposition of these factors can be achieved with a single cartographical representation, since all the evidence suggests that exposure to diverse etiological factors can be distributed at different scales.

If interest is in factors which vary locally, the map would be expected to define zones in which the incriminated exposure can be found. In this case, a detailed subdivision is adopted to obtain relatively homogeneous zones with respect to the exposure under consideration. For example, mesothelioma is particularly frequent in Italy in coastal areas where naval construction, known as a source of exposure to asbestos, is concentrated [2] (Figure 3.2).

If, on the other hand, interest is in factors which are distributed more widely over the spatial map (such as cultural and regional behaviour, or climatic conditions), the objective will no longer be to show the level of risk in a particular area compared to adjacent areas but to provide a more homogeneous representation of broad pat-terns in the phenomenon. If the intensity of the phenomenon varies progressively from one region to another across all or part of the country under consideration, the differentiation of the areas should visually show this gradient. Such a progression

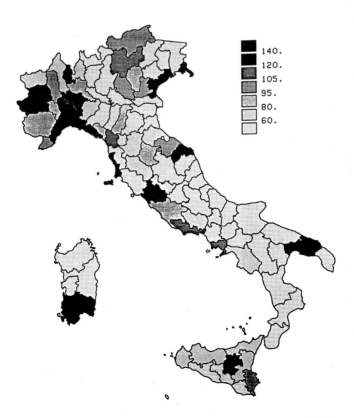

Figure 3.2   Mesothelioma mortality, men, 1975 – 1977
Source : Cislaghi et al. [2]

could in fact suggest a dose-response relationship with the level of exposure, whereas a finer subdivision could be influenced by local variations which are irrelevant to the phenomenon under consideration. An interesting example of geographical variation on a large scale is provided by mortality for malignant melanoma of the skin [3,4]. In the USA (Figure 3.3a), mortality due to this cancer increases as the latitude decreases, while in Europe (Figure 3.3b), the phenomenon is inverted. In the USA, increased exposure to ultraviolet light in the more southern regions results in a detectable increase in melanoma mortality. The way in which this country has been populated by migrants of different origins has led to an unplanned adjustment for ethnicity. Immigrants from different ethnic backgrounds are effectively distributed randomly throughout the country. In Europe, in contrast, factors linked to ethnicity are the most important determinant of melanoma risk and mask the effect of place of residence; individuals most susceptible to ultraviolet light have remained in the north, while recently adopting a life style involving significant exposure to the sun.

Beyond the objectives illustrated by these examples, cancer atlases which have appeared so far have been works of general scope destined for a wide readership. Thus their authors have often made compromises such that the atlases do not necessarily answer the needs of etiological researchers. Nevertheless, the techniques which they apply are fundamental tools which have been used for a long time in descriptive epidemiology to solve etiological problems. As early as 1848, John Snow identified the source of the epidemic which ravaged London by using a map by district of mortality rates due to the disease. Joint study of this map and that of the areas covered by different water suppliers revealed similarities which convinced Snow to follow his investigations at the level not only of the district but also of individual houses [5]. This more detailed approach was rendered necessary because the old part of London was served by two companies, the Lambeth Society and the Southwark and Vauxhall Society. Analysis of the water showed among other things differences between the companies not only in the content of organic material but also its acidity, which undoubtedly affected the conditions for bacteria growth. These geographical observations led Snow to identify the vehicle of the then unknown agent of the disease, *Vibrio cholerae*.

Since that time, the representation of risk or exposure by means of a geographical map and the tools for analysing geographical distributions have advanced considerably. The following sections describe both aspects.

Methods

Geographical division

Geographical representation of cancer frequency is provided by the juxtaposition of areas of different colours or shades, each of which represents a level of frequency. The boundaries and especially the number of the areas determine the degree of detail of the map and thus its overall appearance. As has been indicated, the issues are different when the goal is to produce a series of maps fulfilling a purely descriptive need, such as an atlas of selected cancer sites, or to indicate regions corresponding to a risk or to a given exposure in the context of a specific etiological investigation. The geographical level at which data are available (numerator and denominator) is not always the most important constraint. In practice, difficulties are more likely to occur because of the need to ensure statistical stability for the risk estimates in each, or at least most, areas. It is important to maintain an appropriate ratio between the incidence or mortality from one region to another and the corresponding random variation. For example, it would be unreasonable to define areas which only include four expected cases on average, if the objective is to classify areas into categories representing relative differences of 25%. In this situation, the coefficient of variation of the rate is of the order of $1/\sqrt{4} = 50\%$ (see Chapter 2, page 53). Accordingly, geographical units which are sparsely populated are often grouped together.

If data are available, it is sometimes preferable not to work with administrative subdivisions. For example, in the Finnish study on the relationship between life style and cancer incidence, communities have been grouped together to form areas of 10 000 people, characterized by their geographical proximity as well as their similarity with respect to appropriately selected socioeconomic variables [6].

In some situations, the definition of areas is in response to a specific etiological problem. The goal of cartography is then to illustrate a specific hypothesis, for example, to evaluate the effect of radiation around a nuclear power station or of pollution on the frequency of respiratory cancer. The objective then is to form one or more areas in which the exposure being studied is homogeneous. Recording information from small geographical units becomes essential. Because of this requirement, many countries have introduced systems by which data from population censuses and periodic reports (such as death by cause) are available for geographical units defined by appropriate cartesian coordinates [7]. When the source of risk is at a specific point, the usual approach would be to define the area as all squares located within a circle around this point (Figure 3.4) or between concentric circles, in order to demonstrate a dose-response relationship.

In other examples, the whole region is divided into areas depending on the intensity of exposure, as determined by measurements made at specific points in the region (e.g., measurement of ultraviolet light at meteorological stations). The aim is to divide the region into homogeneous areas around points where measurements have been carried out. Dirichlet's mosaic provides a simple and elegant solution [8]: the region to be mapped is divided into areas such that each point in a specific area is closer to the measurement point situated in it than to any other measurement point. This tiled area is obtained by connecting the perpendicular bisectors of the sides of triangles formed by the measurement points. A more sophisticated solution is based on interpolation from the measurements using polynomial regression. Division into areas of homogenous exposure can be constructed from contour lines of the resulting surface. This method can also be used after having artificially localized a regional measurement (e.g., rate per resident) at the centre

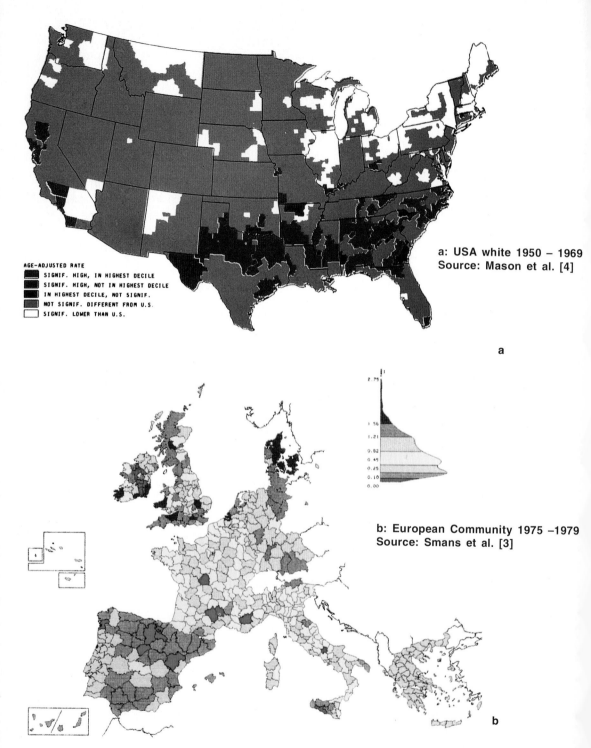

AGE-ADJUSTED RATE
◼ SIGNIF. HIGH, IN HIGHEST DECILE
◼ SIGNIF. HIGH, NOT IN HIGHEST DECILE
◼ IN HIGHEST DECILE, NOT SIGNIF.
◼ NOT SIGNIF. DIFFERENT FROM U.S.
☐ SIGNIF. LOWER THAN U.S.

a: USA white 1950 – 1969
Source: Mason et al. [4]

a

b: European Community 1975 –1979
Source: Smans et al. [3]

b

Figure 3.3   Melanoma mortality; women

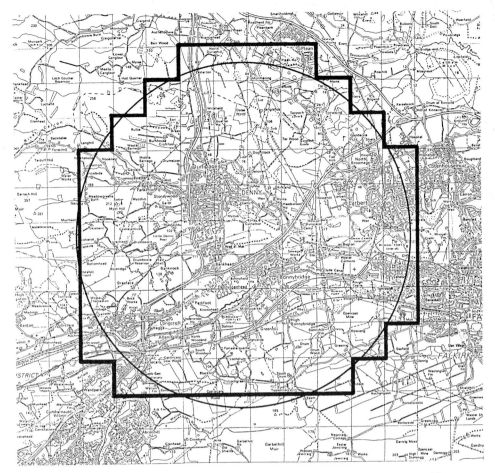

Figure 3.4   Construction of a circle with a radius of 5 km from a 1 km-grid square
Source: Carstairs et al. [7]

of gravity of the region, which is obtained by weighting according to population density.

When small adjacent geographical areas are grouped together to create homogeneous aggregates with respect to exposure, it is obviously important to check that the level of exposure can be considered equal in the areas which have been grouped together. One method of grouping based on the statistical significance of the differences in exposure between adjacent regions will be discussed below (see page 134).

The first objective of these diverse techniques is thus to create areas of more homogeneous risk by departing from the constraints of the politico-administrative subdivisions. Note that when the techniques involve grouping or interpolation, they have the additional advantage of smoothing the exposure data, eliminating the inconvenience of large random fluctuations which usually affect small area statistics.

This is even more evident when the methodology is used for the description of incidence or mortality; for example, a polynomial regression has been used to represent curves of stomach cancer mortality in Italy [9] in a purely descriptive context (Figure 3.5).

Choice of a risk indicator

When the objective is to show variation in risk as opposed to crude rate or number of cases, the graphical representation should use a risk indicator which is adjusted for age. Both direct and indirect standardization methods have been used for this purpose in published atlases.

For direct standardization, either the world or European population is most often used. This choice undoubtedly reflects the desire to expand the atlas's role to international comparisons. Nevertheless, the various atlases which have appeared are seldom comparable, because of the large variation in the choice of the risk categories and colours. None is based on the cumulative rate (Chapter 2, page 60) which would be the most readily interpretable index on a probability scale and make the various maps directly comparable.

Many authors have chosen indirect standardization. This option is justified if the primary objective of a cancer atlas is to represent risk variations within a country. Geographical areas are then classified by their standardized mortality or morbidity ratio (SMR). This index generally has the advantage of providing more precise statistical estimates than the directly standardized rate (Chapter 2, page 100). The reference rate adopted for the calculation of the SMR is in general the incidence or mortality estimated in the region being mapped.

Definition of risk classes

We have already seen that the number of risk classes cannot be determined without taking into account the statistical precision of the risk indicator. Precision is equally relevant in the choice of scale and class limits, as we shall see below.

A priori, a larger number of classes should provide a more detailed picture of risk variation. However, dividing the area too finely diminishes the effect of the colour or shading contrasts required to distinguish the risk variation clearly. Moreover, as a general rule, the homogeneity of classes is proportional to their number: if there are few classes, differences between values in the same class could be much larger than those existing between the central values of two adjacent classes, which are nevertheless represented by different colours.

The colours chosen to represent the various levels of risk differ substantially from one atlas to the next. A principle generally applied is to make the zone representing average risk the least coloured. Zones of increasing (or respectively decreasing) risk are represented by colours which are arbitrarily chosen, but sufficiently contrasting visually. The chromatic intensity progressively decreases from extreme risk classes to intermediate classes.

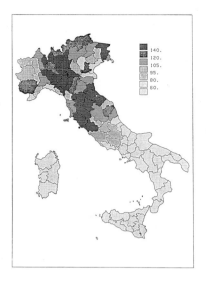

a: SMR,

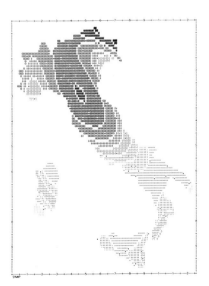

b: Linear model,

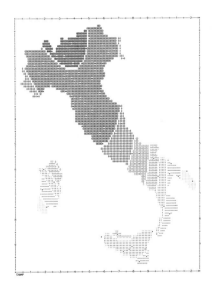

c: Quadratic model,

d: Quintic model

Figure 3.5   Stomach cancer mortality in Italy; men, 1975-1977
Source: Cislaghi et al. [2] and personal communication

It is not surprising that many authors choose red and green to characterize respectively an increase or a decrease compared to a standard risk. Culturally, red indicates danger while green represents ecology. Note also that the range of shades is not obligatorily centred on the average index value but can be distributed asymmetrically around the average index value such that those classes representing risk increase are broken down more finely, as has been done in the Chinese cancer atlas [10]. The subtlety of options used in the various atlases reveals an intention to use the physiology of visual perception, particularly in the choice of colours, to best communicate the desired message [11, 12].

The simplest procedure involves setting the limits of the classes based on an equal division of all risk index values after disregarding extreme values when they are outliers. Under this method, the scale depends on the data, and does not lend itself to comparison between maps of different cancer sites or the two sexes.

When the index is a relative measure (for example, an SMR), the same scale is adopted for all sites. Transition between colours is then immediately interpretable in terms of relative risk increases: for example, a relative risk scale increasing by steps of 25% from left to right open-ended categories. These categories at the extremities of the scale are defined by the maximum number of classes to be used in mapping. This approach has been frequently used in atlases, as it has the advantage of allowing comparisons to be made between sites and between sexes. In the French atlas [13], for example, it can be seen that stomach cancer mortality is one and a half times higher in Brittany than in the rest of the country for both men and women, and that the maps for both sexes are similar. However, this type of comparison is of little value when the standard levels used in the maps being compared (SMR = 1) are very different from each other. For example, for lung cancer in France, the comparison of zones characterized by values between 125 and 150 of the SMR for men and women is not directly informative, because of the difference in background risk between the two groups.

An examination of maps using fixed limits for risk categories shows that the geographical variation in risk is extremely variable between sites. Thus in the French atlas, maps representing oesophageal cancer are more variegated than those for colon cancer. This methodology may be better suited to a public health perspective than to etiological research, in which all real risk differences can be of interest.

The proportion of each colour on the map is directly dependent on whether or not a fixed scale is adopted. If distribution of risk is narrow, the map will be largely monochromatic. If the distribution tends to be bimodal, the map will be largely made up of colour zones representing high and low risk respectively. If the distribution is equally spread, all the selected colours will be almost equally used.

In order to describe all observed variability, the original scale has been replaced in some atlases by grouping together risk classes based on percentiles. For example, in the Scottish atlas directly standardized rates have been divided into seven classes with limits determined by the 5, 15, 35, 65, 85 and 95 percentiles [11]. The middle class therefore includes 30% of the values. By definition, this method leads to the use of a different scale for each site and for both sexes. Each of these scales is a function not only of the risk values but also of the shape of their distribution.

For a given number of classes, the use of percentiles makes the apparent variability of the risk index equal and maximal. It is thus impossible to judge the size of this variability visually, as each map makes the same use of the different colours and extreme values are no longer apparent. On the other hand, when variations in risk are small, any contrasts, gradients or autocorrelative phenomena can be clearly appreciated.

In order to reconcile the advantages of a relative measure with those of a measure expressed on an absolute scale, a division based on a logarithmic scale has been used in the Chinese atlas. All maps can then be built with one scale regardless of site or sex. In this system, the increase in risk for a class compared to the level of risk of the class immediately preceding it is represented on a multiplicative and not an additive scale, so that only pronounced variations are apparent; this is well illustrated by the map of oesophageal cancer in China (Figure 3.6) [10].

We have noted on several occasions that risk estimates are subject to statistical fluctuations that can be of different magnitude in different regions. Taking this variability into account will modify the interpretation of the map. For example, little significance will be attached to the high value of female mortality for cancer of the buccal cavity in France in the département of Cantal [13]: the value of the SMR is equal to 1.75 but its confidence interval (0.98; 2.88) does not exclude unity.

It is generally accepted that maps produced by the principles described above are usefully complemented by information on variability of the risk indices. In some situations, maps can be simply accompanied by an appended table providing the required data, such as the standard error or the confidence interval of the index. Others attempt to give a geographical view of variability by juxtaposing a map of risk with a map of degree of significance for the same areas [14]. Interpreting the two maps together is not always easy, but it can demonstrate that differences can be significant without being large, if the number of cases is high and/or the populations under study large. Thus the majority of European atlases show significant differences between regions for colon cancer, even though the variation in risk for this cancer is generally relatively small.

Some maps attempt to combine the size of the variation and its degree of significance on one single scale. The atlas of cancer mortality in England and Wales used the following four categories [15]: significantly increased risk; increased risk, but not significant; not increased risk; significantly decreased risk. Such a scale allows all rates significantly increased with respect to the reference rate to be placed at the top of the colour hierarchy even if the increase is in reality very small. Risks which are substantially increased, but not significantly so, will appear lower down in this hierarchy. In practice, the procedure is acceptable only if the geographical areas are divided equally (in terms of population), such that the statistical variability is of the same order for a given site.

The difficulties described above can be minimized or avoided in the interest of compromise. However, the study of spatial data, especially for specific problems, requires a more rational approach to account for random variability. The methods described below are more suitable in these situations.

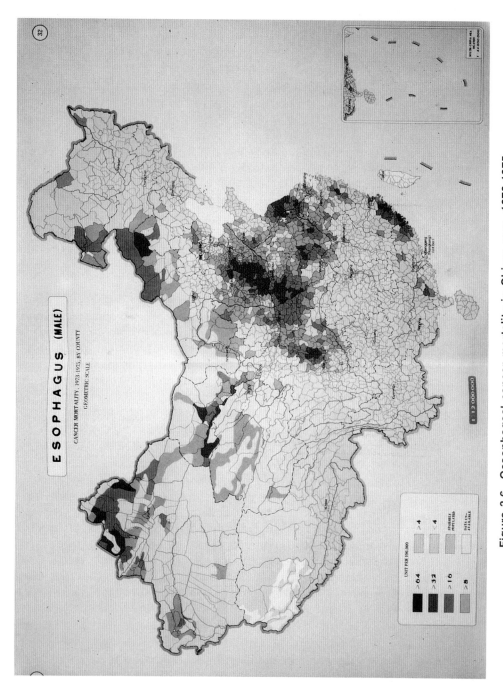

Figure 3.6   Oesophageal cancer mortality in China; men, 1973-1975
Source: China Map Press [10]

Tools to interpret geographical data

Autocorrelations

Graphical representation of disease frequency is not the only objective of the geographical study of the disease. Although this objective is important, quantitative answers to certain simple questions should also accompany the presentation of the data, to facilitate their interpretation.

The first of these questions concerns geographical variability: are rates different from one region to another? A homogeneity test such as that given in Chapter 2 (page 87) can obviously be carried out, but is of little value because it does not take into account the spatial structure of the geographical units being studied. As has been suggested previously, neighbouring regions are often subject to similar cancer risks: exposure to factors influencing the level of incidence or mortality is often more similar in neighbouring regions than in distant regions. Exposure can also vary continuously in a particular direction, resulting in a risk gradient such as those cited for melanoma mortality in the USA and Europe (Figures 3.3a and 3.3b) [4]. When the direction of the gradient is already known, as in this example, the significance of the variation in risk can be evaluated using a test on one degree of freedom (Chapter 2, page 90). However, in the majority of situations, no assumptions can be made about the direction of the gradient and the validity of the test can be questioned if the direction was suggested by observation of the map.

The spatial distribution of risk factors leading to local correlations in disease rates will generally be more complex than the risk factor distributions which determine larger-scale geographical patterns described above. For small areas it is of interest to measure and test the similarity of disease rates on a much finer scale. Local variations in processes which determine cancer incidence or mortality in the area under study are the focus of interest rather than overall trends. We therefore need to evaluate the correlation of risks in adjoining regions, also referred to as the spatial autocorrelation of the random process which gives rise to the observed geographical variations of incidence. A significant autocorrelation is frequently found. Taking this correlation into account using methods described below results in a more satisfactory description of the spatial distribution of risks and thus a better representation of incidence.

Even when the risks are the same over all regions studied, their estimation can result in a spatial correlation simply because the most accurate estimates, which are those in the most populated regions, are also found most often in neighbouring regions. The values observed in these regions will therefore be close simply because they estimate the common risk value better. This autocorrelation of the population sizes in the different geographical units is common and should be kept in mind, since, in this situation, the spatial autocorrelation observed is not in the risks but only in their estimates.

If there is no autocorrelation in risks, the test of geographical homogeneity reduces to the classical comparison of several groups. The presence of spatial correlation in risk establishes heterogeneity *de facto*, but its absence does not confirm homogeneity.

Finally, it is possible that a substantial variation on a large scale and spatial autocorrelation on a finer scale can be observed simultaneously. Methods described below for modelling spatial processes can be used in this situation. Here, we will simply show how to evaluate spatial autocorrelation from risk estimates based on the SMR. We first describe the different indices available, as if the risks were directly observable.

Suppose that the spatial structure of the geographical units is defined by a matrix of weights **W**, the elements w_{ij} of which measure the geographical proximity of the regions i and j. Most often, **W** will be an adjacency matrix whose elements w_{ij} are equal to 1 if i and j are adjacent and zero otherwise. Moreover, let X_i be the spatial process defined by the relative risks of disease ρ_i in the different regions (i = 1,...,n) (for example, $X_i = \log(\rho_i)$ or $X_i = \text{rank } (\rho_i)$]. Moran's coefficient [16] measures autocorrelation of the spatial process X_i using an index which is very close to the classical correlation coefficient :

$$I = \frac{n \sum_{i \neq j} w_{ij} (X_i - \overline{X}) (X_j - \overline{X})}{S_0 \sum_{i} (X_i - \overline{X})^2} \qquad (3.1)$$

where S_0 is the sum $\sum_{i \neq j} w_{ij}$ which, in the case of an adjacency matrix, is the number of pairs of areas with a common border.

Geary's coefficient [17] measures the average squared difference between risks observed in adjacent areas, and should be small in the case of spatial correlation:

$$C = \frac{n-1}{2 S_0} \frac{n \sum_{i \neq j} w_{ij} (X_i - X_j)^2}{\sum_{i} (X_i - \overline{X})^2} \qquad (3.2)$$

Two other indices have been used for investigating the geographical distribution of cancer risks. Ohno [18] suggested using the number of adjacent areas of the same colour on a map of incidence or mortality. Smans [19] recommended calculating the average difference in ranks of adjacent areas. As we shall see below, these statistics are in fact similar to the statistics used to evaluate time-space clustering. The first is similar to that introduced by Knox to analyse time-space clustering (see page 131) [20] and the second can be written:

$$D = \frac{1}{S_0} \sum_{i \neq j} w_{ij} |\text{rank } (\rho_i) - \text{rank } (\rho_j)| \qquad (3.3)$$

Assuming that X_i have independent and identical normal distributions (under the null hypothesis of no autocorrelation), the means and variances of I and C are given by the formulae:

$$E(I) = - \frac{1}{n-1}$$

$$Var(I) = \frac{n^2 S_1 - n S_2 + 3 S_0^2}{(n-1)(n+1) S_0^2} - \left[- \frac{1}{n-1} \right]^2 \qquad (3.4)$$

$$E(C) = 1$$

$$Var(C) = \frac{(2S_1 + S_2)\,(n-1) - 4\,S_0^2}{2\,(n+1)\,S_0^2} \qquad (3.5)$$

where S_1 and S_2 are functions of w_{ij} defined by

$$S_1 = \frac{1}{2} \sum_{i \neq j} (w_{ij} + w_{ij})^2$$

$$S_2 = \sum_i (w_{i.} + w_{.i})^2 \text{ with } w_{i.} = \sum_j w_{ij} \text{ and } w_{.i} = \sum_j w_{ji}$$

The means and variances of the statistics proposed by Ohno and Smans can be obtained directly from the formulae given by Mantel in the context of detecting time-space clustering (see page 133, formulae (3.22) and (3.23)).

Unfortunately, these formulae which only depend on the spatial structure **W**, are of little more than theoretical interest. As we saw above, spatial autocorrelation in risk estimates caused by heterogeneity in population sizes can be detected by these tests even if the risks are identical across areas. These theoretical values would only be valid if the population density was constant.

In practice, spatial autocorrelation in risks can only be tested by randomization procedure using the correct null hypothesis described below.

Let k_{xi}, m_{xi} be the number of cases and the person-years in the population of age x of area i. To test the existence of spatial autocorrelation against the null hypothesis of homogeneity. The total number of cases $k_{x.}$ in the different areas are distributed proportionally to the populations m_{xi} according to the multinomial model (Chapter 2, page 87). The estimates of p_i in each area are calculated for each simulation and, from these, the autocorrelation statistic and its distribution under the null hypothesis are calculated. Table 3.1 gives the mean and the standard error of the statistics I and D obtained by the above method for some cancer sites in the département of Isère in France [21].

Several patterns emerge from this analysis : in men, testicular cancer has a distribution with a significantly positive autocorrelation, while the homogeneity test detects no difference. This finding is noteworthy, given that this cancer is of such low incidence that the homogeneity test has in any case little power. Autocorrelation

Table 3.1   Autocorrelation of risks for selected cancer sites in the département of Isère in France

	K	Moran statistic: I ([a])				Smans statistic: D				Homogeneity ([c])
		Observed	Expected ([b])	Standard error	Z	Observed	Expected ([b])	Standard error	Z	
Males										
Testis	87	30.72	8.17	9.26	2.44	11.75	14.10	0.93	−2.53	42.1
Brain	164	12.34	1.37	9.58	1.15	13.44	14.88	0.96	−1.50	70.9
Kidney	217	−6.53	−1.08	9.33	−0.58	14.89	15.07	0.96	−0.18	43.4
Mouth	431	−6.76	−1.86	9.39	−0.52	13.54	14.89	0.93	−1.45	60.1
Colon-rectum	1 081	14.47	−1.81	9.28	1.75	13.63	14.98	0.93	−1.45	60.3
Females										
Brain	119	8.45	3.78	9.52	0.49	14.12	14.50	0.95	−0.40	56.1
Kidney	124	8.09	1.77	9.41	0.67	12.93	14.83	0.96	−1.98	49.9
Colon-rectum	985	0.30	−1.70	9.37	0.21	14.30	14.94	0.93	−0.69	97.6
Breast	2 208	39.44	−1.76	9.52	3.96	11.60	14.91	0.94	−3.52	100.1

([a]) I is the autocorrelation of the logarithm of the SMRs, multiplied by 100
([b]) Under the assumption of a uniform risk in the département. Under the assumption of a normal distribution with uniform variance but no autocorrelation, the mean and standard error of I would be −2.27 and 9.12; those of D would be 15.33 and 0.93
([c]) This column gives the value of χ^2 for homogeneity (Chapter 2, page 89); the critical value at the 5% level is 60.5.

indicated by high values for I and D is illustrated in Figure 3.7 showing the geographical variation of testicular cancer incidence in the département of Isère. In males, oral and brain cancers have nonhomogeneous distributions without autocorrelation; the distribution of kidney cancer seems completely random. In females, brain cancer also has a random distribution. The statistic D detects a significant autocorrelation for kidney cancer, suggesting that in this case it is more powerful than I, which detects no autocorrelation. Colorectal cancer has geographical variation without significant autocorrelation while breast cancer shows both heterogeneity and autocorrelation. It is worth noting that the means of I and D can deviate from their theoretical values obtained by formulae (3.4) and (3.22) considerably when the number of cases is small but only slightly for more frequent cancers such as colorectal and breast. At the same time, the variances of I and D remain approximately constant and close to their theoretical values (see table 3.1, note ([b])).

Identifying risk clusters

The preceding sections have shown how to describe and interpret the spatial distribution of incidence or mortality using the basic geographical unit from which the data are usually collected. The aim of this section is to present methods for studying spatial distribution on a finer scale. These methods may require a knowledge of the place of incidence for each case.

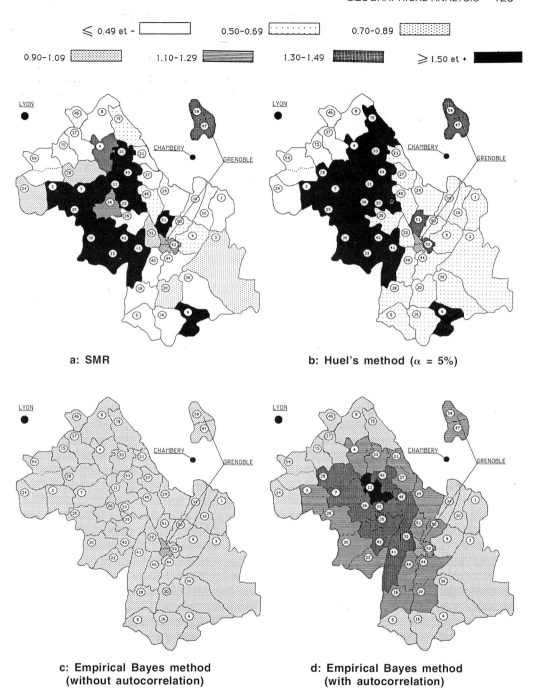

Figure 3.7   Testicular cancer incidence in Isère (France), 1979-1984
Source: Colonna [21]

Methods for studying the spatial distribution of biological or economical phenomena have been developed principally in the specific context of ecology and geography. In the medical area, this type of research has been carried out mainly for communicable diseases, with the goals of identifying clusters of infection and describing routes of transmission. The use of these methods in the epidemiology of noncommunicable diseases is relatively new. It is due mainly to the recognition of a geographical component among the risk determinants of these diseases.

The existence of apparently unusual clusters of cases in some regions and the concern caused by such aggregations among the resident populations are at the basis of this type of epidemiological research. Thus, the observation of a cluster of leukaemia cases around the nuclear installation at Sellafield in the UK [22] has led to much controversy and used as a further argument for the creation of a national system for collecting incidence and mortality data from small geographical areas [7]. Many epidemiologists were dissatisfied that the cluster had not been detected by the existing surveillance system and that it was ultimately revealed to the public by the lay press. Although the causes of this increased incidence remain to be established, the resulting research has led to new results, in particular concerning the spatial distribution of leukaemia.

Before describing the methods of analysis, the notion of case aggregation or clustering should be clearly defined. A number of clusters are nothing more than a misinterpretation of the observations, often as a result of confusing random phenomenon with regular or uniform phenomenon. This difficulty arises because of our frequently inaccurate picture of what is taken to be the normal reference situation, against which unusual rates of incidence are judged.

The problem of demonstrating the existence of a cluster often arises in the following circumstances:

• a geographical region exists in which disease incidence is *a priori* homogeneous over all areas within it.

• the disease is of unknown etiology and rare in each unit of the geographical region.

• the number of units in the region is sufficiently large to allow the geographical distribution of the disease to be studied.

A cluster is thus made up of one or more adjacent units in which the number of cases observed is inconsistent with the possibility of an homogeneous risk in the region under study, that is, of a random distribution of cases in all units of the region. Thus testicular cancer incidence in Isère [21], discussed in the preceding section and on page 140 clusters around canton 11, as demonstrated by bayesian methods given in this section (Figure 3.7 d).

It is necessary to distinguish the situation in which data are collected to test the possible excess of cases around the source of exposure that is, the hypothesis is proposed *before observing* the data, from that in which the hypothesis about the origin of the observed increase in risk is formulated *after making the observations*. In the latter situation, study of the distribution of cases in the whole geographical region can provide the basis for confirming or denying the unusual nature of the observation. This approach, which inevitably leads to statistical tests on a large number of degrees of freedom, is extremely conservative. On the other hand, tests on one degree of freedom, based on a more specific alternative, are not acceptable as they are designed for the situation in which the hypothesis precedes the observation (for example, variation of risk with distance from a source of exposure). Thus, specific methods are required.

The distinction between the two situations cited above is not always obvious. For example, the existence of a nuclear reactor or a toxic waste outlet in the vicinity of a leukaemia cluster might not always provide an *a priori* hypothesis. A systematic study of suspect environmental situations and the bias caused by the selective publication of significant results can lead to confusing interpretations. In the following section we provide a brief survey of the principal methods used to examine such clustering.

When the hypothesis precedes the observation, we would generally attempt to verify that risk increases with proximity to the source of the exposure. A trend test, in which the weights are the distances between the study areas and the source of exposure, can be used for this purpose [23]. The test's power nevertheless depends on the way in which risk decreases with distance and on the distribution of population density according to distance. Schulmann and coworkers [24] have suggested transforming the distances in such a way that the population density remains constant while still maintaining the topological structure of the area (sometimes known as isodemographical maps). There has been little research on the influence of the choice of proximity measurement on the power of corresponding tests.

Stone has proposed a method which is largely independent of the relationship between risk and distance [25]. Although it could be presented in a rather theoretical framework (estimation of risk under the constraint that it decreases with increasing distance), the method is based on a fairly intuitive principle; the essential idea is to construct a sequence of areas of increasing size around a source of exposure using available incidence or mortality data, then to choose the area for which the ratio between observed and expected cases or deaths is highest. In other words, the SMR is evaluated for that area for which the effect is maximum. The statistic thus accumulates the information available to test the assumption of homogeneity of the risk. This function of the observations no longer follows a Poisson distribution, given the way in which the area on which it is based was selected. Stone has shown how the level of significance of the test can be calculated exactly. In practice, it is often simpler to proceed by simulating the multinomial distribution of the number of cases observed in the constructed sequence of non-overlapping areas, conditional on the total number of cases observed in the region under study.

When several identical sources of exposure can be studied, the fact of living close to one of these sources can be considered a potential risk factor and the statistical significance of its effect can be evaluated in a geographical analysis. For example, the risk of leukaemia in small geographical areas as a function of the proportion of people living near a nuclear installation has been studied using a log-linear model [26] or more traditional approaches based on the SMR [27]. These methods can nevertheless suffer from methodological weaknesses inherent in ecological studies (see page 148). Kinlen [28,29] has shown that other conditions, such as living in a 'new town' created in the middle of a rural area, can also be linked to a high risk of childhood leukaemia. This factor could be confounded with the proximity of nuclear installations in the evaluation of leukaemia risk; its effect might be difficult to separate from the potential effect of radiation in an ecological study.

The problem of spatial aggregation of leukaemias and lymphomas has often been raised. In particular, an attempt has been made to evaluate the hypothesis that these diseases have a viral etiology, by assessing whether the spatial distribution of cases is random or is a cluster distribution. In this approach it is implicitly accepted that the viral hypothesis automatically leads to clustering; this latter inference can be questioned today in the light of recent findings on viral mechanisms and of the existence of a long latency period between infection and disease. Irrespective of any specific hypotheses, however, such studies are of value: beyond the test of randomness of the spatial distribution, it is of interest to identify clusters of disease, which can lead to further investigation in the geographical areas thus identified. A better understanding of the aggregative structure of the spatial distribution of a disease results in a more objective analysis of any supposed excess in risk.

The methods proposed rely on the study either of the distribution of cases in small geographical areas defined *a priori* or of the distribution of distances between cases observed over the whole geographical area under consideration. Generally speaking, the studies of homogeneity in risk are based on geographical areas with small populations and limited numbers of cases. Usually, about half the areas do not contain a single case. The test of homogeneity described in Chapter 2 (see page 87) is clearly inappropriate. An acceptable test should be able to detect deviations from randomness, which could either result from the preferential occurrence of excess cases in geographical units where there were already subjects with the disease, or be the consequence of small excess risk in several areas, the overall distribution of risk having however a small variance. In this second situation, few excess cases would be found in each unit, but cases in excess of the expected number would be found in the units where risks were higher. These alternatives to randomness are known as contagious distributions; the second differs however from the strict concept of contagion for which it is the presence of a subject with the disease which increases the probability of healthy subjects developing the disease. A powerful test against the alternative of heterogeneous risks with a small variance distributed around a common value has been proposed by Potthoff and Whittinghill [30,31] and used in the above context by Muirhead and Ball [32].

Recall that heterogeneity is demonstrated when the g multinomial distributions corresponding to g age groups (or more generally to g risk categories)

$$\left(k_{x.}, p_{xi} \; ; \; p_{xi} = \frac{p_i \, m_{xi}}{\sum\limits_i p_i \, m_{xi}} \; , 1 \leq i \leq n \right) \qquad 1 \leq x \leq g \qquad (3.6)$$

are not compatible with the hypothesis $\rho_i = 1$, $1 \leq i \leq n$. Potthoff and Whittinghill have shown that for such a distribution a powerful test against the alternative of small variation of ρ around 1 is based on the statistic [30]

$$U_x = \left(\sum_{i=1}^{n} \frac{k_{xi} (k_{xi} - 1)}{p_{xi}^*} \right) \tag{3.7}$$

where p_{xi}^* is the value specified by the null hypothesis $\rho_i = 1$, $1 \leq i \leq n$

$$p_{xi}^* = \frac{m_{xi}}{\sum_i m_{xi}}$$

Thus, U_x in this situation becomes:

$$U_x = \left(\sum_{i=1}^{n} m_{xi} \right) \left(\sum_{i=1}^{n} \frac{k_{xi} (k_{xi} - 1)}{m_{xi}} \right) \tag{3.8}$$

Note that U_x is based on the number of pairs of cases observed in different units, weighted by the inverse of the number of person-years accumulated by the corresponding population. This weighting has an intuitive explanation, the occurrence of a pair of cases being all the more indicative of clustering if the population is small. Note also that units with only 0 or 1 case make no contribution to this statistic. It can be shown that the mean and variance of U_x, under the null hypothesis, are:

$$E (U_x) = k_{x.} (k_{x.} - 1)$$

$$Var (U_x) = 2 (n - 1) E (U_x) \tag{3.9}$$

The test of homogeneity is thus constructed by summing the information from different age groups as has been done several times previously:

$$T_1 = \frac{\sum_{x=1}^{g} [U_x - E (U_x)]}{\sqrt{\sum_{x=1}^{g} [Var (U_x)]}} \tag{3.10}$$

Table 3.2 shows brain cancer incidence in five cantons of the département of Isère and Potthoff and Whittinghill's test applied to these data. Numbers in parentheses have been observed while those which precede them correspond to a fictitious incidence, constructed to provide an example of a contagious distribution.

With T_1 equal to 3.488, the distribution of cases does not appear to be random, even though the classic test of homogeneity gives the value 1.63 for a χ^2 on four

Table 3.2   Potthoff and Wittinghill's test using data on brain cancer from five cantons of the département of Isère, France ([a])

Age group	Canton					Potthoff and Whittinghill's test				
	1	2	3	4	5	$k_{x.}$	U_x	$E(U_x)$	$Var(U_x)$	T_1 ([b])
1	0 (1)	0 (0)	2 (0)	1 (2)	0 (0)	3	13.803	6	48	1.1263
	4 766	4 139	7 876	26 102	11 473					
2	0 (0)	2 (1)	0 (0)	0 (1)	0 (0)	2	24.265	2	16	5.5661
	8 038	5 345	9 162	28 438	13 864					
3	1 (1)	0 (0)	0 (0)	1 (1)	0 (0)	2	0.000	2	16	−0.5000
	9 934	5 959	10 666	29 424	15 131					
4	0 (1)	0 (0)	0 (0)	2 (1)	0 (0)	2	4.478	2	16	0.6195
	9 860	5 908	13 312	34 772	14 004					
5	0 (1)	0 (0)	0 (0)	3 (4)	2 (0)	5	27.084	20	160	0.5601
	8 688	5 284	19 200	48 835	12 133					
6	2 (2)	0 (0)	0 (1)	3 (3)	2 (1)	7	50.445	42	336	0.4607
	6 923	5 070	14 641	49 304	12 529					
7	0 (0)	2 (1)	0 (1)	2 (2)	0 (0)	4	31.384	12	96	1.9783
	7 557	5 639	10 260	39 611	14 392					
8	1 (1)	0 (0)	0 (0)	4 (4)	0 (0)	5	25.699	20	160	0.4506
	8 245	5 335	8 377	30 233	12 557					
9	0 (2)	1 (1)	2 (0)	0 (0)	0 (0)	3	14.627	6	48	1.2453
	7 844	4 517	7 456	24 795	9 919					
10	0 (0)	0 (0)	3 (3)	2 (2)	1 (1)	6	47.298	30	240	1.1166
	7 452	4 285	7 427	24 400	9 590					
11	2 (2)	0 (0)	0 (0)	1 (1)	2 (2)	5	26.911	20	160	0.5464
	6 557	4 044	6 507	25 420	9 364					
12	2 (2)	0 (1)	0 (0)	3 (3)	2 (1)	7	39.077	42	336	−0.1595
	5 746	3 445	5 287	24 103	8 746					
13	0 (3)	0 (0)	0 (0)	5 (5)	3 (0)	8	71.089	56	448	0.7129
	4 250	2 352	3 510	18 189	6 272					
14	0 (1)	0 (0)	2 (0)	2 (3)	0 (0)	4	25.114	12	96	1.3385
	2 880	1 498	2 384	14 341	4 566					
15	2 (2)	0 (0)	0 (0)	1 (1)	0 (0)	3	18.192	6	48	1.7597
	2 626	1 304	1 931	13 502	4 523					
16	0 (1)	0 (0)	2 (0)	0 (1)	0 (0)	2	25.628	2	16	5.9070
	1 867	805	1 269	9 094	3 226					
17	0 (0)	0 (0)	0 (0)	0 (0)	0 (0)	0	0.000	0	0	0.0000
	1 153	442	743	5 319	1 892					
18	0 (0)	0 (0)	0 (0)	0 (0)	0 (0)	0	0.000	0	0	0.0000
	643	233	300	2 886	892					
Total	10 (20)	5 (4)	11 (5)	30 (34)	12 (5)	68	445.1	280	2 240	3.488
	105 029	65 604	130 308	448 768	165 073					

([a]) Fictitious incidence corresponding to a contagious distribution. The number of cases which were actually observed are in brackets; the second line gives the person-years of observation.
([b]) This column gives the T_1 test for each age group separately. The total value of T_1 is calculated from formula (3.10).

degrees of freedom (p = 0.80). On the other hand, this test statistic is equal to 25.1 when applied to observed data (p = 0.00005). The Potthoff and Whittinghill test on these same data gives a value of T_1 equal to 0.55. As the value is not significant it shows that this test is not powerful enough to detect certain types of heterogeneity. It is important to realize that T_1 is a powerful test only against the alternative of risk dispersion discussed at the beginning of this section. The statistic is constructed to detect a trend towards contagion and cannot detect even substantial heterogeneity in the absence of aggregation of this type. In particular, it can be shown that the application of this method to testicular cancer data does not provide a significant result (T_1 = 1.405; p = 0.16) despite clustering of cases (Table 3.1; Figure 3.7d).

The test does not take into consideration the spatial structure of the geographical units being analysed. It is therefore not constructed specifically for geographical analyses. Muirhead and Butland [33] have suggested that the test be applied to several different levels of geographical grouping in order to define the scale on which the phenomenon of aggregation occurs.

A related approach to that described above consists of regrouping the geographical units in such a way that the expected numbers based on a homogeneous distribution of risk are identical in the newly-formed groups. The problem of heterogeneity of populations is thus removed. The randomness of the distribution of the number of cases can then be tested simply by verifying that it follows a Poisson distribution. Such a test based on the same principle as above [31] is given by a statistic known in plant ecology as the dispersion index, defined as the ratio of the observed variance to the observed mean [34]. When ϕ is calculated over n units and n is large, $(n - 1) \phi$ is approximately distributed as a χ^2 on $(n - 1)$ degrees of freedom. Then :

$$T_2 = \sqrt{2(n-1)\phi} - \sqrt{2(n-1) - 1} \qquad (3.11)$$

can be considered to be a standard normal random variable. When several risk groups are to be distinguished (for example, age groups), stratification can be used, as before.

Urquardt and coworkers [35] developed this approach further, including an algorithm to group units. This procedure takes into account the variations in population density, to construct study units which lead back to the simple case of the Poisson distribution. This idea has also been used in the dual approach, which involves working with distances between cases. If the population density is uniform in the geographical area under study, the distribution of the number of cases in each unit of area would be Poisson, with the mean given by the product of the surface area and the average number of cases per unit surface area. Thus, the number of cases in a circle with a radius r would follow a Poisson distribution with mean $\lambda\pi r^2$. The probability that the distance from a given point to the closest case was less than r would be equal to the probability that the corresponding circle only contained one case, that is $e^{-\lambda\pi r^2}$. In other words, the square of the distance from a given point to the nearest case has an exponential distribution with parameter $\pi\lambda$. More generally, when distances are ranked, if R_j is the distance from a given point to the jth nearest case (neighbour of order j), it can be shown by using the same principle (see Chapter 2, page   the relationship between χ^2 and Poisson distributions) that $2\pi\lambda R_j^2$ has a χ^2 distribution on 2j degrees of freedom. Thus, study of the distribution of distances between neighbouring cases (from the first or jth order) provides a means of evaluating the randomness of a spatial distribution. Unless distances are transformed appropriately, population density cannot be considered constant and the distance to the jth case will not have the stated property. Nevertheless, the method still provides a useful statistic to define a test of randomness or to characterize the geographical units which are at excess risk and which need further investigation.

Cuzick and Edwards [36] have proposed to comparing the proximity of n_0 cases to that of n_1 controls representing of the population residing in the region under study. For example, for a childhood disease, these controls could be births of the same sex preceding and following the case in the regional birth register. A test of spatial aggregation is constructed by determining the pairs of subjects (cases and controls) which are neighbours of order j, and counting among these pairs those in which both members are cases. An excess of such pairs compared to the expected number under the assumption of no aggregation (i.e., if the labels 'case' or 'control' are randomly distributed among the $n_0 + n_1$ subjects) will indicate spatial aggregation of cases. The statistic is then defined by:

$$T_k = \sum_{i \neq j} X_{ij} Y_{ij}$$

where $X_{ij} = 1$ if j is the label of a kth order neighbour of i, and 0 otherwise, and $Y_{ij} = 1$ if i and j are cases, and 0 otherwise.

Cuzick and Edwards also suggest other statistics to analyse the structure of distances in the group of cases and controls. They describe the distribution of these statistics under the null hypothesis of no spatial aggregation, and analyse their power to detect certain types of spatial aggregation. The controls in this approach are used to evaluate the density of people at risk in the area under consideration. A similar approach would be possible if this density was known from other sources : the expected number could then be calculated and it would not be necessary to resort to a sample of controls.

Besag and Newell [37] suggested defining areas of investigation around each case by circles with radius given by the distance to the nearest neighbour of order j. The possibility of a cluster around the case under consideration can then be identified from the evaluation of the population at risk in this circle, and hence the number of expected cases, under the hypothesis of homogeneity of risks. In fact, because of the nature of the available data, the region being examined around a given case is not exactly a circle : it is constructed by successive accumulation of small areas of known population. At each stage, the centre of gravity of the area being added is the closest one to the area added at the previous stage. The procedure stops when j cases are obtained in the resulting region (the initial case being excluded) and the expected number is calculated. A circle around the case under consideration is then drawn on the map each time that the probability of observing j cases in the region is less than a specified probability level (for example $\alpha = 5\%$). The number of expected cases in the region at the level α can obviously be calculated taking into account the presence of several risk classes (e.g., age, sex, urban or rural residence) if the population at risk can be characterized according to the values of these parameters. The method is well suited to detect potential clusters in a region for which the population is known on a small geographical scale. In particular, it can be used to identify clusters when the contagious nature of the distribution has already been demonstrated (this last condition is in fact necessary because if $\alpha = 5\%$, Besag and Newell's test will identify 5% of cases as defining a cluster in a purely random distribution).

In practice, these methods are limited by the imprecise information available on the location of cases, and the necessity of placing them at the centres of gravity of the geographical units being studied. The references cited in the bibliography provide more details in this regard.

Time-space clustering

If differences in demographic structure and the prevalence of risk factors across regions are sufficiently stable over time, the spatial distribution of incidence tends to remain constant. Further, time trends will tend to be identical between geographical units. This baseline situation corresponds to the absence of time-space interaction. One possible disruption to this state of equilibrium is the occurrence of change in risk at a given time in one area of the geographical region being studied. The resulting excess of cases defines *time-space clustering*. In investigation of cancer, for which the latency period between the start of exposure and the onset of disease is usually very long, it is uncertain that the identification of such clusters has led to meaningful epidemiological results. Nevertheless, the statistical methods suggested for this type of data merits a brief review.

One of the first studies in this area was by Knox [20] who examined the distribution in space and time of 96 cases of childhood leukaemia. He assumed that any two cases within a kilometre of each other were spatially close and that any two cases occurring within a month of each other were close in time. He then noted 152 pairs which were close in time and 25 pairs close in space. The observation of five pairs close in both time and space led him to the conclusion that there was time-space interaction. He based his conclusion on an analysis of the 2×2 table, classifying the 4560 pairs of subjects ($96 \times 95/2$) into four categories according to their spatial and temporal proximity. Under the assumption of absence of interaction between these two variables, the expected number of subjects close in space and time was estimated as $25 \times 152/4560 = 0.83$. Furthermore, considering that the number of occurrences of such pairs follows a Poisson distribution, he calculated that the probability of observing a value greater than or equal to five was 0.0017, and thus highly improbable under the null hypothesis.

In fact, David and Barton [38] have shown that the mean and variance of the number of pairs belonging simultaneously to two distinct and independent relationships (for example, time and space) can be derived from the number of subjects N and the number of edges a_i and b_i $1 \leq i \leq N$ connecting related subjects in the respective graphs[1] of the two relations S and T which define proximity in space and

---

[1] A relationship can be represented graphically by a set of points (subjects, $1 \leq i \leq N$), and by a set of segments linking points which are in the relation. The subjects are the vertices of the graph and the segments are its edges. When the relationship is not symmetrical, the segments are replaced by vectors when (i,j) is in the relation and (j,i) is not.

time. Specifically, by characterizing the graph of a relationship by a matrix with elements equal to 1 if the pair (i,j) is in the relationship and 0 when it is not, U, the number of pairs which are in both relationships S and T, can be written in the form:

$$U = \sum_{i \neq j} X_{ij}Y_{ij} \tag{3.12}$$

where X_{ij} and Y_{ij} are the elements of the matrices of the graphs of S and T. Let P be the number of edges of a relationship and Q be the number of pairs of edges of this same relationship, then the number of edges connecting i, the total number of edges and the number of pairs of edges in the relation S can be written in the form:

$$a_i = \sum_{i \neq j} X_{ij} ; \quad P_s = \frac{1}{2}\sum_{i=1}^{N} a_i ; \quad Q_s = \sum_{i=1}^{N} \frac{a_i(a_i - 1)}{2} \tag{3.13}$$

with similar relationships holding for P_T and Q_T as functions of Y_{ij} through b_i, the number of edges connecting i in the realation T. David and Barton's result can then be written:

$$E(U) = \frac{2P_sP_T}{N(N - 1)} \tag{3.14}$$

$$E(U^2) = \frac{2P_sP_T}{N^{(2)}} + \frac{4Q_sQ_T}{N^{(3)}} + \frac{4(P_s^{(2)} - 2Q_s)\,(P_T^{(2)} - 2Q_T)}{N^{(4)}} \tag{3.15}$$

where

$$N^{(k)} = N\,(N - 1) \,.....\, (N - k + 1)$$

In the example given by Knox, we have $P_s = 25$, and $P_T = 152$; Barton and David calculate Q_S and Q_T to obtain a variance of 0.802, showing that the hypothesis of Poisson variation is acceptable and that consequently Knox's conclusions are correct.

This approach can obviously be applied to situations other than the evaluation of time-space clustering. For example, to test the homogeneity of risk in a series of g families, each of size n_j and including k_j subjects with a genetic defect, we calculate the number of pairs of affected subjects in the same family

$$U = \sum_{j=1}^{g} \frac{k_j\,(k_j - 1)}{2} \tag{3.16}$$

if S denotes the relationship of belonging to the same family and T is the relationship of sharing a genetic defect, then $a_i = n_j - 1$ for all members of family j. If, in addition,

K is the total number of cases, then $b_i = K - 1$ when i is a case and $b_i = 0$ for other subjects. Application of formulae (3.13) then gives:

$$P_s = \frac{1}{2} \sum_{j=1}^{g} n_j (n_j - 1) \qquad P_T = \frac{1}{2} K (K - 1) \qquad (3.17)$$

$$Q_s = \frac{1}{2} \sum_{j=1}^{g} n_j (n_j - 1) (n_j - 2) \qquad Q_T = \frac{1}{2} K (K - 1) (K - 2) \qquad (3.18)$$

which immediately gives the mean and variance of U, from formulae (3.14) and (3.15) above.

The statistic U has been generalized by Mantel [39] by allowing X_{ij} and Y_{ij}, the indicators of proximity in space and time of the pair (i, j), to assume values other than 0 and 1. Furthermore, Mantel's method does not require the relationships S and T to be symmetric, so that it can account for very general situations such as the relationship of proximity discussed in the previous section. Cuzick and Edwards' method [36], presented earlier, is within the scope of this approach. Mantel's result is discussed by Cliff and Ord [40], whose work we will return to in more detail. Below, the method for calculating the moments of the statistic U are given.

First, the quantities S_0, S_1, S_2, defined by the following formulae, are calculated:

$$S_0 = \sum_{i \neq j} X_{ij} \qquad (3.19)$$

$$S_1 = \frac{1}{2} \sum_{i \neq j} (X_{ij} + X_{ji})^2 \qquad (3.20)$$

$$S_2 = \sum_{i} (X_{i.} + X_{.i})^2 \qquad (3.21)$$

The quantities T_0, T_1 and T_2 are defined by similar formulae as functions of Y. Mantel has shown that under the hypothesis of no correlation between X_{ij} and Y_{ij}, the expected value and variance of U are given by:

$$E(U) = \frac{S_0 T_0}{N(N - 1)} \qquad (3.22)$$

$$E(U^2) = \frac{S_1 T_1}{2N^{(2)}} + \frac{(S_2 - 2S_1) (T_2 - 2T_1)}{4N^{(3)}} + \frac{(S_0^2 + S_1 - S_2) (T_0^2 + T_1 - T_2)}{N^{(4)}} \qquad (3.23)$$

where $N^{(k)}$ is defined as in formula (3.15). Smans and Ohno's statistics given in the previous section are of this kind. In particular, the mean and the variance of D is derived from formulae (3.22) and (3.23) in the case of uniform population density.

Smoothing and the empirical Bayes method

Data from small geographical areas can be more informative in the analysis of disease occurrence than those for larger geographical areas, for example by allowing more homogeneous risk groups to be constructed. However, the size of the populations in these areas being studied then implies that most statistics, in particular measures of incidence and mortality, are subject to large random variability that makes the direct interpretation of data difficult. Use of a smoothing procedure then becomes necessary.

Although numerous smoothing methods have been proposed, their statistical properties have been relatively poorly investigated. The polynomial regression method discussed above (Figure 3.5) and the moving average method used in the Finnish cancer atlas [41] and elsewhere do not totally address the problem of inhomogeneity of populations. These methods can therefore produce extreme risk estimates for areas with small populations.

When sufficient information is available, groups of contiguous geographical zones can be formed by objectively defining similarity based on determinants of risk as geographical or socioeconomic variables. The SMR can then be calculated in the resulting areas to obtain more stable estimates, as was done for the atlas of cancer incidence in the Isère [42]. In a related approach, Huel [43] proposed grouping geographical zones based on similarity of incidence or mortality itself. This method assumes an extremely strong autocorrelation since it is based on the idea that contiguous geographical zones are *a priori* alike, in the absence of evidence to the contrary. Contiguous zones are grouped according to the following algorithm :

• Define a *coefficient of similarity* or *distance* between areas which measures their proximity with regard to the variable being considered (e.g., the Mantel-Haenszel statistic comparing incidence or mortality in two neighbouring areas; see page 77).

• Choose a cut-off point in the coefficient beyond which two areas cannot be grouped (e.g., significant difference at level α).

• Group two contiguous areas when their similarity is greater than that between each of the two areas with all other neighbours.

Iteration of step 3 leads to a unique solution if, at each step, all distances between neighbouring areas formed at the previous step are different. In this situation, one area can be grouped with only one of its neighbours.

This method has several advantages. It can eliminate spurious excesses of risk that a simple description using SMRs might produce. It can also reveal the minimal spatial structure compatible with the precision of the observations. On the other hand, the method suffers the inevitable arbitrariness of the choice of the cut-off point for similarity. The variability in the number of neighbours across regions raises another problem: a region with few neighbours probably has a greater chance of remaining isolated and thus attracting attention. This method has been systematically used in the atlas of cancer incidence in the Isère in France and the results appear to confirm this point. Figures 3.7a and 3.7b show the map of testicular cancer incidence based on SMRs and the smoothed map using Huel's method as applied by

Colonna [21]. The method confirms the existence of a spatial structure which had previously been detected by Moran and Smans' coefficients of autocorrelation. Furthermore, it shows a high-risk region. Note that the SMRs do not provide any clear indication of spatial structure because of the small observed numbers available in each geographical unit.

As noted previously, the description of risk in a group of geographical units raises the problem of simultaneous estimation of a series of values for which the available statistical information is of variable precision. Furthermore, a series of comparisons of geographical units taken two at a time does not necessarily lead to a ranking. It is likely that Huel's method provides the best solution that can be obtained using a series of tests of this kind.

The preceding discussion has also shown that the construction of a map implicitly or explicitly involves two steps: firstly, the establishment of a class of geographical units by risk level, then a grouping of these units into large risk categories from which the scale of the map is constructed. If this grouping is carried out on the basis of centiles, two methods to estimate incidence or mortality which rank the geographical units in the same order, or almost the same order, are equivalent and lead to the same graphical representation. As a consequence, the choice between various methods of standardization is not a major problem, since the rank correlation between the resulting measure of risk is usually high. Similarly, the fact that the random variability of the estimators is large compared to that of the underlying risks that they estimate only causes difficulty when the units contain populations of varying sizes: in this situation, estimates of risk in small population units based on small numbers are likely to be misclassified and have an unjustified weight in the final definition of risk categories. In this case, the classification of regions by incidence or mortality level should take into account not only the estimated value of the risk, but also the precision with which risk is estimated.

The empirical Bayes approach is probably the most satisfactory solution which has been proposed to date for this problem. Basically, this method [44] does not allow imprecise estimates to appear among the extreme values simply on the basis of their imprecision.

Suppose the map is defined by n geographical units in which O_i cases have been observed and E_i cases were expected under the hypothesis of equality of risk in different units. Then the relative risk ρ_i of each area compared to the standard risk is classically estimated by the SMR, O_i/E_i (see Chapter 2, page 100). We have seen that O_i can be considered to have a Poisson distribution with mean $\rho_i E_i$. Up to this point, in the classical approach, ρ_i was considered fixed and totally unknown. Now we suppose that the observations are the result of two successive, random mechanisms. The first, determined by the risk factors for the disease, generates the values ρ_i which then become the n realizations of the same underlying random variable determining the risk levels in different regions. The second mechanism leads to observations O_i from the Poisson distribution with mean $\rho_i E_i$. The geographical variability to be described obviously corresponds to the first of these mechanisms. In practice a model is chosen to describe the distribution of the relative risks ρ_i, which relies on available *a priori* information about them such as the prevalence of the risk factors in the regions, or a possible autocorrelation in risks detected by one of the methods discussed above. Several classes of distribution can appear to be reasonable in this context. If the aim is simply to impose some form of cohesion on the estimates and avoid extreme estimates from lightly populated regions, the gamma distribution is an appropriate choice, for reasons explained below. Its density is:

$$\gamma(\rho) = \frac{1}{s\,\Gamma(r/s)} \left(\frac{\rho}{s}\right)^{r/s-1} e^{-\rho/s} \tag{3.24}$$

where the function Γ is classically defined by the integral

$$\Gamma(x) = \int_0^\infty t^{x-1}\,e^{-t}\,dt \tag{3.25}$$

The mean and the variance of this distribution are r and rs, as can be verified by recalling that $\Gamma(x + 1) = x\Gamma(x)$. Thus r is the mean risk in the group of regions under study and s is a scale factor indicating the size of the geographical variability relative to this mean risk.

If the risks in different regions constitute a sample from this distribution, the probability that k deaths (or cases) are observed in region i is:

$$\Pr(O_i = k) = \int_0^\infty \gamma(\rho)\,e^{-\rho E_i}\,\frac{(\rho E_i)^k}{k!}\,d\rho \tag{3.26}$$

that is

$$\Pr(O_i = k) = \frac{\Gamma(k + r/s)}{k!\,\Gamma(r/s)} \left(\frac{sE_i}{1 + sE_i}\right)^k \left(\frac{1}{1 + sE_i}\right)^{r/s} \tag{3.27}$$

which can be written :

$$\Pr(O_i = k) = \frac{(r/s)\,(r/s + 1)\ldots(r/s + k - 1)}{k!} \left(\frac{sE_i}{1 + sE_i}\right)^k \left(\frac{1}{1 + sE_i}\right)^{r/s} \tag{3.28}$$

Thus, the marginal distribution of O_i is a negative binomial distribution with parameters sE_i and r/s having mean rE_i and variance $rE_i(1 + sE_i)$. This distribution, which serves as a paradigm for cluster distributions, is particularly appropriate here. Effectively, if there is heterogeneity in risks, the distribution of cases in the different geographical units will differ from the random scatter represented by the Poisson distribution, and the cases will tend to group together in higher-risk regions.

Using the distribution of observations in the set of geographical units allows r and s to be estimated by the method of maximum likelihood, thus giving the mean risk and the variance of the distribution of ρ. This marginal distribution is however of limited interest. The main aim of disease mapping in this case is to obtain an estimate of risk in the area i which takes into account both a priori information about the distribution of ρ and a posteriori information provided by the value k taken by O_i. The a posteriori distribution of ρ in this region is used for this purpose, using the fact that the observed value of O_i is k. From Bayes' theorem, the probability density of ρ can be written:

$$\pi(\rho|k) = \frac{\gamma(\rho)\,Pr(O_i = k|\rho)}{Pr(O_i = k)} \tag{3.29}$$

$$\pi(\rho|k) = \frac{1}{u_i\,\Gamma(k + r/s)}(\rho/u_i)^{k + r/s - 1}\,e^{-\rho/u_i} \tag{3.30}$$

where

$$u_i = \frac{s}{1 + s\,E_i}$$

This is the density of a gamma distribution with parameters $k + r/s$ and u_i. The *a posteriori* mean and the variance of ρ are therefore:

$$\hat{\rho}_i = \left(\frac{r}{s} + k\right)\left(\frac{s}{1 + s\,E_i}\right) = \frac{r + ks}{1 + s\,E_i} \tag{3.31}$$

$$\hat{v}_i = \hat{\rho}_i\left(\frac{s}{1 + s\,E_i}\right) \tag{3.32}$$

If r and s are known, these formulae will provide a Bayesian estimate of ρ_i, that is, both a value for ρ_i and the variance of the chosen estimator. In fact, r and s must be estimated from the marginal distribution as indicated above, explaining the use of the term 'empirical' in this method. Similarly, the variability of the estimator cannot be characterized by $\hat{v}_i$, since, the estimation of r and s introduces additional variation which is not taken into account in $\hat{v}_i$.

Replacing k by O_i in (3.31), the estimator $\hat{\rho}_i$ can be written

$$\hat{\rho}_i = \frac{r/s + (O_i/E_i)E_i}{(1/s) + E_i} \tag{3.33}$$

that is, as the weighted average of the mean risk r and of the ratio O_i/E_i, the SMR of the region i. Since s is the parameter characterizing the variance rs of the *a priori* risk distribution, the following observations can be made:

• For a given variance of the geographical distribution, the estimates will be closer to the SMR as E_i increases; however, on the other hand, less precise estimates are moved closer to the mean risk (r).

• If the variance of the geographical distribution (s) is very large, there is effectively no *a priori* information and the empirical Bayes estimates are close to the SMRs.

• When all the SMRs are equally precise, the only effect of their collective estimation will be to reduce the range of the estimates by bringing them all closer to the mean risk.

In spite of its attractive features, the gamma distribution can still be questioned as the only constraint it imposes on the estimates is in their variances. Generally, it would be of interest to incorporate in the *a priori* distribution of ρ additional data concerning the spatial structure under study or a series of covariables characterizing the geographical units being described. These objectives could be achieved by making the parameters r and s of the gamma distribution depend on the spatial structure and covariables. However, because of technical difficulties in incorporating the spatial structure, studies of this type have generally resorted to the arsenal of autoregressive Gaussian spatial processes used in other areas of investigation.

In this context, suppose that the variables X_i = Log ρ_i are Gaussian, with mean depending on a number of covariables (**z**) and correlation depending on the spatial structure (**W**). Besag [45] has shown that such a model can be specified using the conditional expectation of X_i in the form:

$$E\,(X_i \mid X_j,\, j \neq i) = \mu_i + a \sum_{j \neq i} w_{ij}\,(X_j - \mu_j) \tag{3.34}$$

$$\mathrm{Var}\,(X_i \mid X_j,\, j \neq i) = \sigma^2 \tag{3.35}$$

$$\mu_i = \boldsymbol{\beta}\,\mathbf{z}_i \tag{3.36}$$

where **W**, with elements w_{ij}, is most often the indicator matrix of proximity and $\boldsymbol{\beta}$ is a set of parameters to be estimated. More precisely, this specification is equivalent to a Gaussian model with mean μ and variancecovariance matrix $\sigma^2(\mathbf{I} - a\mathbf{W})^{-1}$.

This model is especially appropriate for regular geographical subdivisions in which each unit has the same number of neighbours. In practice, this condition is rarely met, and it seems more satisfactory to suppose that the conditional variance of X_i increases as the number of neighbouring regions decreases. A model proposed by Besag and Kempton [47] and examined in detail by Mollie [48] fulfils this objective. This model (mixed model) assumes that the observations result from the sum of two processes : the first T_i is a normal random process with mean μ_i, constant variance σ^2 and without autocorrelation. The second, U_i, which has zero mean and maximal autocorrelation, is obtained by supposing that the conditional expectation of the U_i is the mean of observations U_j in the neighbouring units, and that the conditional variance of U_i is $\tau^2/w_{i.}$, where $w_{i.} = \sum_j w_{ij}$ is the number of neighbours of unit i. The conditional variance of X_i then depends on the number of neighbours, and the autocorrelation of the process $X_i = T_i + U_i$ depends on the relative size of the variances σ^2 and τ^2. The bigger the ratio σ^2/τ^2, the smaller is the spatial autocorrelation, while it is maximized for $\sigma^2 = 0$.

The use of such an *a priori* model for the distribution of risks requires numerical methods, because the marginal and *a posteriori* distributions are no longer expressed in a simple analytical form [44, 46].

In practice, the method gives estimates influenced not only by the mean risk of the region under study but also mean risks in areas neighbouring the unit where the risk is being estimated. This method is especially useful in preventing undue attention being focused on areas with small numbers and randomly raised SMR, when they are surrounded by areas of low risk.

Mollié [48] provides a particularly convincing example of the effectiveness of these methods, using gall bladder cancer mortality in French men. Figure 3.8 shows the SMR for 94 French départements, as well as smoothed estimates produced by the methods described above. The gamma distribution provides little insight into the spatial structure while this structure becomes apparent using models which take into

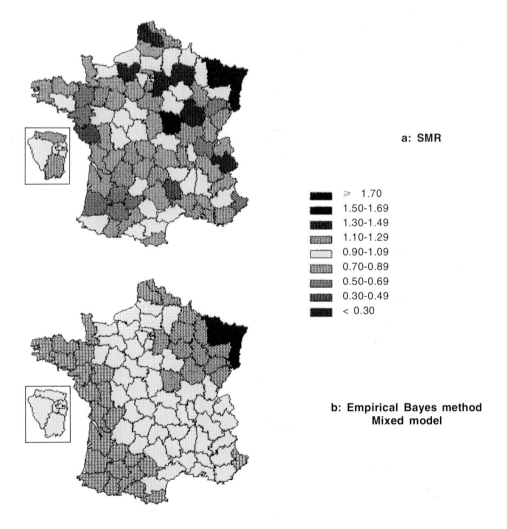

a: SMR

≥ 1.70
1.50-1.69
1.30-1.49
1.10-1.29
0.90-1.09
0.70-0.89
0.50-0.69
0.30-0.49
< 0.30

b: Empirical Bayes method
Mixed model

Figure 3.8   Gallbladder cancer mortality in France; men, 1971-1978
Source: Mollié [48]

account the strong autocorrelation of the spatial process. It is worth noting that the indicated gradient continues beyond the regional borders, the mortality rate for this cancer being particularly high in north east Europe.

The example of testicular cancer in the Isère used above [21,42] is also helpful in demonstrating how this method may incorporate the *a priori* information. The SMRs by canton vary from 0 to 628.7 but are considered not to differ from 1 by the homogeneity test (Table 3.1). The choice of the gamma distribution as the *a priori* description of risk is not justified because of the autocorrelation demonstrated previously. Its use gives risk estimates between 96.9 and 101.6 within the département; they are much more compatible with homogeneity of risk than the crude estimates but they completely ignore the local characteristics of the risk process. On the other hand, using the above model (formulae 3.34, 3.35, and 3.36) as *a priori* distribution provides estimates with a strong spatial autocorrelation and suggests the existence of higher-risk areas. This is reflected in the range of estimates (95.4; 162.0) which is larger than that obtained from the *a priori* gamma distribution. The second set of estimates should be preferred because the data are not compatible with an absence of autocorrelation. It is clearly more logical in this case to use an estimation method which takes into account the spatial organization of the geographical units, to allow a better appreciation of the geographical variation in risk.

Concluding remark

We conclude this section on geographical methods with a cautionary remark. The recent rapid development of these methods results more from a preoccupation with the environment than from new biological knowledge generating hypotheses to be examined. Although legitimate, these preoccupations have led to the introduction of some confusion and may well generate substantial report bias. The increase in the number of situations in which excess risk is investigated has tended to invalidate the statistical methods used in this context which are not designed to deal with this multiple test of randomness.

In these situations, epidemiologists can be caught between two extreme positions : either they may accept as having been stated *a priori* a hypothesis which was in reality suggested by the observations; from this point on, the hypothesis will be confirmed simply by a suitably chosen test. Alternatively, they can deny the existence of any excess risk in the particular case presented to them and look in the armoury of available tests for the most conservative one which will simply show that their own *a priori* ideas cannot be disproven by statistics. This ambiguity emphasizes the need to adopt an approach dictated by a biological hypothesis which integrates research from other disciplines. When there are no data of this kind, a good theoretical knowledge of the tools being used is the only support available. With this knowledge, wrong conclusions resulting from excessive confidence in statistical significance alone can be avoided. Thus, for many reasons, the contribution of geographical studies to etiological research is uneven, and depends on the context in which they are applied. Although they are useful, a number of these methods are at best tools of preliminary investigation.

Ecological studies

Aim and methodological principles

Correlation studies, also called *ecological studies*, have fundamentally the same objective as the methods of analytical epidemiology, that is, to detect associations between risk and exposure levels and then suggest, or preferably confirm, explanatory hypotheses. As with all methods in descriptive epidemiology, it is the group rather than the individual which constitutes the basic statistical unit.

Correlation studies are often seen as equivalent to geographical analyses of the determinants of risk. Indeed, the procedure is frequently used with groups that are geographically defined, whether by region or by country. It is a logical development of the studies described in the previous sections, and represents the most straightforward approach to try to explain geographical heterogeneity. Nevertheless, the methods have a much wider use, applying to all situations which involve investigating the relationship between the frequency of an event in several groups and a parameter characterizing the average exposure of individuals in the groups, no matter how the groups are defined.

Ecological studies also represent a natural extension of the pairwise comparisons often made in descriptive epidemiology, in that they provide a synthesis of the information obtained from these comparisons. Their advantage is especially obvious when many factors are presumed to act simultaneously and the average exposure of the group can be determined for each one of them. In this situation, it is not particularly informative to simply examine rates and levels of exposure to different factors. In theory, the specific effects of each factor could be assessed by simultaneously accounting for them in a multivariate analysis. In addition, correlations across groups should offer a further opportunity to confirm the existence of a relationship between exposure and risk if it is possible to demonstrate a dose-response relationship. In the following section, however, it will be seen that ecological studies are subject to a number of weaknesses which limit their value and make their interpretation difficult.

Correlation studies are often justified on the grounds that they use available data on groups which have been formed for other reasons, but nevertheless reflect different levels of the exposure being studied. As with other methods in descriptive epidemiology, ecological studies are based on the implicit assumption that the groups on which the study is based correspond to a categorization of exposure of acceptable specificity. It will be seen later that the homogeneity of exposure within groups is an important determinant of the method's success.

When groups are not defined *a priori*, the way in which they are formed using available data is obviously of crucial importance. In an ideal situation where these data are available at an individual level, groups could be formed by categorizing individuals with respect to increasing, if not homogeneous, exposure levels. The situation arising in this case is then strictly identical to that of an analytical study.

In general, study of the relationship between exposure and risk level is based on a graphical representation, in which each group under consideration appears as a point, situated on two axes characterizing respectively the two measures in question. For example, in Figure 3.9, data on tobacco consumption and the cumulative risk of lung cancer are shown for European countries. An important feature is the shape of the resulting scatter of points : concentration of points around a simple, especially linear, function tends to support the determining role of the exposure in the statistical explanation of risk level.

The effect of exposure can be quantified by fitting a regression line which predicts incidence or mortality as a function of the level of exposure. Later, we will see that this method is more appropriate than the calculation of the correlation coefficient, which is nevertheless the procedure most often used.

Technical aspects of the calculation and interpretation of regression and correlation are presented briefly below.

Figure 3.10a shows the linear function $Y = 2X + 1$ when X is between 0 to 1; the value of Y depends only on X and its variability is similarly defined by that of X:

$$Var(Y) = 4 \ Var(X)$$

Figures 3.10b, c and d show how such a relationship is changed when a random component of increasing variance is added to the deterministic element $2X + 1$ defining Y. Table 3.3 provides numerical values corresponding to these figures and details of the calculations for Figure 3.10c. In this example X is assumed to be

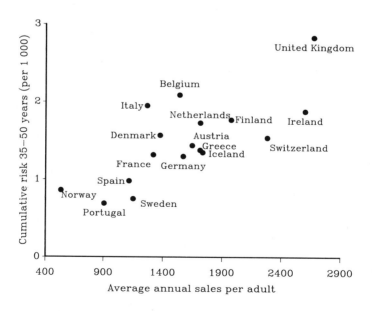

**Figure 3.9   National sales of cigarettes (1955-1964)
and risk of lung cancer in European countries
(average risk in males and females born around 1925; see Table 1.1)**

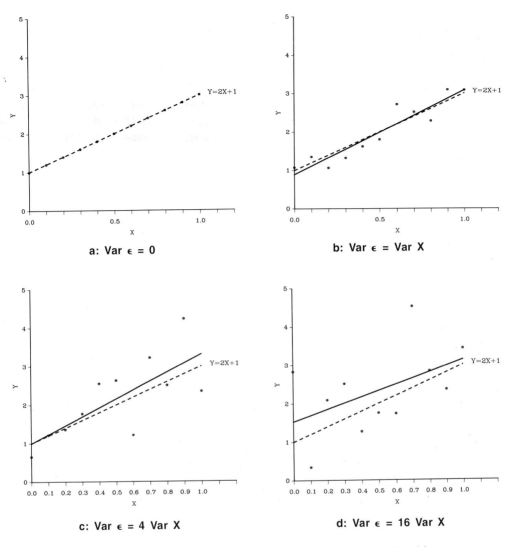

Figure 3.10   Least squares estimate of the linear relationship
Y = 2X + 1 + ε, simulated data

controlled, that is, it takes the values x_i, i = 1, n defined *a priori* (here from 0 to 1 by steps of 0.1). The classical model used to represent this type of data is

$$Y = aX + b + ε$$

where the errors ε are assumed to be independent with the same normal distribution

$$ε \rightsquigarrow N(0, σ_ε^2) \tag{3.37}$$

It expresses a relationship in which the mean of the normal variable Y depends linearly on the variable X and the conditional variance σ_ε^2 is the same for all values of X. The variability of Y is thus the result of its structural variability due to the relationship with X and the random variability added by the error ε, which may be due to other determinants of Y not accounted for by the model:

$$Var(Y) = a^2 \, Var(X) + \sigma_\varepsilon^2 \tag{3.38}$$

In Figure 3.10, σ_ε^2 respectively has the value Var(X) (Figure 3.10b), 4Var(X) (Figure 3.10c) and 16Var(X) (Figure 3.10d). In Figure 3.10c, only half of the variance of Y is due to the structural relationship linking X and Y.

The accuracy of the prediction of Y that can be made from knowing X is often measured by the percentage of the variance of Y which is due to its relationship with X. This relationship is written as $\rho^2 = a^2 Var(X)/Var(Y)$. Its values are respectively 100%, 80%, 50% and 20% in the four diagrammes of figure 3.10 above. This figure show that the accuracy of the prediction, therefore ρ^2, depends on the random variability σ_ε^2. The above formula indicates that it is also a function of the structural variance. The less the slope, the smaller the value of ρ^2, for given random variability and variance of X; ρ^2 is obviously zero when the slope is horizontal, because X no longer provides any information on Y.

In practice, a and b are not known. They can be estimated by the maximum likelihood method which, for the model (3.37), is equivalent to the method of least squares: the estimates $\hat{a}$ and $\hat{b}$ of a and b are the values which minimize the deviance D(a,b), that is, the sum of squares of the differences in the model

$$D(a, b) = \sum_{i=1}^{n} (Y_i - aX_i - b)^2 \tag{3.39}$$

A simple rearrangement shows that

$$\hat{a} = \frac{\sum_{i=1}^{n} (X_i - \overline{X})(Y_i - \overline{Y})}{\sum_{i=1}^{n} (X_i - \overline{X})^2} = \frac{\hat{Cov}(X, Y)}{Var(X)} \tag{3.40}$$

$$\hat{b} = \overline{Y} - \hat{a}\overline{X}$$

where $\overline{X}$ and $\overline{Y}$ are the observed averages of X and Y.

Calculation of the regression line from data shown in Figure 3.10 c is given in Table 3.3.

**Table 3.3   Data from Figures 3.10(b,c,d)
and calculation of the regression line for Figure 3.10c**

Unit	Y^b (1)	Y^c (2)	Y^d (3)	X (4)	X^2 (5)	$(Y^c)^2$ (6)	XY^c (7)	$\hat{Y}^c$ (8)
1	1.07	0.65	2.83	0.0	0.00	0.422	0.000	0.99
2	1.35	1.21	0.34	0.1	0.01	1.464	0.121	1.22
3	1.06	1.36	2.09	0.2	0.04	1.850	0.272	1.46
4	1.32	1.77	2.51	0.3	0.09	3.133	0.531	1.69
5	1.62	2.55	1.27	0.4	0.16	6.502	1.020	1.92
6	1.80	2.63	1.75	0.5	0.25	6.917	1.315	2.15
7	2.71	1.21	1.73	0.6	0.36	1.464	0.726	2.38
8	2.51	3.22	4.51	0.7	0.49	10.368	2.254	2.62
9	2.28	2.50	2.83	0.8	0.64	6.250	2.000	2.85
10	3.09	4.23	2.35	0.9	0.81	17.893	3.807	3.08
11	3.08	2.34	3.42	1.0	1.00	5.476	2.340	3.31
Total	21.89	23.67	25.63	5.5	3.85	61.739	14.386	23.67

The regression of Y^c on X is obtained from columns 5, 6 and 7 of Table 3.3 using the following calculation:

$$\overline{X} = 0.5 \qquad \sum (X_i - \overline{X})^2 = 1.1$$

$$\overline{Y} = 2.15 \qquad \sum (Y_i - \overline{Y})^2 = 10.81$$

$$\sum (X_i - \overline{X})(Y_i - \overline{Y}) = \sum (X_iY_i - n\overline{X}\overline{Y}) = 2.55$$

$$\hat{a} = \frac{2.55}{1.10} = 2.32$$

$$\hat{b} = 2.15 - (2.32)(0.5) = 0.99$$

Then, column 8 gives estimated values of Y which define the observed regression line:

$$\hat{Y}_i = \hat{a}X_i + \hat{b}$$

By writing:

$$\sum_{i=1}^{n} (Y_i - \hat{Y}_i)^2 = \sum_{i=1}^{n} [Y_i - \overline{Y} - \hat{a}(X_i - \overline{X})]^2$$

and by developing the second member of the equation, the relationship analagous to (3.38) is obtained:

$$\sum_{i=1}^{n} (Y_i - \overline{Y})^2 = \hat{a}^2 \sum_{i=1}^{n} (X_i - \overline{X})^2 + \sum_{i=1}^{n} (Y_i - \hat{Y}_i)^2 \qquad (3.41)$$

which explains the fact that the observed variance of Y is made up of the variance due to the regression and the residual variance; in the present example, this is written:

$$10.81 = (2.32)^2 \times 1.1 + 4.89$$

The value 4.89 obtained for $D(\hat{a}, \hat{b})$ can be calculated in principle from the formula $\sum_i (Y_i - \hat{Y}_i)^2$. In practice, rounding errors prevent a precise result from being obtained in this way and the value is obtained by subtraction using formula (3.41). The percentage of variance explained by the regression is therefore:

$$\hat{\rho}^2 = \frac{\hat{a}^2 Var(X)}{\hat{Var}(Y)} = \frac{5.92}{10.81} = 0.55$$

this equation provides an estimate of the exact value ρ^2 which, in this example, was set *a priori* to 0.50.

The correlation coefficient, classically defined by the formula:

$$\rho = \frac{Cov(X, Y)}{\sqrt{Var(X) \cdot Var(Y)}} \tag{3.42}$$

is estimated by:

$$\hat{\rho} = \frac{2.55}{\sqrt{10.81 \times 1.1}} = 0.74$$

which is the square root of the percentage of variance explained, and has the same sign as a.

Variations of $\hat{a}, \hat{b}$ around their respective expected values a = 2 and b = 1 are described by a bivariate normal distribution. In particular, the variance of the estimate of the slope can be shown to be

$$Var(\hat{a}) = \frac{\sigma_\varepsilon^2}{\sum_i (X_i - \bar{X})^2} \tag{3.43}$$

this result, which can be easily obtained from formula (3.40), shows that the estimate of a is more precise when the variance of X is large. In other words, a is estimated more accurately when the range of values of X is wide, as intuition would suggest.

Further, $D(\hat{a}, \hat{b})/\sigma_\varepsilon^2$ can be shown to follow a χ^2 distribution on n − 2 degrees of freedom, leading to an estimate of σ_ε^2 (which has a value in this example of 4Var(X) = 0.40) equal to

$$\hat{\sigma}_\varepsilon^2 = \frac{D(\hat{a}, \hat{b})}{n - 2} = \frac{4.89}{9} = 0.54$$

A 1 − α level confidence interval around â can be constructed as

$$[\hat{a} - t_{\alpha/2}(n - 2) S_{\hat{a}} \; ; \; \hat{a} + t_{\alpha/2}(n - 2) S_{\hat{a}}]$$

where

$$S_{\hat{a}} = \frac{\hat{\sigma}_\varepsilon}{\sqrt{\sum (X_i - \bar{X})^2}} = 0.70$$

is the standard error of $\hat{a}$ and $t_{\alpha/2}(n - 2)$ is the value exceeded with probability $\alpha/2$ by a Student t distribution on $n - 2$ degrees of freedom. From data in Figure 3.10c where $n = 11$ and $t_{0.025}(9) = 2.26$, the confidence interval of a is equal to [0.74 ; 3.90].

From data in Figures 3.10 b and d, a calculation not shown here leads to estimates of ρ^2 respectively equal to 0.88 and 0.23, as compared to the true values which are 0.80 and 0.20.

Now suppose that the data in Figure 3.10 c give an incidence or mortality rate Y calculated in n groups characterized by the proportion X of subjects exposed to a risk factor; such a relationship obviously expresses a positive association between risk and exposure. The statistical significance of the increase in this risk is evaluated by testing the hypothesis a = 0. This test is simply carried out by calculating:

$$t = \frac{\hat{a}}{S_{\hat{a}}} = \sqrt{(n - 2)} \frac{\hat{\rho}}{\sqrt{1 - \hat{\rho}^2}} = 3.3 \tag{3.44}$$

which can be compared to the critical value of a Student t distribution on $n - 2 = 9$ degrees of freedom. In this example, the test leads to rejection of the hypothesis a = 0. On the other hand, in Figure 3.10 d, although the estimate of a is 1.61, the hypothesis a = 0 cannot be rejected as the formula above provides a value of t equal to 1.64 for $\rho^2 = 0.23$. The random component has blurred the structural relationship between X and Y. Here, the confidence interval of the slope [-0.60 ; 3.82] is probably more informative than the probability associated with Student's t test (p = 0.14), which reveals nothing about the power of the test carried out and a fortiori about the precision of the estimate obtained.

This model is nevertheless not really suitable for describing random fluctuations of incidence or mortality, which are a function of the number of expected cases. It may seem preferable to suppose that k_i, the number of cases (or deaths) observed in each group, follows a Poisson distribution with mean $M_i(aX_i + b)$, where M_i is the corresponding number of person-years, and to account for the heterogeneity in the variances implied by this distribution, if the sizes of the groups being studied are very different. This would be particularly relevant if the relationship were log-linear instead of linear; calculation of the regression line could then be modified by taking the predicted variable as $Y = Log(k/M)$ and by supposing that the error variance is proportional to that predicted by the Poisson distribution. This leads to a weighted regression in which the function D(a,b) becomes:

$$D(a, b) = \sum_{i=1}^{n} w_i [Y_i - (aX_i + b)]^2 \tag{3.45}$$

where the weights w_i are proportional to the information provided by each observation, or, as a first approximation, proportional to the number of cases observed. In fact, it is unfortunately unlikely that the random component of the number of cases is limited to its Poisson part: other factors which have not been taken into account possibly play a more important role. Consequently the difference between $Y = Log(K/M)$ and $aX + b$ is the sum of a first component due to the random variation of K/M and a second attributable to geographical variation in risk associated with factors other than X. In practice, this second error, sometimes called *extra-Poisson variation*, renders the suggested weight insufficient and its advantages debatable (see page 182 for a discussion of this problem in the context of time trends). Furthermore, in practice, Y is often the logarithm of a directly standardized rate; its random variability can then no longer be of the Poisson type.

Examples of the use of this method will be given later. Firstly, we turn attention to a specific problem raised by the inherent nature of ecological studies.

Strengths and limitations of a measure of group exposure

Group versus individual exposure

The effect of errors in the measurement of exposure on the risk estimates has been largely studied in the context of analytical studies. It has been shown that these errors lead systematically to underestimation of risk when they are nondifferential, ie, independent of the status – case or non-case – of the individuals being studied. The problem is just as common, but rarely discussed in the context of ecological studies. In this situation, exposure is most often estimated from data collected for other reasons, which generally provide only an indirect measure of possible risk factors. For example, sales of a given product only partially reflect its consumption, because losses and unregistered imports are not taken into account. Furthermore, exposure is only characterized by a single value for the whole group, leading to more or less serious consequences depending on the type of exposure being considered.

When the exposure is collective by definition, it is often reasonable to assume that this single collective value is a good measure of individual exposure for all members of the group. Thus, in the study already cited of the association between water hardness and the incidence of cardiovascular disorders, there is little doubt that the quality of the local water is a good indicator of individual exposure for the residents of the district. A similar situation would apply in a study of the effects of sun exposure or natural radiation. A descriptive study in this case is conceptually the same as an analytical study. In the examples given, research carried out on individuals would rely on exactly the same data.

Most often, exposure is individual in nature and rarely homogeneous within a group, either because all members are exposed but at very different levels, or because exposure is either present or absent and the exposure of the group therefore amounts to the proportion of exposed individuals. In practice, distribution of exposure can often have both characteristics. Cigarette consumption represents an example of a heterogeneous distribution of individual exposure, but the heterogeneity may be even more marked as, for example, in the study of occupational risks. In fact, heterogeneity of exposure is the norm in ecological studies, generally as a result of the fact that groups are defined using available data, which usually characterize the exposure only indirectly.

Under these conditions, it is not appropriate to assume that all individuals classified as belonging to a given group have actually experienced the same extent of exposure, as is done in an analytical study: as a consequence, when it is stated that group A is defined as more exposed than group B, it is actually known that group B will include subjects more exposed than some subjects in group A and vice versa. Most often in an ecological study, hierarchical classification of groups based on the degree of exposure is thus only valid for the averages.

Intuitively, the quality of the information that can be derived from an ecological study based on group measurements depends on the relative magnitude of the variability of exposure within groups with respect to its variability between groups. For example, it is doubtful whether a correlation study of the relationship between meat consumption and colon cancer, conducted in districts of the same country, could provide an interpretable result because variations in average consumption between districts would probably be too small in comparison to individual differences within districts.

On the other hand, the more the groups formed for the study can provide a representative classification of individual exposure, the more one is tempted not only to establish the existence of a relationship between exposure and risk, but also to quantify the relationship.

Risk estimation in the context of an ecological study

Consider the situation in which individual exposure is characterized by a dichotomous variable (exposed/unexposed) and where therefore the exposure in each group is defined by the proportion of exposed subjects.

In contrast to a study based on individual follow-up (cohort study), a correlation study cannot use the distribution of events (whether deaths or incident cases) in exposed and unexposed subjects to calculate risk in the two subgroups and the relative risk of exposure. Nevertheless, it is still possible to estimate the relationship between risk and the factor under study when event data are available for a series of n groups. Table 3.4 presents data for the ith group.

**Table 3.4 Distribution (^{a}) of events (deaths or incident cases)
and person-years in a cohort study and a correlation study**

	Exposed	Unexposed	Total
Events	d_{1i}	d_{0i}	$\mathbf{D_i}$
Person-years	$\mathbf{m_{1i}}$	$\mathbf{m_{0i}}$	$\mathbf{M_i}$

(^{a}) Data available from correlation study are in bold type.

If λ_{1i} and λ_{0i} are the unknown rates for the exposed and unexposed, the expected number of events in group i can be written:

$$E(D_i) = m_{0i}\lambda_{0i} + m_{1i}\lambda_{1i} \tag{3.46}$$

If $p_i = m_{1i}/M_i$ characterizes the proportion of exposed subjects in a group i, the rate in this group is:

$$\mu_i = \lambda_{0i} + p_i(\lambda_{1i} - \lambda_{0i}) \tag{3.47}$$

that is, the sum of the baseline risk and the additional risk attributable to exposure for a subset of the group. If risk in the different groups depends entirely on whether or not an individual is exposed, it is independent of other individual characteristics. λ_{0i} and λ_{1i} then do not depend on i and the incidence rate μ_i is a linear function of p_i, the proportion exposed in the group. In fact, if $\delta = \lambda_{1i} - \lambda_{0i}$, we have the model:

$$\mu_i = \mu_0 + \delta p_i \tag{3.48}$$

where δ is independent of i. In other words, if the baseline risk is constant ($\lambda_{0i} = \mu_0$), and if the relative risk ($R = \lambda_{1i}/\lambda_{0i}$) of exposed subjects does not depend on the group, the relationship (3.47) can be written:

$$\frac{\mu_i}{\mu_0} = (R - 1)p_i + 1 \tag{3.49}$$

and thus R can be estimated by:

$$\hat{R} = 1 + \frac{\hat{\delta}}{\hat{\mu}_0} \tag{3.50}$$

This estimate of relative risk is based on the assumption that the expected number of cases in each group depends only on the proportion of exposed and on absolutely no other characteristic of the group. Although this condition is often accepted implicitly, it is not routinely satisfied: hence the limited value in practice of this type of relationship (see the following section). On the other hand, these calculations have a theoretical value in showing that when the assumption is true, the relationship between risk and exposure is linear and the slope of the regression line is the important parameter.

The ecological fallacy

A number of authors have noted that the study of the association between exposure and risk based on grouped data can lead to false conclusions. An example frequently cited in this context [49] is Durkheim's study on suicide rates in four areas of western Europe in the nineteenth century [50]. Durkheim relied on the observation that the suicide rate increased with the proportion of Protestants in a given region to conclude that Protestants committed suicide more often than Catholics. Was this conclusion valid? It may have been that suicide was in fact more frequent among Catholics and increased the more they found themselves in the minority and experienced social pressures predisposing to suicide. This explanation is nevertheless unlikely, because it would require an extremely rapid increase in the suicide rate among Catholics as the proportion of Protestants increased. Indeed, Durkheim ultimately showed that this was not the case. Logically, it was not implausible and reveals one of the major contradictions in the ecological approach: the average level of an exposure factor can have a positive association with the incidence rate in the group, even when the same factor is associated negatively with individual risk within the group. This paradox has many causes. As an example, imagine that the increases in the average income of a group can lead to increased risk behaviour among the poorest of the group. The study of cervical cancer in Finland illustrates this situation (see below, page 157). This intrinsic weakness of correlation studies is known as *the ecological fallacy*.

Secondly, it should be emphasized that the ecological approach is particularly vulnerable to the effects of confounding variables; not only does the approach not allow for control as does a study carried out at an individual level, but it also tends to transform other risk factors into confounding variables, even when they are independent of the factor being studied at an individual level. For example, in an investigation of the relationship between the proportion of wood workers and lung cancer incidence using data from 25 Swiss cantons, smoking will induce confounding if consumption changes with the proportion of wood workers in each canton, even if the two factors in question are independent at the individual level.

To illustrate this point, consider the situation of two dichotomous factors given in Table 3.5. In an ecological study, only the data in bold type are known for each group in the study. If the two factors are independent and there is no interaction (on a multiplicative scale), it is clear that the relative risk for one of them can be estimated from the complete data without taking account of the other.

The marginal estimate of relative risk corresponding to the first factor $(d_{1.}/m_{1.})/(d_{0.}/m_{0.})$ is equal to the estimate obtained after stratifying by the second;

Table 3.5   Distribution ([a]) of events (d) and person-years (m)
in the presence of two risk factors

Factor No 1	Factor No 2		Total
	Exposed	Unexposed	
Exposed	$d_{11}/\mathbf{m_{11}}$	$d_{10}/\mathbf{m_{10}}$	$d_{1.}/\mathbf{m_{1.}}$
Unexposed	$d_{01}/\mathbf{m_{01}}$	$d_{00}/\mathbf{m_{00}}$	$d_{0.}/\mathbf{m_{0.}}$
Total	$d_{.1}/\mathbf{m_{.1}}$	$d_{.0}/\mathbf{m_{.0}}$	$\mathbf{D_i/M_i}$

([a]) Data available from correlation study are in bold type.

since the independence of the exposure factors implies an equal distribution of per-son-years, we can write:

$$\frac{m_{01}}{m_{11}} = \frac{m_{00}}{m_{10}} = \frac{m_{0.}}{m_{1.}}$$

furthermore, as an absence of interaction between the two factors implies that the relative rates are equal in the groups exposed and unexposed to the second factor, the above formula shows that the relative rate which would be obtained after strati-fication is also the marginal relative rate.

This property is important for the validity of analytical studies where there are several risk factors under study which are independent within groups, but which have a different distribution from one group to another. Membership in the group can then be taken as a categorical confounding variable. In such studies where data for a given factor are available at an individual level, it is possible to calculate an unbiased estimate of the overall relative risk after adjusting for the group as a factor, in the absence of precise information about any other factors. In an ecological study, where the group itself is the unit of analysis, it is by definition impossible to proceed in this way.

Using the example in Table 3.5, let the relative risks corresponding to the two factors be R_1 and R_2, and the proportions exposed to each factor in group i be p_{1i} and p_{2i}. Then the relationship previously established between baseline risk and risk in the group becomes (see 3.49):

$$\mu_i = \mu_0 [1 + (R_1 - 1)p_{1i} + (R_2 - 1)p_{2i} + (R_1 - 1)(R_2 - 1)p_{1i} p_{2i}] \qquad (3.51)$$

This relationship shows not only the need to introduce p_{2i} in the regression equation despite the independence of the two factors at an individual level but also the inadequacy of linear adjustment[2].

Table 3.6 illustrates this situation from fictitious data. Five groups, each com-prising 100 000 person-years, are divided according to level of exposure to a factor for which the relative risk is constant and equal to 2 in each group. The regression of the death rate against the proportion exposed leads to estimates:

$$\hat{\mu}_0 = -0.1367 \quad \text{and} \quad \hat{\delta} = 7.56$$

these values are not meaningful, because they provide a negative value for the estimated relative risk $\hat{R}$ (3.50). If the baseline risk is taken to have the value $\mu_0 = 1$, which was used to generate the data for Table 3.6, the relative risk estimated from equation (3.49) is 4.43, a number much greater than its true value of 2.

In reality, the data have been generated assuming that two factors distributed independently in each group act multiplicatively on the risk of death. The proportions

---

[2] Formula (3.51) is only valid for two independent factors with a multiplicative effect. It can be checked that, in general, the last term of (3.51) is $p_{12i} [R_{12} - (R_1 + R_2 - 1)]$; it is equal to zero only when the effects are additive.

Table 3.6   Correlation study. Example of a possible relationship between mortality rate and percentage of exposed subjects

Group	Deaths		Person-years (thousands)		Relative risk	Rate (per 1000)
	Exposed	Un-exposed	Exposed	Un-exposed		
1	56	112	20	80	2	1.68
2	84	98	30	70	2	1.82
3	220	110	50	50	2	3.30
4	360	120	60	40	2	4.80
5	420	90	70	30	2	5.10
Total	1 140	530	230	270	1.96	3.34

of subjects exposed to the second factor in the five groups were respectively 10%, 10%, 30%, 50%, 50% and the relative risk corresponding to the second factor was 5.

If a linear model with two factors is fitted to the data, by an extension of the procedure used above (see page 158 and formula (3.56) for the method to estimate coefficients), the following relationship is obtained:

$$\mu_i = 0.67 + 1.67\,p_1 + 6.33\,p_2$$

which does not provide correct relative risks. Only fitting p_1, p_2 and $p_1 p_2$ would in principle result in an exact estimation of the coefficients of the relationship (3.51), respectively 1, 1, 4, 4. In fact, models of this type are rarely fitted, either because the factors to be taken into consideration are not known or because the necessary data are not available.

In addition, factors associated with the group which act on the variable of interest are not necessarily dichotomous, but are often defined by a number of categories or are of a quantitative nature. Equation (3.46) can be generalized to account for these situations if the distribution of exposure is known in each group, through a model linking exposure and incidence. In the same way as before,

$$E(D_i) = \int_e m_i\,(e)\,\lambda_i\,(e)\,de$$

$$= M_i\,\lambda_i\,(0)\left[1 + \int_e (r_i\,(e) - 1)\,dp_i\right] \qquad (3.52)$$

where $M_i = \int_e m_i(e)\,de$ is the total number of person-years of exposure and $dp_i = \dfrac{1}{M_i}\,m_i(e)\,de$ characterizes the distribution of exposure e in group i.

If the baseline risk $\lambda_i(0)$ and the relative risk $r_i(e)$ are not dependent on the group, we have, as before:

$$E(D_i) = M_i\,\mu_0\left[1 + \int_e (r(e) - 1)\,dp_i\right] \tag{3.53}$$

Moreover, if risk is a simple function of exposure (for example, $r(e) = 1 + \alpha e$), the incidence rate in group i can be written as a function of the mean exposure in the group (in the preceding example: $\dfrac{\mu_i}{\mu_0} = 1 + \alpha\bar{e}_i$). Again, this relationship is only valid in the absence of confounding factors.

In conclusion, caution is required in the interpretation of correlation studies, as a number of risk factors which are known to be independent at the individual level can be associated at the group level. It is only under particular conditions of independence of the factors at a group level, such as when they are equally distributed throughout the groups, that this confounding effect is no longer present. For example, failure to account for sex would produce substantial bias in an analytical study of health in relation to an occupational exposure but would probably be without consequence in a geographical correlation study of the same exposure, because the sex ratio varies little from one population to another.

Despite these critical remarks, ecological studies can play an important role in epidemiological research. Some factors exhibit weak interindividual variation within populations, whereas the populations differ substantially in terms of mean levels of exposure. In this situation, the ecological approach can be very informative if carried out in conjunction with study on individuals. In addition to environmental factors, culturally determined behavioural factors, such as diet or sexual practice, can sometimes lend themselves to group studies with regard to exposure measurement. Ecological studies are not necessarily less accurate than studies of individuals. Some biases due to self-reporting, such as interviewer bias and recall bias, may even be avoided.

A review of the literature in this area shows the wide diversity in the applications of the basic principle. In most situations, the method is justified by the need to control for the effects of potential confounding factors. Some of the techniques used will be described in the following section.

Specific techniques and examples

Definition of groups

An example of the grouping of the subjects is provided by an ecological study of occupational risk of nasal cancer by Gardner and Winter [51]. The population census in England and Wales (carried out by sampling) provided the percentage of the male population employed in different occupations for each of 1366 local ad-

Table 3.7 Number of deaths from nasal cancer in the male population as a function of the percentage of workers employed in the furniture and upholstery industry [51]

Category	Percentage of workers	Number of workers in the industry [a]	Total number of workers [b]	Number of districts	Observed number of deaths	Observed expected radio [c]
1	0.00	0	73 488	75.5	76.5	0.98
2	0.00	0	65 245	130.6	63.5	0.82
3	0.00	0	58 166	323.2	71.0	0.91
4	0.06	47	73 268	51.4	64.1	0.82
5	0.12	85	71 684	44.3	67.9	0.87
6	0.16	111	70 414	43.0	82.0	1.05
7	0.19	134	70 781	34.8	90.8	1.17
8	0.21	147	68 675	48.9	75.9	0.98
9	0.26	177	68 690	48.2	57.9	0.74
10	0.30	191	64 456	39.4	70.6	0.91
11	0.34	228	67 382	64.6	84.5	1.09
12	0.39	265	68 832	54.3	67.0	0.86
13	0.44	305	69 480	47.9	75.6	0.97
14	0.50	336	67 943	50.6	67.0	0.86
15	0.59	392	66 500	51.8	75.3	0.97
16	0.72	474	66 176	28.8	91.4	1.17
17	0.82	557	68 219	54.9	94.6	1.22
18	0.98	680	69 571	45.7	100.2	1.29
19	1.40	963	68 940	63.1	68.2	0.88
20	3.12	2 153	68 958	65.0	111.9	1.44

[a] Furniture and upholstery.
[b] Based on the 1971 census of 10% of the male population aged between 15 and 64 years.
[c] Expected number of deaths in each group is 77.8.

ministrative districts. The authors grouped these geographical units into a small number of areas which would have had the same risk for the cancer under study if age had been the only determinant of the disease. This grouping was carried out using the following procedure for each occupational category for which the risk was to be investigated. First, the districts were ranked according to the percentage of the population employed in the category. The number of expected deaths was then calculated for each district based on national age-specific rates. Finally, the districts were grouped such that each of the newly formed units had the same number of expected deaths from nasal cancer. In order to get this result, the total expected cases in some districts could not be allocated to one unit and had to be divided between two successive units. The observed numbers in these districts were then allocated to the two units in proportion to the expected number of cases. The 20 new units thus formed were then considered to have the same *a priori* risk, with age no longer having a confounding effect in the correlation study.

Having formed the groups, the authors carried out a regression of the observed number of deaths on the percentage exposed in the 20 groups, and tested the significance of the slope. As a result, they showed an association between mortality due to nasal cancer and employment in the furniture and upholstery industry, and the leather industry, which is free of the confounding effect of age.

The classical regression of age-adjusted rates on the proportion of people employed in a given sector of activity may appear *a priori* equivalent and simpler than the above procedure.However,while adjusting for age takes account of the differing proportion of younger people across districts, it does not account for the fact that the proportion of the population employed in the relevant sector of activity is highest in groups with the largest proportion of younger people (see formula 3.51). This method of forming groups thus has specific advantages from the point of view of eliminating the effect of age. In addition, combining groups can in some circumstances eliminate other confounding factors, especially those which have geographical autocorrelation.

The detailed results given by the authors (Table 3.7) illustrate the calculation of relative risk by fitting a regression line of risk against the proportion exposed, as described above. For the furniture and upholstery industry, the mortality rate of group i is defined by the fitted line (using the notation in formula 3.48):

$$\hat{\mu}_i = 0.9133 + 0.1640p_i$$

where p_i is the proportion of workers in this occupational category. The increase in risk with this proportion is highly significant ($\chi^2 = 20.02$ on one degree of freedom). Note that the authors could have estimated the relative risk by:

$$\hat{R} = 1 + \frac{0.1640}{0.9133} = 1.18$$

This relatively small increase in risk is surprising, especially as it relates to an industry for which the association with nasal cancer has already been established. It is possible that the percentage of workers actually exposed to the carcinogens (such as wood dust and leather dust) represents only a small fraction of the workers employed in this sector; this dilution effect is the most likely explanation for the underestimation of true risk.

The authors of this study propose that the idea of combining groups into homogeneous units could be extended to the situation where control for confounding factors, such as socioeconomic status, is required. They recognize, however, that the combination is much more difficult to achieve, and that true homogeneity of groups cannot be attained. Generalizability of the approach is, in any case, limited by the requirement that data are available for small geographical units.

In some situations, exposure is so poorly characterized by the defined exposure variable that erroneous conclusions can result. The study of breast and cervical cancer incidence in Finnish municipalities as a function of a socioeconomic indicator illustrates this phenomenon. Teppo and coworkers grouped 500 Finnish communes into five categories by percentage of inhabitants in the upper social class. When they examined variations in breast cancer incidence, they found, as expected, an increase in risk with the proportion of women 'exposed' according to the above definition. It is known that women at higher risk of breast cancer are generally from the well-off classes (where risk factors such as lower parity and later marriage are more prevalent). On the other hand, the gradient observed for cervical cancer was in the same direction as that for breast cancer (Figure 3.11), and contrary to the relationship between high incidence and lower socioeconomic classes established in previous studies.

Discussing later the results of this ecological study in the light of an analytical study of the above association, the same authors [52] concluded that the risk factors for cervical cancer are more difficult to identify by the ecological approach than those of breast cancer. Under the assumption that cervical cancer is primarily associated with sexual history, it is possible that the diversity of individual exposure resulting from different sexual behaviour is greater than for breast cancer risk factors like parity and dietary factors even in small geographical units such as municipalities. In other words, the ratio between inter- and intra-municipality variation in exposure to breast cancer risk factors could be greater than the corresponding ratio for cervical cancer. This explanation is, however, only partially satisfactory, and raises questions about the characterization of exposure in the ecological study. In particular, the reduction to two social classes undoubtedly yields a measure of low specificity for exposure to risk factors for cervical cancer, and it is likely that in the group defined as exposed, there is in fact a heterogeneous exposure to the true risk factors for cervical cancer. In addition, this heterogeneity can differ from one municipality to another. Finally, it can be assumed that the population subgroups for which cervical cancer risk is particularly high (marginal groups, prostitutes) are generally more represented in urban municipalities. Given that these municipalities are defined as most exposed on the basis of having a large proportion of residents from the upper social class, an apparently positive relationship between cervical cancer risk and upper social class is the result. In fact, the number of subjects actually exposed to

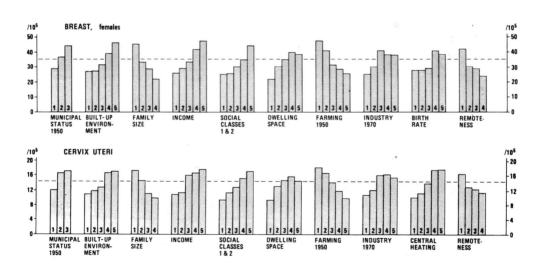

Figure 3.11 Standardized incidence rates of breast and cervical cancer by socioeconomic characteristics in Finnish municipalities, 1955-1974 (Finnish population as standard) Source: Teppo et al. [6]

risk factors for cervical cancer increases with the proportion of persons in the upper social class, at the same time as the heterogeneity of the group increases.

The exposure indicator used is therefore doubly inadequate: not only does it not define the populations at risk, but it cannot characterize exposure to cervical cancer risk factors. We are faced here with the same type of problems as were discussed above in the context of Durkheim's study of the relationship between suicide and religion. Subjects actually exposed cannot be those identified by the defined exposure criteria. In this situation, a hasty interpretation of observed relative risk will inevitably lead to an ecological fallacy.

Multivariate analysis

When potential confounding factors cannot be controlled for by an appropriate grouping, the necessary adjustment must be carried out in the statistical analyses. The regression method described on page 142 for a single variable can be extended without difficulty to several variables, and appear, a priori, to be an appropriate tool for studying the relationship between cancer risk and multiple environmental factors. This method has been used often, mainly in exploratory epidemiological analyses. Its methodological principles will be explained using an example in which the method discussed on page 142 is extended to two variables. The only new concept required when going from one variable to two or more is that of *partial correlation*, which expresses the specific association between a single exposure variable and the risk measure, that is, the association which would be observed if all other factors were held constant.

Firstly, suppose that we wish to estimate the association of Y with two variables X_1 and X_2. As previously, the estimates of a_1 and a_2 in the relationship:

$$Y = a_1X_1 + a_2X_2 + b + \varepsilon \qquad (3.54)$$

are obtained by minimizing the deviance $D(a_1,a_2,b)$ corresponding to the sum of the squares of the deviations in the model:

$$D(a_1, a_2, b) = \sum_{i=1}^{n} (Y_i - a_1X_{1i} - a_2X_{2i} - b)^2 \qquad (3.55)$$

If Var and Cov are the estimates of variance and covariance, then:

$$D(a_1, a_2, b) = n[Var(Y) + Var(a_1X_1 + a_2X_2) - 2 \, Cov(Y, a_1X_1 + a_2X_2)]$$

From this last expression, and setting the derivatives with respect to a_1, a_2 and b equal to zero, it can be verified that $\hat{a}_1$, $\hat{a}_2$ and $\hat{b}$ are given by the equations:

$$\hat{a}_1 \, Var(X_1) + \hat{a}_2 \, Cov(X_1, X_2) = Cov(Y, X_1)$$

$$\hat{a}_1 \, Cov(X_1, X_2) + \hat{a}_2 \, Var(X_2) = Cov \, Y, X_2)$$

$$\hat{b} = \bar{Y} - \hat{a}_1\bar{X}_1 - \hat{a}_2\bar{X}_2 \qquad (3.56)$$

Letting:

$$S_X = \begin{bmatrix} Var(X_1) & Cov(X_1, X_2) \\ Cov(X_1, X_2) & Var(X_2) \end{bmatrix}$$

and

$$S_{YX} = \begin{bmatrix} Cov(Y, X_1) \\ Cov(Y, X_2) \end{bmatrix}$$

we can write:

$$\hat{a} = S_X^{-1} S_{YX} \tag{3.57}$$

a formula which, when added to the third of the equations (3.56) above forms the analogue of formula (3.40). The minimum value of $D(a_1, a_2, b)$ can similarly be written with the same notation:

$$D(\hat{a}_1, \hat{a}_2, \hat{b}) = n[Var(Y) + Var(\hat{a}_1 X_1 + \hat{a}_2 X_2) - 2 Cov(Y, \hat{a}_1 X_1 + \hat{a}_2 X_2)]$$

$$D(\hat{a}_1, \hat{a}_2, \hat{b}) = n[Var(Y) + S'_{YX} S_X^{-1} S_{YX} - 2 S'_{YX} S_X^{-1} S_{YX}]$$

$$D(\hat{a}_1, \hat{a}_2, \hat{b}) = n[Var(Y) - S'_{YX} S_X^{-1} S_{YX}]$$

which leads to the relationship:

$$n \, Var(Y) = n \, S'_{YX} S_X^{-1} S_{YX} + D(\hat{a}_1, \hat{a}_2, \hat{b}) = n \, S'_{YX} \hat{a} + D(\hat{a}_1, \hat{a}_2, \hat{b}) \tag{3.58}$$

This formula, analogous to formula (3.41), shows how the total variance can be decomposed into two terms: the variance due to regression and the residual variance. As before, the quantity:

$$\hat{\rho}^2_{YX} = \frac{S'_{YX} \hat{a}}{Var(Y)} = 1 - \frac{D(\hat{a}_1, \hat{a}_2, \hat{b})}{n \, Var(Y)}$$

is the percentage of variance explained by the regression. Its positive square root, called the *multiple correlation* between Y and X_1, X_2, is the correlation between Y and the function $\hat{a}_1 X_1 + \hat{a}_2 X_2$; it is equal to the maximum correlation that can be obtained between Y and all functions of the form $a_1 X_1 + a_2 X_2$. Table 3.8 uses data from Figure 3.10c (Table 3.3) to which is added a second predictor X_2 of Y.

Columns 4, 5 and 6 are obtained directly from columns 1, 2 and 3. The data from Table 3.3 combined with these results gives:

$$\sum_{i=1}^{11} (X_{2i} - \bar{X}_2)^2 = 104.3 - \frac{(29.5)^2}{11} = 25.14$$

$$\sum_{i=1}^{11} (X_{1i} - \overline{X}_1)(X_{2i} - \overline{X}_2) = 17.05 - \left(\frac{5.5 \times 29.5}{11}\right) = 2.30$$

$$\sum_{i=1}^{11} (Y_i - \overline{Y})(X_{2i} - \overline{X}_2) = 76.08 - \left(\frac{23.67 \times 29.5}{11}\right) = 12.60$$

the value of the other coefficients of equation (3.56) have been obtained previously (see Table 3.3). Ignoring the factor 1/11, the first two equations can be written:

$$1.10\,\hat{a}_1 + 2.30\,\hat{a}_2 = 2.55$$

$$2.30\,\hat{a}_1 + 25.14\,\hat{a}_2 = 12.60$$

leading to the estimates:

$$\hat{a}_1 = 1.57 \text{ and } \hat{a}_2 = 0.36$$

The third of these equations gives:

$$\hat{b} = 2.15 - 1.57(0.50) - 0.36(2.68) = 0.40$$

From (3.58), the component of variation explained by the regression can then be calculated:

$$n S'_{YX}\,\hat{a} = (2.55 \times 1.57) + (12.6 \times 0.36) = 8.54$$

and similarly the square of the multiple correlation coefficient:

$$\hat{\rho}^2_{YX} = \frac{8.54}{10.81} = 0.79$$

Table 3.8 An example of the calculation of multiple regression (Y and X_1 are columns 2 and 4 in Table 3.3)

Unit	X_1 (1)	X_2 (2)	Y (3)	X_1X_2 (4)	X_2Y (5)	X_2^2 (6)	$\hat{Y}$ (7)
1	0.0	0.0	0.65	0.00	0.00	0.00	0.40
2	0.1	1.6	1.21	0.16	1.94	2.56	1.14
3	0.2	1.2	1.36	0.24	1.63	1.44	1.13
4	0.3	2.8	1.77	0.84	4.96	7.84	1.88
5	0.4	5.4	2.55	2.16	13.77	29.16	2.97
6	0.5	4.5	2.63	2.25	11.83	20.25	2.80
7	0.6	1.6	1.21	0.96	1.94	2.56	1.92
8	0.7	3.7	3.22	2.59	11.91	13.69	2.83
9	0.8	2.3	2.50	1.84	5.75	5.29	2.48
10	0.9	3.9	4.23	3.51	16.50	15.21	3.22
11	1.0	2.5	2.34	2.50	5.85	6.25	2.87
Total	5.5	29.5	23.67	17.05	76.08	104.25	23.67

In the same way, from (3.58) it can be verified that[3]

$$D(\hat{a}_1, \hat{a}_2, \hat{b}) = 10.81 - 8.54 = 2.27$$

It is then important to be able to evaluate the role of each variable in the prediction of Y and in particular, the improvement in this prediction when the variable X_2 is added to the variable X_1 in the regression equation. The correlation of Y and X_2 (r = 0.76) shows that X_2 is a predictor of Y. However, as X_1 and X_2 are correlated (r = 0.44), it is probable that X_1 and X_2 provide partially the same information about Y. The independent relationship between X_2 and Y should therefore be evaluated.

When X_2 is added to the model equation, the deviance is reduced by 2.62, the difference between the deviance of the model not containing X_2 $(D_1 = D(\hat{a}_1, 0, \hat{b}) = 4.89)$ and that of the model above $(D_2 = D(\hat{a}_1, \hat{a}_2, \hat{b}) = 2,27)$. This reduction expresses the additional role of X_2 after taking X_1 into account. By expressing the reduction in relation to the deviance of the initial model, a measure of the specific contribution of X_2 is obtained:

$$\hat{\rho}^2_{YX_2 \mid X_1} = \frac{D_1 - D_2}{D_1} = \frac{2.62}{4.89} = 0.53 \tag{3.59}$$

Dividing by $\hat{\text{Var}}(Y)$ shows that:

$$\hat{\rho}^2_{YX_2 \mid X_1} = \frac{\hat{\rho}^2_{YX} - \hat{\rho}^2_{YX_1}}{1 - \hat{\rho}^2_{YX_1}} = \frac{0.79 - 0.55}{0.45} = 0.53 \tag{3.60}$$

where $\hat{\rho}^2_{YX_1} = 0.55$ is the square of the correlation of Y with X_1.

The square root of $\hat{\rho}^2_{YX_2 \mid X_1}$ with the same sign as $\hat{a}_2$ is called the *partial correlation* of Y with X_2, holding X_1 constant. Furthermore, it is the correlation between the residuals of the regressions of Y on X_1 and of X_2 on X_1, and is given by the formula:

$$\rho_{YX_2 \mid X_1} = \frac{\rho_{YX_2} - \rho_{YX_1} \rho_{X_1 X_2}}{\sqrt{(1 - \rho^2_{YX_1})(1 - \rho^2_{X_1 X_2})}} \tag{3.61}$$

from which we get the estimate

$$\hat{\rho}_{YX_2 \mid X_1} = \frac{0.76 - 0.74 \times 0.44}{\sqrt{0.45 \times 0.81}} = 0.72 \quad (= \sqrt{0.53} \text{ up to rounding errors})$$

Many authors have used the techniques of multivariate analysis to try to distinguish the roles of multiple factors or to better estimate the effect of a given factor by controlling for confounding effects. Two examples illustrating the use of these methods are given below.

---

[3] Note that the direct application of the formula $\Sigma (Y_i - \hat{Y})^2$ would lead to the value 2.29.

Blot and Fraumeni [53] estimated the effect of industrial exposure on lung cancer mortality using data from 3056 US counties, attempting to control for sociodemographic factors. Firstly, they estimated the total number of workers in each of 18 industrial sectors in each county, based on the census of industrial employment. For each of the 18 sectors, they then grouped the 3056 counties into three exposure categories: those in which less than 0.1% of the total residential population worked in the sector; those in which between 0.1 and 1% were so employed; and thirdly those with more than 1% of the population employed in the sector.

The estimation of risk associated with the 18 industrial sectors was carried out using a weighted multiple regression model including the exposure variable as well as the main factors to be controlled for. The dependent variable to be fitted was age-standardized lung cancer mortality for the period 1950 to 1969. The exposure variable was included in the model as a categorical variable with three levels defined as above by the proportion of the population working in the sector. The factors to be controlled for were population density, degree of urbanization and proportion of non-whites. A further indicator, situating the county in one of seven broad areas reflecting differences in lung cancer mortality in the USA, was introduced to take large-scale geographical variation into account. The model was thus intended to evaluate the risk associated with industrial activities after adjusting for potential confounding factors. Examination of the residuals, after initially fitting linear terms, led the authors to add quadratic factors to the regression. The weighted regression method was used, with weights defined by the square roots of the number of person-years accumulated in each county during the period under study, giving weights inversely proportional to the standard errors of the mortality rate estimates. The authors did not explain why they chose this type of weighting.

On the basis of the fitted models, the authors concluded that, after accounting for sociodemographic factors, the lung cancer mortality rate increased significantly for four of the 18 industrial sectors: paper, chemicals, petroleum and transport (Table 3.9)

Results of this kind should obviously be interpreted with caution. It is particularly advisable to question the ability of this multivariate analysis to effectively control for the known etiological factors for lung cancer. The authors considered that differ-

Table 3.9   Regression coefficients (^{a}) of the standardized rate (^{b}) of lung cancer by percentage of workers employed in four manufacturing industries

Industry	Percentage employed in industry	
	0.1-1%	≥ 1%
Paper	0.24 (0.36)	1.02 (0.50)
Chemical	1.49 (0.31)	2.26 (0.49)
Petroleum	0.98 (0.45)	1.32 (1.00)
Transportation	1.22 (0.32)	0.84 (0.46)

(^{a}) Estimated coefficients (standard error).
(^{b}) Standardized with respect to the white male population of USA.

ences in tobacco consumption between counties were partially associated with the degree of urbanization, which was accounted for in the model. It should also be noted that the classical approach adopted by Blot and Fraumeni considers each county as a statistically independent unit. It takes large-scale geographical variation into account in a way that differs from Gardner's approach described above. The integration of areas into non-contiguous zones, as in Gardner's method, can, to a certain extent, be thought of as a random assignment of spatially autocorrelated factors. On the other hand, the approach described here can be interpreted as an attempt to adjust the risk for confounding factors using large geographical zones in which they remain approximately constant; thus it indirectly accounts for the correlation in risk which might exist between geographically neighbouring units.

Other approaches which avoid the difficulties of interpretation created by spatial autocorrelation have been described; that proposed by Richardson [54] is described here. First, remember how confounding factors intervene in the equation relating the exposure of interest and the risk of disease in an ecological study.

It has been shown previously (3.53) that the relationship between risk and exposure, under general assumptions, can be written:

$$E(D_i) = M_i \, \mu_0 \, (1 + \alpha \bar{e}_i)$$

where $\bar{e}_i$ characterizes the average exposure in group i, M_i and D_i are the numbers of person-years and deaths in the group, and μ_0 is the baseline mortality rate.

If only this exposure plays a role in the determination of risk, the observations D_i would have independent Poisson distributions and estimation of the parameters μ_0 and α would not present any particular difficulty. In practice, other factors confound their effect with that of the exposure under study and should in principle be included in the equation. As they are generally not measured, the equation becomes:

$$E(D_i) = M_i \, \mu_0 \, (1 + \alpha \, \bar{e}_i) + f_i \qquad (3.62)$$

where f_i is a random variable which is included as an error term, in the absence of more specific data on the confounding variables. Thus, we are led back to the estimation of a regression equation with correlated errors if, as is generally the case, the unmeasured confounding factors have spatial autocorrelation. If we do not take this correlation into consideration in the analysis, the result will be excessively liberal tests of significance, because the improvement in the deviance will be evaluated with respect to an underestimated error. This phenomenon will be systematic if the Poisson distribution is used as an error model. It will also occur in the situation of positive autocorrelation if the normal approximation for the distribution of incidence or mortality rates is used.

Some authors have proposed regression models with correlated errors [55,56]. However, fitting these models is often unduly complicated in relation to the importance of the results which are expected. In contrast, Richardson's approach is appealing because of its simplicity and the fact that it provides a rapid means of evaluating the significance of an association.

The test of the association is based on the variance σ_r^2 of the empirical correlation coefficient r between incidence (or mortality) and exposure, considered as two spatially autocorrelated processes X and Y. It can be shown that:

$$\sigma_r^2 \approx \frac{\text{Var}(S_{XY})}{E(S_X^2)\,E(S_Y^2)} \tag{3.63}$$

where S_{XY}, S_X^2, S_Y^2 are the empirical covariance and variances of the two processes.

In the absence of autocorrelation, $\sigma_r^2 = 1/(N-1)$, where N is the number of observations X_i, Y_i. In the presence of autocorrelation, σ_r^2 is estimated from the observations and used to calculate $N^* = 1 + 1/\hat{\sigma}_r^2$ from which the significance of the correlation is tested with the statistic:

$$T = \frac{r\sqrt{N^* - 2}}{\sqrt{1 - r^2}} \tag{3.64}$$

considered as a Student's variable on $N^* - 2$ degrees of freedom. The method thus proceeds as if the number of autocorrelated observations made were equivalent to a smaller number N^* of independent observations. In the same article the author showed that the method can be extended to any number of variables. If, for example, the significance of the association between X and Y after adjustment for Z is to be evaluated, the correlation of residuals of the regressions of X and Y on Z could be assessed directly by the method.

In practice, S_X^2 and S_Y^2 are used to estimate their expected values. The calculation of the variance of S_{XY} requires an additional assumption; by calculating this variance conditional on X, we obtain:

$$\text{Var}(S_{XY}) = \frac{\sum_{i,j} (X_i - \bar{X})(X_j - \bar{X})\,\text{Cov}(Y_iY_j)}{N^2} \tag{3.65}$$

that is, S_{XY}^2 as an estimate of the variance of S_{XY}. When the Y_i are independent, $\text{Cov}(Y_iY_j) = 0$ if $i \neq j$. $\text{Var}(S_{XY})$ has the value $\frac{1}{N^2}\sum (X_i - \bar{X})^2\,\text{Var}(Y)$ and we find that $r\sqrt{N-1}$ is the standard normal variable corresponding to S_{XY}. When the Y_i are not independent, formula (3.65) is only informative under specific assumptions about the structure of the covariance of the Y_i. Accordingly, suppose that $N(N-1)/2$ pairs of geographical units can be stratified into subgroups in which the covariances of the X_i and the Y_i are constant. This grouping is generally based on the distance between the administrative centres of the geographical units being studied, under the assumption that the intensity of the autocorrelation only depends on distance.

The estimate of σ_r^2 is then written, using (3.63), (3.65) and the constancy of the covariances:

$$\hat{\sigma}_r^2 = \frac{\sum\limits_k N_k \, C_{X_k} \, C_{Y_k}}{N^2 \, S_{X^2} \, S_{Y^2}}$$

where

$$C_{X_k} = \frac{\sum\limits_{i,j} (X_{ik} - \bar{X}_k)(X_{jk} - \bar{X}_k)}{N_k}$$

and

$$C_{Y_k} = \frac{\sum\limits_{i,j} (Y_{ik} - \bar{Y}_k)(Y_{jk} - \bar{Y}_k)}{N_k}$$

are the respective empirical covariances of the X_i and the Y_i in subgroup k and N_k is the number of pairs of units in this subgroup.

Applying these principles to the study of the association between lung cancer and occupational exposure, Richardson [54] showed that the percentage of men employed in the metal industry was correlated with lung cancer mortality across French departments (Table 3.10). The classical test overestimates the intensity of the association but the corrected test is highly significant and remains so even after adjustment for cigarette sales. Since adjustment for a confounding variable partially accounts for autocorrelation of errors, it should be expected that the total corrected

Table 3.10 Correlation between risk of dying from lung cancer (^{a}) and employment in selected industries (^{b}) in France [54]

	Correlation	Classical test (N = 82)		Corrected test		
	r	t	p	t	p	N*
Metal industry						
Crude	0.63	7.16	10^{-9}	3.00	0.010	16
Ajusted (^{c})	0.52	5.46	10^{-6}	3.46	0.002	34
Mining Industry						
Crude	0.33	3.16	0.003	2.37	0.020	47
Adjusted (^{c})	0.24	2.26	0.030	2.42	0.020	94
Textile industry						
Crude	0.28	2.57	0.010	1.52	0.140	30
Adjusted (^{c})	0.26	2.40	0.020	1.91	0.070	53

(^{a}) Lung cancer mortality rate (35-74 truncated rate) for 1968-69.
(^{b}) As measured by percentage of men employed in the industry indicated.
(^{c}) Adjusted for the sales of cigarettes (number per inhabitant in 1953 ; source : SEITA).

number of observations in the test increases after this adjustment, which is in fact the case. Correlations with the mining and textile industries are weaker and the second is eliminated altogether by the corrected test. Richardson shows that the first of these two associations also disappears after adjustment for a geographical gradient. However, it might be questioned whether such a procedure might have led to overadjustment, and hence the elimination of the real associations, if the variable being studied has a large geographical autocorrelation, and possibly a strong covariation with the variable describing the geographical gradient.

Migrant studies

Migrant studies are based on the idea that immigrants are, by their life style and culture, exposed to risk factors which differ from those prevailing in the host country. Thus evidence for risk levels specific to immigrants can indirectly suggest or confirm etiological hypotheses. In general, the risk to which immigrants are subject is recognized by comparison with the risk in the host country, but it is sometimes compared with the risk in the country of origin.

Immigrants are identified by their nationality when they keep it, or by their place of birth. Some studies are exclusively based on surname. In certain situations, first-generation immigrants (born in the country of origin), can be distinguished from their children, often born in the host country, who are described as second-generation immigrants. This distinction sometimes provides information on the effects of behaviour changes resulting from the cultural integration, which act more profoundly on the second generation.

This technique has been used by Buell and Dunn [57] in their study of Japanese migrants living in California. The incidence of common forms of cancer in first and second-generation migrants was compared with the corresponding rates for California and Japan. The main results, shown in Figure 3.12 have been discussed by Cairns [58]. They show that the risk to which migrants are exposed converges towards the risk in the host country, passing through intermediate risk levels. These findings demonstrate the importance of environmental factors over factors linked to ethnicity. The change in risk is shown to differing degrees for cancers at four sites, the stomach, liver, colon and prostate. Incidence of colon cancer, much rarer in Japan than in the USA, increases markedly for first-generation migrants; the second generation has approximately the same rate as Californians. The transition is much slower for stomach cancer. The risk is extremely high in Japan, and remains much higher for Japanese migrants, even those of the second generation, than for Californians. This phenomenon can obviously be explained by the maintenance of risk behaviour or the failure to adopt protective behaviour, for example, dietary habits. On the other hand, based on these data, the hypothesis of an ethnic susceptibility for stomach cancer cannot be completely excluded.

The principle of migrant studies has been extended to cultural and religious minorities. Cancer risk has been studied among Mormons and Seventh Day Adventists, who are recognized as consuming little or no alcohol, tobacco, coffee or other

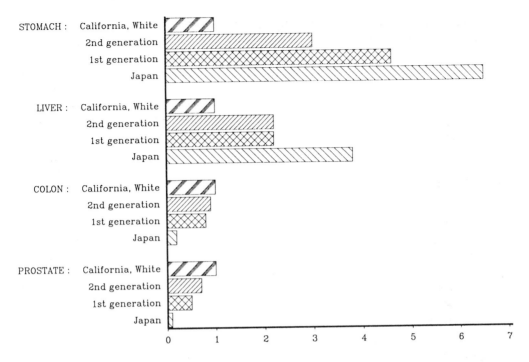

**Figure 3.12   Relative risk of death from various cancers
for male Japanese migrants to California compared to white Californian males
Source: Buell and Dunn [57]**

stimulants. Research of this kind has largely confirmed the importance of lifestyle on cancer risk. For example, it has been shown that cancers of the upper aero-digestive tract were much less frequent in Californian Seventh Day Adventists than in the Californian population as a whole [59].

This type of study has sometimes allowed the effects of closely associated factors to be distinguished. In Chapter 1, it was noted that the apparent effect of urbanization on lung cancer disappeared when the association was studied in Mormons who were living in the same environment but were nonsmokers. The effect originally observed was thus largely due to the fact that smoking is more frequent in urban populations (see page 10).

In terms of methodology, migrant studies can be classified according to whether or not denominators are available. Given the numbers in each group for which risk is to be estimated, the appropriate analysis is the calculation of rates and their comparisons (see Chapter 2, page 85). In practice, the groups being studied are often small and indirect age standardization using the SMR or log-linear modelling based on the Poisson distribution is used. When denominators are not available, study of the relationship between risk and membership in specific groups can be carried out by the PMR method described on page 96 in Chapter 2. As we have seen, it is actually preferable to carry out the analysis using logistic regression identical to that used in case-control studies. A study of Italian migrants in Geneva illustrates this double approach[4].

The Geneva cancer registry has been operating since 1970 and identifies cases by nationality. Swiss nationality is not granted automatically after a certain length of residence, even for foreigners born on Swiss territory. Therefore most immigrants keep their original nationality for one or more decades, as do their descendants. Numbers of foreigners by sex, age and nationality living in Geneva have been estimated regularly since 1976.

Standardized morbidity ratios for immigrants of Italian nationality were first calculated for the main digestive tract cancers over the period during which denominators were available (1976-1987). The calculation was carried out by comparison with the incidence rates established for the total resident population of the Geneva canton. Although this population includes Italians who represented 9% of all residents, the potential diluting effect in the risks was not considered to be large. Table 3.11 shows that significant differences only emerged for gastric cancer, therefore subsequent investigations were restricted to this site alone.

Although the etiology of stomach cancer is not well understood, research has focused mainly on dietary factors. Consumption of salted or smoked food, particularly in places where refrigeration is not widely available, might be a risk factor; fresh fruit and vegetables, on the other hand, could have a protective effect. An often observed increase in risk in lower socioeconomic classes could simply be a marker of dietary practice associated with access to refrigeration. Relatively marked geographical differences have nevertheless been observed between countries, apparently independent of living standards. In Italy, in particular, differences in mortality are substantial from one province to another, with the highest rates observed in regions in the centre of the country. It is also widely accepted, notably from Buell

Table 3.11   **Standardized incidence ratio ([a]) for Italians living in Geneva, Switzerland, by sex and site (1976-1987)**

ICD-9	Site	Men		Women	
		Relative risk	95% CI	Relative risk	95% CI
150	Oesophagus	0.79	[0.43 ; 1.33]	0.83	[0.10 ; 2.99]
151	Stomach	1.61	[1.18 ; 2.14]	1.81	[0.92 ; 2.33]
153	Colon	0.97	[0.71 ; 1.30]	0.71	[0.45 ; 1.05]
154	Rectum	0.88	[0.56 ; 1.32]	0.94	[0.56 ; 1.49]
155	Liver	1.21	[0.75 ; 1.85]	0.85	[0.18 ; 2.48]
156	Gall-bladder	1.48	[0.60 ; 2.84]	1.12	[0.41 ; 2.55]

([a]) Geneva resident population incidence rates as standard rates.

---

[4] See Sarti et al. chapter 16 in [60]

and Dunn's study [57] described above, that the period of induction of gastric cancer is particularly long.

In Geneva, several characteristics routinely recorded for each registered case enable the role played by the above factors in gastric cancer carcinogenesis to be studied. They include socioeconomic status, country of birth and duration of residence since migration. Other information relating to the above hypotheses, such as province of birth and spouse's nationality, was obtained from local files of residents by *ad hoc* inquiries. Because it was not feasible to construct denominators for these additional variables, study of their effects could be carried out only by using an analysis of relative frequencies.

This analysis was carried out with 100 cases of stomach cancers occurring between 1970 and 1978 among Italian nationals residing in Geneva and 300 controls drawn randomly from 1161 cancers of other sites registered among Italian nationals during the same period. The number of controls was kept to three per case to minimize the manual investigation of data files. No matching was carried out. Analyses were carried out by unconditional logistic regression (see Chapter 2, page 98).

The evaluation of living standard was based on three socioeconomic categories (manual labourers; clerical workers; management and professional) and from a variable distinguishing five regions of birthplace (southern Italy; central Italy; northern Italy; Switzerland; other), which defined a gradient of socioeconomic status from most socioeconomically deprived to most socioeconomically privileged, that is, from southern Italy to Switzerland. For men, after taking age into account, neither of these variables significantly modified gastric cancer risk; a nonsignificant increase in risk was noted for central Italy. For women, no significant variation in risk was observed with social class, but the risk was significantly higher for women born in central Italy.

The degree of cultural integration was measured by the number of years of residence and by the fact of being married to a Swiss national. No significant association was found from the analysis of these two variables, despite a decreasing trend in risk with duration of residence (both sexes), and with a Swiss spouse (men only).

To investigate differences in risk with place of birth, the 95 Italian provinces were grouped by relative mortality rates, available for the period 1975 to 1977 into three categories: less than 80% of the national average (low); between 80 and 120% of the national average (medium); and more than 120% (high). Separate scales were constructed for both sexes. This breakdown was completed by a fourth class corresponding to cases born in Geneva, where stomach cancer mortality is particularly low, and this category was used as the reference.

This indicator was shown to be highly significantly associated with risk (after accounting for age). For provinces of birth characterized by the highest mortality rates, relative risk was estimated as 4.0 for men and 6.8 for women. The trend of increasing risk across categories was also significant.

In order to judge their effects in the presence of other factors, the variables under study were introduced simultaneously in the same model, with the exception of social class which was assumed to be represented largely by the place of birth. Because no interaction between these factors and sex was significant, an analysis was undertaken with both sexes combined. The results of this analysis (Table 3.12) confirmed the importance of province of birth as a risk factor for gastric cancer. There remained, however, an independent effect of region of birth (highest risk for central and southern Italy), which may reflect a residual role of the birth province, if this factor was too broadly categorized. The dominant role of birth province supports the results of analytical studies, which have demonstrated the local specificity of dietary habits in central Italy, suggesting that they play an important role in the mechanism of gastric cancer [61]. The apparent absence of effect of variables measuring the degree of integration (length of residence and Swiss spouse) is not surprising, considering that gastric cancer has a long latency period.

Table 3.12   Distribution of cases and controls and risk estimates associated with selected factors (both sexes combined) [60]

	Cases (100)	Controls (300)	Relative risk [a]	p
Level of risk of Italian province of origin				< 0.001
Low [b]	43	182	1	
Medium	23	76	1.4	
High	34	42	4.3	
Italian region of origin				< 0.05
North [b]	68	228	1	
Central and South	32	72	2.3	
Length of residence	–	–	1.1	NS
Spouse				NS
Non-Swiss	84	238	1	
Swiss	16	62	0.8	

[a] Adjusted for age and the other factors in the table.
[b] Includes those born in Switzerland and elsewhere, except Italy.

Time trends

Objectives

In the context of descriptive epidemiology, there are many reasons for studying time trends. Firstly, information on the historical evolution of risk (incidence or mortality) can generate etiological hypotheses or confirmation of suspected associations between risk factors and disease. While the existence of geographical variation in incidence between populations might be explained by genetic differences, changes in incidence in single populations imply the introduction or disappearance of environmental risk factors much more clearly. Comparison of the development of environmental factors with the development of the frequency of different types of cancer should therefore be profitable. For example, the increase in lung cancer mortality parallels the progressive introduction of cigarette smoking, while its decrease quickly follows a decrease in the proportion of smokers.

However, in etiological research, the interpretation of chronological covariation remains delicate. It would be simple to show that the incidence of melanoma has undergone an increase identical to that of many changes in lifestyle which cannot be incriminated in the etiology of this cancer. Similarly, the general decrease in frequency of stomach cancer could be related to the modification of many environmental factors which accompany higher living standards; its etiology nevertheless remains largely unexplained. The existence of a direct link between the evolution in risk of a given cancer and that of a suspected etiological factor may be less questionable when they both show the same inversions of trend. For example, the parallel trends in incidence of larynx and oesophageal cancers (Figure 1.3) clearly suggests a common etiology, in this case alcohol consumption. Alcohol consumption has in fact declined substantially in the period when the generations at lowest risk of these cancers were between 20 and 25 years of age (Figure 3.13). When the joint evolution of a cancer and a risk factor are studied, it

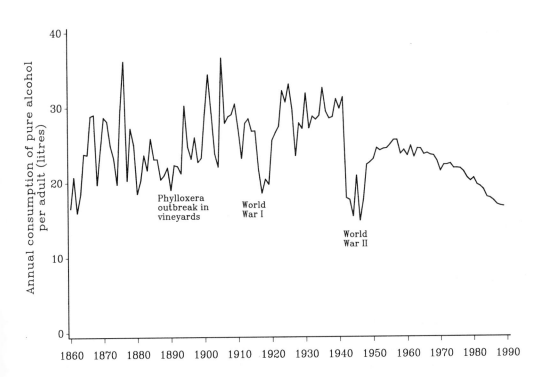

Figure 3.13   Change in alcohol consumption in France between 1860 and 1989
Source : Hill et al. [64]

is necessary to consider the mechanism of action of the risk factor and particularly the latency period. Thus, in contrast to the previous observation on alcohol-related cancers, the large decrease in tobacco consumption during the second world war did not have a marked effect on lung cancer mortality. In fact, it is difficult to detect joint evolution : risks and etiological factors generally undergo a slow, steady evolution.

The observation of time series can also be seen as an instrument for epidemiological surveillance of the population with the aim of detecting new risk factors. However, in addition to the difficulties created by the delayed effects of the latency period, it should be emphasized that rapid detection of changes in trends is not easily achieved. In particular, when monitoring relates to a relatively small population or a small risk, observed variations are often simply a reflection of purely random fluctuations.

The study of time trends is of particular interest in the evaluation of *primary prevention*, which involves the reduction in exposure to risk factors, and of *secondary prevention* (screening) which is aimed at reducing mortality. It is anticipated that the intervention will cause a more or less generalized shift in the existing trend in incidence or mortality. Before-and-after designs, aimed at identifying such shifts, have generally been used for this purpose.

The study of time trends is not limited to incidence or mortality. Descriptive epidemiology is increasingly concerned with the overall assessment of progress made through improved treatment or earlier detection of disease. This requires methods for quantifying the corresponding increase in survival rates calculated for all cases in the population in which the evaluation is being carried out.

Finally, from the public health viewpoint, the observation of changes in risk in the recent past leads naturally to a desire to predict its future development, in order to determine budget priorities and plan necessary services.

The following sections are devoted to definitions and basic concepts, which are of fundamental importance in the development of modelling methods, particularly those used in identifying age, period and cohort effects.

Methods

Components of temporal evolution

From 1955 to 1959, 417 438 deaths from cancer were registered in France. Twenty-five years later, between 1980 and 1984, these deaths numbered 638 012. In other words, cancer deaths increased 53% over 25 years, or 1.7% per year (see formulae 3.68 and 3.69). To varying degrees, the same phenomena occurred in other Latin countries (Table 3.13). The increase concerned not only numbers of deaths for each type of cancer but also their proportion in all-cause mortality and crude rates.

**Table 3.13 Changes in number of deaths (^{a})
for cancer between 1955 and 1984 in selected European countries**

	Men			Women		
	1955-59	1980-84 (^{b})	Variation (^{c}) (% per year)	1955-59	1980-84 (^{b})	Variation (^{c}) (% per year)
Spain						
Number	77 438	172 957	3.2	74 036	121 350	2.0
Crude rate	108.1	187.3	2.2	97.29	126.6	1.1
Proportion (^{d})	11.2	22.6	3.0	10.9	17.6	2.0
France						
Number	212 718	382 883	2.4	204 720	255 129	0.9
Crude rate	198.4	288.2	1.5	179.0	183.6	0.1
Proportion (^{d})	16.1	26.8	2.0	16.1	19.3	0.7
Italy						
Number	173 405	369 232	3.0	157 638	258 172	2.0
Crude rate	143.9	266.4	2.5	125.6	177.0	1.4
Proportion (^{d})	14.1	25.4	2.4	14.2	19.9	1.4
Switzerland						
Number	25 800	41 552	1.9	23 213	32 860	1.4
Crude rate	207.8	267.1	1.0	175.2	200.4	0.5
Proportion (^{d})	19.8	26.8	1.2	19.0	23.1	0.8

(^{a}) WHO mortality data bank.
(^{b}) Spain 1980-81; Italy: 1980-83.
(^{c}) Average annual rate of change over the period of n = t_1-t_0 years, calculated according to formula (3.69).
(^{d}) Proportion of deaths from cancer among deaths from all causes in the period.

These observations are important from the public health viewpoint. However, they do not reveal anything about the way in which cancer risk evolved over the course of the 25 years, and can even lead to errors in interpretation. The proportion of deaths due to cancer increases partly because of a decrease in the number of deaths from competing causes, while the increase in crude rates is largely explained by the ageing of the population. An examination of trends in the net risk of cancer mortality which leaves aside competing causes ends up with rather different conclusions (Table 3.14). In particular, net cancer mortality decreases when cancers associated with tobacco use are excluded. Similar conclusions were reached by a study carried out some years ago in the USA: while the number of cancer deaths increased 181% between 1930 and 1970, an analysis of the components of the increase shows that 10% was due to change of risk, 74% to population growth, 46% to the ageing of the population, 17% to the amplification of changes in risk resulting from demographic changes and finally 34% to interactions between demographic factors (62). A recent study carried out for the European Community predicted that cancer mortality would increase 48% for men and 20% for women between 1980 and 2000, with approximately half of this variation due to demographic changes expected during this time.

Table 3.14 Change in net risk (^{a}) of dying from cancer between 1955 and 1984 in selected European countries

Country	Men			Women		
	1955-59	1980-84 (^{b})	Variation (^{c}) (% per year)	1955-59	1980-84 (^{b})	Variation (^{c}) (% per year)
Spain						
Tobacco-related (^{d})	3.5	7.2	3.1	0.6	0.7	0.7
Other	9.3	9.9	0.3	8.3	8.0	−0.2
Total	12.8	17.1	1.2	8.9	8.7	−0.1
France						
Tobacco-related (^{d})	6.2	10.8	2.2	0.7	0.9	1.0
Other	11.9	12.0	0.03	10.8	9.0	−0.7
Total	18.1	22.8	0.9	11.5	9.9	−0.6
Italy						
Tobacco-related (^{d})	4.3	10.2	3.5	0.8	1.1	1.3
Other	11.2	11.8	0.2	10.4	9.8	−0.2
Total	15.5	22.0	1.4	11.2	10.9	−0.1
Switzerland						
Tobacco-related (^{d})	6.9	8.9	1.0	0.8	1.1	1.3
Other	12.5	10.7	−0.6	12.3	9.9	−0.9
Total	19.4	19.6	0.04	13.1	11.0	−0.7

(^{a}) Net risk is measured by the cumulative risk from 0 to 75 years ; source : WHO mortality data bank.
(^{b}) Spain: 1980-81; Italy: 1980-83.
(^{c}) Average annual rate of change over the period of n = t_1-t_0 years, calculated according to formula (3.69).
(^{d}) Sites for which the effect of tobacco use has been established (mouth and pharynx, oesophagus, lung, larynx and bladder).

In etiological research, the focus should be on the risk of disease and not only the risk of death. Unfortunately, trends in incidence can be studied in only a few countries, because of the relatively recent establishment of cancer registration. In addition, results can rarely be generalized because registries often cover subpopulations chosen by circumstance, not necessarily corresponding to regions that would have been selected for the study of specific hypotheses. Therefore, we are often forced to rely on mortality data, which are available over long time periods for both national and regional populations. Nevertheless, it should be kept in mind that the risk of death is only an indirect, and even a biased measure, of the risk of cancer occurrence, particularly because of the increase in survival.

The methods proposed in Chapter 2 for comparing incidence between populations should in principle be suitable for studying changes over time. However, most of these methods rely on the assumption that ratios of incidence (or mortality) remain more or less constant with age. In fact, it is far from certain that risk alters in the same way for all age groups in a changing environment. Indeed, there are, in general, good reasons to assume that different age groups behave in different ways.

The epidemic of lung cancer illustrates this point. At first, the older age groups were unaffected and the increase in risk was observed only in younger age groups. Signs that the epidemic is declining are now obvious, for example, in the UK and the USA, and again in the youngest age groups which are decreasingly exposed to the carcinogenic effects of tobacco. In the oldest groups, on the other hand, the increase in risk is sustained for much longer, as they are still experiencing the consequences of high tobacco consumption twenty years ago. In France, where the smoking epidemic occurred later, there is still an increase in risk in the younger age groups (Figure 3.14). In such circumstances, neither crude nor standardized rates can provide an appropriate assessment of trend. Calculations based on age-adjusted rates, which in principle control for the effects of population ageing, provide an incomplete picture of the phenomenon, and hide its more interesting components.

This example underlines the importance of observing changes in risk in young adults when the consequences of a new risk factor or protective agent are to be assessed (or predicted). For cancer, as for most non-transmissible diseases, etiological factors are often linked to forms of social behaviour which come and go with passing generations.

These considerations are illustrated in Figure 3.15, which shows cancer mortality over time in Scotland. If we only consider overall trends, the patterns in three usual standardized rates (African, European and world standards) are similar and indicate a regular and relatively small increase in risk. On the other hand, examination of rates calculated for less than and greater than 65 years of age shows that the trend in standardized rates is due to changes which diverge with age, with an

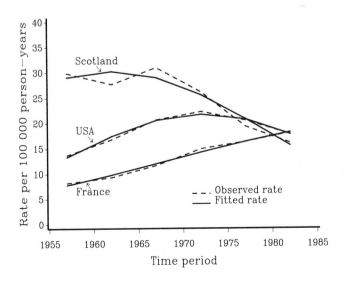

Figure 3.14 Lung cancer mortality trend in France, the USA and Scotland in 40–44-year-old men

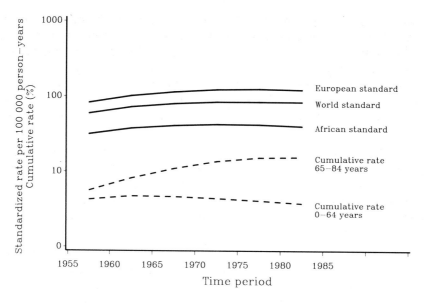

Figure 3.15 Lung cancer mortality trend in Scotland; men, 1955-1984

increase in risk for the oldest age groups and a decrease for the youngest. It is likely that this decline signals an inversion of trend which will ultimately affect other age groups.

Effect of data quality

In addition to real trends in risk and random variations, changes in data quality over time affect the observed trend in incidence or mortality. These effects can create apparent increases or decreases in risk, when the true risk is actually completely stable.

For incidence data, time series partially reflect progressive improvements in the registration rate, whether resulting from the development of diagnostic techniques or improved reporting systems for the registry. The newer the registry, the stronger this effect is likely to be. In some situations, the very existence of the registry creates an awareness which increases the proportion of cases diagnosed (such as through post-mortem examinations). In most registries, there has been a progressive decrease in the proportion of registered cases on the sole basis of death certificates. In Connecticut, the proportion declined from 35% in the first years after the registry was established (1935) to 1% in the 1980s [63]. This improvement in the rate of registration of cases during their lifetime has led to a temporary and artificial increase in the number of incident cases. It has been proposed that the standard indices calculated to assess the completeness of registration (proportion of cases registered from death certificates only and frequency of autopsy) be used to correct incidence rates.

As a registry develops, there is also an improvement in the quality of diagnostic information obtained for each cancer registered, and a consequent increase in the precision in coding of the site and type of the tumour. Codes corresponding to poorly defined sites are progressively less used as the percentage of histologically confirmed cases rises. An artificial increase in the frequency of well specified sites will therefore be seen. In the Connecticut registry, the percentage of histologically confirmed cases increased from 73% to 93% during the period mentioned above [63].

Finally, incidence can fluctuate as a result of changes in the stage at which cancer is detected, particularly for slow-growing tumours. For example, it is known that the incidence of *in situ* cervical tumours can increase explosively during cytological screening campaigns, because of the inclusion of prevalent cases which are not detected clinically. The detection of early stage disease has an even greater effect in the study of time trends in survival.

The quality of cancer mortality data has undoubtedly also improved over time, but the improvement has occurred more in the precision of diagnosis than in the number of registered deaths. As with incidence, there have probably been artificial increases in the number of deaths from better defined causes. Thus, increased mortality from ovarian cancer observed in France between 1950 and 1985 in women over 50 years might be due partially to the introduction of systematic surgical investigation of abdominal masses. Previously, some ovarian cancers discovered at an advanced stage were wrongly classified as peritoneal cancer [64].

Problems in classification have been discussed too extensively elsewhere to justify detailed review here. We simply note that all changes in classification, or even coding practices, can affect the number of cases at a given site or due to a specific cause of death and distort trends. The decision to register papillomas or non-infiltrating lesions has clearly played a role in the apparent increase in the incidence of bladder cancer. Also well known are the difficulties which arise in the study of trends in non-Hodgkin lymphoma, which is sometimes coded according to topographical site and other times as a tumour of the haematopoietic system.

The problem of imprecise data is accentuated by the differences in the evolution of precision with region or age. Errors in diagnosis are generally more serious in older people, and improvements in diagnostic precision can therefore have a fundamental effect on incidence rates in this age group. The phenomenon is probably a partial explanation for the recent increase in multiple myeloma in the elderly [65]. As a final point, it should be noted that chronological patterns in incidence or mortality rates depend on the quality of the denominators over time. Population estimates provided by statistical services may be increasingly distorted the further they are from the date of the census. This distortion often results in an underestimation of the denominators, because enumeration is not as accurate for persons leaving the population as it is for those arriving.

Role of modelling

Observed time trends should be evaluated in the context of the problem under study : sometimes it is sufficient to describe long-term trends; in other situations, interest might focus on variation over a more limited time period, in particular the recent past, if the goal is to predict new directions of the phenomenon. Apart from the simple description of changes in risk over time, the study of trends should therefore involve the search for models which can describe observed data via plausible hypotheses about the causes of observed changes. Under this approach, the relevant components of the time trend can effectively be separated from the random or systematic (e.g., seasonal fluctuations), allowing a more complete interpretation of the observed data.

Models of risk evolution over successive generations have a particularly important place in the study of cancer incidence, because of the long latency period between the start of exposure to a risk factor and the occurrence of the disease. When interest focuses on the *generation effect*, also known as the *cohort effect*, the inevitable presence of *period effects* created by, for example, changes in diagnostic practice or the appearance of an environmental risk factor which could simultaneously affect all age groups, necessitates the combined analysis of both the cohort and period components of risk. In other situations, the period effect may be of primary interest and the cohort effect is only a confounding factor that must be controlled for. An example of this situation is the evaluation of the effect of screening for cervical cancer (see page 202).

The use of models in the study of trends has not been widespread, because of two fundamental problems which will be discussed in this section.

The first is the difficulty of separating meaningful variations from those which can be considered to be random fluctuations. Simpler models might be discarded because the random component is in fact greater than that predicted by the Poisson distribution which is used to assess significance of the terms included in the model. In such a situation, it might be wrongly concluded that specific factors play a significant role in the explanation of the observed phenomenon.

The second difficulty lies in the impossibility of satisfactorily separating cohort and period effects from the data alone, when hypotheses on the nature of these components cannot be formulated *a priori*. It is for this reason that some authors have questioned the value of modelling over traditional graphical approaches to carry out this type of investigation [66]. This point of view, however, ignores the fact that exclusive use of graphical methods can also lead to subjective interpretations which an appropriate model may avoid.

The following section presents the tools required for the quantitative description of trends and the evaluation of the adequacy of the underlying models. Data on lung cancer in young adults are used to show how the analysis of trends in the logarithms of age-specific rates can display several types of time trend, and ultimately allow different components of this evolution to be revealed. This analysis naturally leads to a discussion of age-period, age-cohort and age-period-cohort models.

Description of trend by period

First, recall the concept of rate of change, which summarizes exponential increase in incidence or mortality. If $N(t_0)$ cancers were observed in year t_0, and $N(t_1)$ cancers in year $t_1 = t_0 + n$, the relative change is measured by:

$$\tau = \frac{N(t_1) - N(t_0)}{N(t_0)} \qquad (3.66)$$

or by the corresponding percentage $100 \times \tau$.

To derive the constant annual rate of change r that must apply each year to observe this relative change after n years, write:

$$N(t_1) = N(t_0)(1 + r)^n \qquad (3.67)$$

or

$$1 + r = (1 + \tau)^{\frac{1}{n}} = \left(\frac{N(t_1)}{N(t_0)} \right)^{\frac{1}{n}} \qquad (3.68)$$

given that $t_1 - t_0$ is equal to n, we have

$$\text{Log}\,(1 + r) = \frac{\text{Log}\,[N(t_1)] - \text{Log}\,[N(t_0)]}{t_1 - t_0} \qquad (3.69)$$

in other words, the slope of the line linking the logarithm of incidence at the two time points under consideration is practically equal to the average annual rate of change in incidence, since $\text{Log}(1 + r) \approx r$ when the rate is small. If the rate is not small, and if ß denotes this slope, we have the relationship $r = e^{\beta} - 1$. The calculation above based on number of incident cases can obviously be carried out with all other indices of incidence or mortality.

When the numbers of cases occurring in the intervening years are known and if the logarithm of incidence varies linearly between the two dates, the rate of increase can be estimated by the slope of the line which best represents the logarithm of incidence as a linear function of year of diagnosis or death. Estimation of this regression line can be based on either maximum likelihood or weighted least squares.

As an example, we calculated the annual rate of change in lung cancer mortality among males in the USA, France and Scotland in the 40-44 years age group. The data for six successive five-year periods appear in Table 3.15 and in Figure 3.14.

Let k_t, m_t, λ_t be the numbers of cases and person-years and the incidence rate for the age group under consideration for the period t. As was described above, the rate of change is the value $e^{\beta_1} - 1 \approx \beta_1$ in the equation :

$$\text{Log}(\lambda_t) = \beta_1 t + \beta_0 \qquad (3.70)$$

**Table 3.15   Change in lung cancer mortality over 25 years
for men aged between 40 and 45 years**

	USA			Scotland			France		
	Number	M x Y [a]	Rate [b]	Number	M x Y [a]	Rate [b]	Number	M x Y [a]	Rate [b]
1955-59	3 762	27 599	13.6	242	811.0	29.8	479	5 878	8.2
1960-64	4 900	29 249	16.8	222	803.2	27.6	612	6 586	9.3
1965-69	6 147	29 859	20.6	247	798.8	30.9	968	8 333	11.6
1970-74	6 318	28 416	22.2	195	747.7	26.1	1 265	8 507	14.9
1975-79	5 638	27 590	20.4	138	717.6	19.2	1 308	8 032	16.3
1980-84	5 413	30 569	17.7	116	724.4	16.0	1 349	7 484	18.0
Rate of change [c]		4.95 %			− 10.63 %			17.67 %	

[a] Man-years in thousands.
[b] Death rate per 100 000 man-years.
[c] Five-yearly percentage change $100(e^{\beta_1} - 1)$ estimated by the method of maximum likelihood using the linear model (3.70).

The parameter β_1 is estimated by maximum likelihood, supposing that k_t has a Poisson distribution with mean $m_t e^{\beta_1 t + \beta_0}$, or by using weighted least squares, minimizing:

$$\Delta (\beta_1, \beta_0) = \sum_t w_t \left[Log \left(\frac{k_t}{m_t} \right) - \beta_1 t - \beta_0 \right]^2 \tag{3.71}$$

where w_t is proportional to the inverse of the variance of the logarithm of the observed rate, that is :

$$w_t = \lambda_t m_t \approx k_t$$

The calculations were carried out with the software GLIM, using a program given in Appendix 2. Table 3.16 shows that the estimate of the rate of change and the deviance (an overall measure of the quality of the model's fit) are almost identical for the methods of maximum likelihood and weighted least squares when the model specifies a linear change in rates. On the other hand, the precision of the estimate, as indicated by the standard error, appears much greater when the method of maximum likelihood is used. In fact, this method assumes that the model is appropriate and that the variation observed around the values calculated for each period using equation (3.70) are those predicted by the Poisson distribution. In this situation, the deviance indicates that the differences between observed and expected numbers are too big for the model to be acceptable. This statistic should be of the order of 4 (the mean of a χ^2 distribution on four degrees of freedom), if the logarithms of the rates really varied linearly with time. Figure 3.14 suggests that the linear model

Table 3.16   Modelling of data from Table 3.15

Country	Method ([a])	Model	Coefficients ([b]) β_2	β_1	Deviance	d.f.
USA	ML	Linear	–	0.048 (0.003)	553.1	4
		Quadratic	–0.053 (0.002)	0.428 (0.017)	14.1	3
	LS	Linear	–	0.048 (0.041)	547.2	4
		Quadratic	–0.053 (0.005)	0.428 (0.036)	14.0	3
Scotland	ML	Linear	–	–0.112 (0.018)	15.5	4
		Quadratic	–0.041 (0.012)	0.162 (0.083)	4.1	3
	LS	Linear	–	–0.111 (0.036)	15.8	4
		Quadratic	–0.041 (0.014)	0.164 (0.095)	4.0	3
France	ML	Linear	–	0.163 (0.008)	14.9	4
		Quadratic	–0.016 (0.006)	0.282 (0.042)	6.5	3
	LS	Linear	–	0.163 (0.016)	15.0	4
		Quadratic	–0.016 (0.080)	0.282 (0.061)	6.5	3

([a]) ML = maximum likelihood method based on the Poisson distribution; LS = method of weighted least squares.
([b]) Standard error in brackets.

is quite good for France but not for the USA and Scotland. The measure of fit (deviation) is very bad for the USA (553.1 for a χ^2 on four degrees of freedom) but also poor for Scotland and France (approximately 15 on four degrees of freedom).

In the present situation, the poor fit observed for the USA and Scotland is partly due to the inversion of trends observed in these two countries during the period being studied. A linear model is therefore inadequate, and a second-order term must be added in the model to account for the concave curve representing this phenomenon:

$$\text{Log}(\lambda_t) = \beta_2\, t^2 + \beta_1\, t + \beta_0 \qquad (3.72)$$

Fitting this quadratic model, represented geometrically by a parabola, significantly improves the deviance compared to the linear model, as judged by maximum likelihood. This result suggests that the trend inversion is real.

The validity of this conclusion is difficult to challenge for Scotland because the second-degree model fits the data perfectly (χ^2 = 4.1 for three degrees of freedom). The conclusion is also confirmed by the standard error of the quadratic term obtained from the method of least squares (t test = $-0.041/0.014 = -2.9$). This method assumes that $\log(k_t / m_t)$ has a normal distribution with mean $\beta_2 t^2 + \beta_1 t + \beta_0$ and variance σ^2/k_t. As σ^2 is estimated by the quotient of the deviance and its number of degrees of freedom, it will not be very different from 1 when the model with Poisson error is satisfactory. The result is that, in this situation, the standard error of the parameters obtained with the method of least squares will be close to the standard error estimated under the method of maximum likelihood, as can be seen from the Scottish data. Therefore, when the deviance suggests a good fit, the two methods are practically equivalent.

For the USA, and to a lesser extent for France, the problem of lack of fit remains. The test of the quadratic term based on the standard error obtained from the method of maximum likelihood is therefore not valid. For the French data, the coefficient of the quadratic term is not significant when evaluated by the method of least squares ($F_3^1 = (15.0 - 6.5)/(6.5/3) = 3.92$), but it is highly significant by the method of maximum likelihood ($\chi^2 = 14.9 - 6.5 = 8.4$ on one degree of freedom). Similarly, the standard error obtained using the method of maximum likelihood for the linear coefficient in the US data is obviously incorrect, while that obtained by the method of least squares correctly indicates the poor fit of this model. The two methods thus lead to contradictory results with neither being truly satisfactory.

For the USA and France, a large number of person-years of observation are available from populations that are *a priori* quite heterogeneous with respect to lung cancer risk. It is therefore likely that the randomness predicted by the Poisson distribution accounts only for a small portion of the random variation in the data. In particular, the assumption of a constant risk λ_t for all individuals is an oversimplification which masks a much more complex reality. For these two countries, the size of the populations being studied allows the rates to be estimated more precisely, showing that the observed variability is significantly greater than that predicted by the Poisson distribution.

The fit could certainly be improved by constructing a more complex model, especially by adding higher degree terms to describe observed variations more precisely; however, this approach is contrary to the principle of simplicity which is fundamental to all modelling, and can lead to a good but useless description of purely random variation.

In order to take the excess variability into account, it is preferable to conclude explicitly that λ_t, a fixed parameter to be estimated in the previous calculations, is in fact a random variable describing the distribution of risk in the population under study. Equations (3.70) and (3.72) are then only true on average. Effectively, we have:

$$\text{Log}(\lambda_t) = f(t) + \varepsilon_t = \text{Log}(v_t) + \varepsilon_t \tag{3.73}$$

where f(t) is the model proposed for the change over time in the mean of Log(v_t), the logarithm of the rate, and ε_t is a random variable of unknown distribution and constant variance σ^2 [67,68]. Hinde assumes, in addition, that the distribution of ε_t is normal [67].

As a first approximation, Log(k_t / m_t) can be assumed to have a normal distribution with mean f(t) and variance $1/v_t m_t + \sigma^2$, the sum of the Poisson and extra-Poisson variance.

Calculations not shown here show that estimation of this model by the maximum likelihood method from data given in Table 3.15 gives σ^2 equal to 0.260×10^{-3} for the US data. This value corresponds to extra-Poisson variation of between 30 and 50%, but the likelihood is not significantly improved by the introduction of this additional parameter ($\chi^2 = 2.92$ on one degree of freedom).

The estimate of σ^2 is null for the Scottish data, as would be expected given the excellent fit of the quadratic model without an extra Poisson variation obtained previously (Table 3.16).

The French data are as well described by a quadratic model without extra Poisson variation as by a linear model which includes variation of this type between 30 and 60% ($\hat{\sigma}^2 = 0.144 \times 10^{-2}$). This result proves that the slowing of the increase in lung cancer mortality, suggested by the more recent data, requires further confirmation before being unequivocally accepted.

From this discussion, it is clear that the rate of change alone is rarely sufficient to comprehensively describe the data, even within a single age group. *A fortiori*, a method which describes the evolution of the logarithm of a standardized rate using a linear regression can conceal interesting aspects of a time trend. In the Scottish data (Figure 3.15), it can be seen that standardization leads to an estimated increase of between 0.90 and 1.52% per year, depending on the standard population. However, the cumulative rate between 65 and 84 years of age increases by more than 4% per year, while the rate from 0 to 64 years decreases by nearly 0.6% per year, as shown in Table 3.17. Note that the trend in the cumulative rate between 0 and 84 years depends largely on the trend observed in the elderly and, consequently,

Table 3.17   Change in lung cancer mortality in men in Scotland ([a])

Standard population	Rate of change ([b])	Standard error
European	1.52	0.41
World	1.19	0.42
African	0.90	0.40
Cumulative rate 0-64 years	-0.61	0.32
65-84 years	4.10	0.65
0-84 years	2.70	0.47

([a]) Mortality data in six five-yearly periods from 1955 to 1984 (see Figure 3.15).WHO mortality data bank.
([b]) Estimated by the method of least squares assuming that the logarithm of the standardized rate varies linearly; the result is expressed as a percentage change per year.

completely disregards the important epidemiological fact that the lung cancer rate is decreasing in young people, as might be predicted by the changing smoking habits of this generation.

The preceding discussion underlines the importance of studying time trends with respect to age. Three examples corresponding to different epidemiological situations are shown in Figure 3.16. The first example concerns the incidence of bladder cancer in Birmingham, UK. The incidence of this cancer increased sharply for all age groups from the end of the 1960s, due to the inclusion of papillomas. The calculated rates of change are thus positive and of the same order of magnitude at each age; the curve obtained is approximately a horizontal line. The second example concerns the evolution of lung cancer mortality in Scotland, already discussed on several occasions. The graph shows that the rates of change increase strongly with age, and become positive after 65 years. The third example is provided by the incidence of cervical cancer in Birmingham, UK. The graph is a complex curve with a minimum at around 40 years. This shape could be partially explained by the progressive extension of screening to successive generations, and partly by increased exposure among young women to risk factors linked to sexual behaviour.

To obtain the data in Figure 3.16, rates of change have been calculated for each age group by fitting of the log-linear model :

$$\text{Log} (\lambda_{xt}) = \alpha_x + \beta_x t \tag{3.74}$$

where the rate of change β_x depends on the age group x.

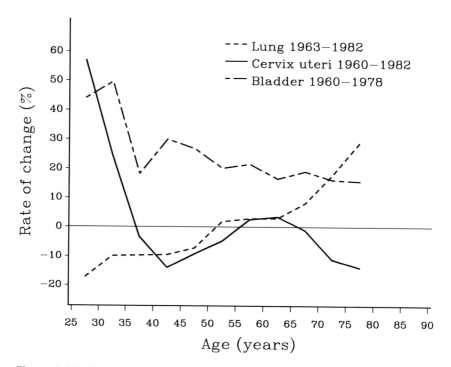

Figure 3.16 Trend in the age-specific incidence of bladder cancer in men and cervical cancer (Birmingham,UK), and of lung cancer in men (Scotland)

For bladder cancer in Birmingham, UK, the constant rate of change with age suggests that a model in which β is constant will provide an equally good description of the data. This model is written:

$$\text{Log}\,(\lambda_{xt}) = \alpha_x + \beta t \tag{3.75}$$

Fitting the models (3.74) and (3.75) gives χ^2 values of 70.28 and 80.69 respectively, on $(4 \times 11 - (2 \times 11)) = 22$ and $(4 \times 11 - (11 + 1)) = 32$ degrees of freedom, showing that the improvement in fit created by introducing a different slope for each age group is negligible. Nevertheless, the size of the deviance indicates that the linear model does not adequately describe the data.

A careful examination of the data given in Table 3.18 and Figure 3.17 shows that the increase, although similar in all age groups, was greater between the second and third time periods. The absence of linearity is not surprising in that it corresponds to a change in the case definition which occurred precisely between the second and third period, and resulted in the inclusion of papillomas, previously considered benign. The constant rate of change observed before indicates that this event has produced an effect which is proportional to the existing incidence. This finding was not obvious *a priori*: the relationship between papillomas and invasive cases could have varied with age. We therefore adopt a multiplicative model, in which the incidence rate is multiplied by a factor independent of age. In addition, the poor fit of the linear model leads us to calculate a relative rate for each period, rather than a single parameter summarizing the increase over the 15 years of reg-

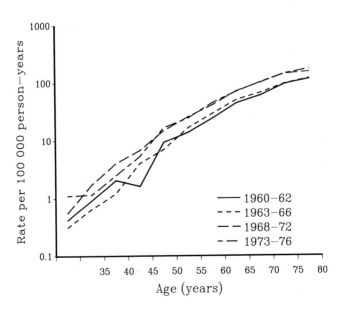

Figure 3.17 Bladder cancer incidence in Birmingham, UK; men, 1960-1976

istration. This way of describing the rates is usually called an *age-period model*. It is written:

$$\text{Log}\,(\lambda_{xt}) = \alpha_x + \beta_t \qquad x_1 \leq x \leq x_g$$
$$t_1 \leq t \leq t_h$$
$$\beta_{t_1} = 0 \tag{3.76}$$

where g and h are respectively the number of age groups and the number of study periods. The term βt in the linear model is thus replaced by a term $\beta_{t,}$ indicating changes of unspecified shape over time which are nevertheless identical in all age groups.

Maximum likelihood estimates of $\mu_x = 100\,000\,e^{\alpha_x}$ and $\rho_t = e^{\beta_t}$ are given in Table 3.18. The values of μ_x provide a smoothed incidence curve for the first registration period and ρ_t provide a description of the increase similar to that given by the SIR in the same Table.

The goodness-of-fit of the multiplicative age-period model can be assessed from the results. For example, incidence for the age group 60 to 64 years in the third period is estimated by:

$$100\,000\,\lambda_{xt} = 100\,000\,e^{\alpha_x}\,e^{\beta_t} = \mu_x\,\rho_t = 43.99 \times 1.62 = 71.26$$

Table 3.18   Incidence of bladder cancer; men, Birmingham, UK, 1960-1976 ([a])

Age (x)	Registration period (t)				Estimated rates ([b]) (μ_x)
	1960-62	1963-66	1968-72	1973-76	
25-29	0.42	0.31	0.55	1.10	0.45
30-34	0.00	0.65	1.73	1.15	0.71
35-39	2.06	1.21	4.02	2.49	1.85
40-44	1.62	4.03	6.74	5.29	3.43
45-49	9.40	7.02	14.95	16.80	8.97
50-54	13.90	16.65	25.73	24.41	15.12
55-59	24.25	29.15	41.06	44.81	25.94
60-64	44.50	50.51	71.39	70.25	43.99
65-69	60.47	66.97	100.69	101.97	61.62
70-74	94.84	95.73	141.96	142.70	87.88
75-79	116.08	118.16	154.19	174.42	103.43
Relative rate ([b]) : ρ_t	1.00	1.09	1.62	1.65	
SIR ([c])	71.47	78.00	115.91	117.98	
Observed cumulative rate 25-79 years	1.84	1.95	2.82	2.93	

([a]) Rates as number of cases per 100 000.
([b]) Estimated using an age-period model (3.76).
([c]) Using observed incidence between 1970 and 1976 as standard.

as compared to the observed number of 71.39. The deviance of this model is 41.17 on $(4 \times 11 - (11 + 3)) = 30$ degrees of freedom. Despite being somewhat large for a χ^2 on 30 degrees of freedom, this value ($p = 0.08$) confirms that the multiplicative model is a good description of the data. As the SIRs have been designed for such a situation, they obviously provide a good description of the time trend. A detailed discussion of the adequacy of this model for the Birmingham incidence data can be found in a recent article which, to a large extent, inspired these developments [70].

At this stage, it is important to ask why an age-period model has been adopted to describe this data set. The presence of a clear change in rates for all ages between the second and third registration period excluded the model (3.75). In other words, it was necessary to introduce the effect of period as a non linear function of time, leading to model (3.76), which has an acceptable fit because of the proportionality of the observed incidence curves.

It is worth dwelling a little longer on model (3.75) which, as we will see below, can be equally well interpreted as an age-period or an age-cohort model. This model, known as an *age-drift* model [70, 71], implies the same linear change in the logarithms of incidence rates over time for all age groups. In this situation, the estimate of the rate of change β (or $e^\beta - 1$, if β is large) is a complete summary of the time trend. This model and an example of its application are presented below in detail.

Table 3.19 gives the incidence rate and the number of observed cases by five-year age group from 30 to 74 years for malignant melanoma in Norwegian women, for five time periods from 1960 to 1980. From the Table, it can be seen that incidence of this cancer has approximately quadrupled between 1960 and 1980 and that the increase has been very regular. This four-fold increase over 20 years corresponds to a growth of approximately 7% per year ($4^{1/20} = 1.07$).

We have seen that under model (3.75), $\text{Log}(\lambda_{xt})$ depends linearly on the period. On the other hand, the age effect is represented by separate parameters α_x for each age group, with no *a priori* assumptions about the shape of the age-incidence relationship. Just as we have considered other assumptions about the relationship with time, there are various ways of incorporating age in the model. Here, an age-drift model of the form:

$$\text{Log}(\lambda_{xt}) = \alpha_0 + \alpha_1 x + \alpha_2 x^2 + \alpha_3 x^3 + \beta t \tag{3.77}$$

where the logarithm of age-specific incidence is modelled by a polynomial of degree 3, provides a satisfactory fit for this data set. The deviance of the model fitted by maximum likelihood is 45.87 on 40 degrees of freedom ($p > 0.20$) and leads to an estimated annual rate of increase of 7.4%.

The age-drift model, shown in equation (3.75) in its age-period form, can be immediately transformed into an age-cohort model by writing:

$$\text{Log}(\lambda_{xu}) = (\alpha_x + \beta x) + \beta u = \alpha'_x + \beta u \tag{3.78}$$

where $u = t - x$ is the year of birth of an individual aged x at time t. Thus, by adopting a different model of age-specific incidence, the age-drift model becomes an age-cohort model in which the change in risk depends linearly on the date of

Table 3.19   Incidence ([a]) of malignant melanoma in Norwegian women
aged 30 to 74 years between 1959 and 1982

Age	Registration period				
	1959-61	1964-66	1968-72	1973-77	1978-82
30-34	3.10	4.84	8.07	12.14	11.71
	(10)	(14)	(42)	(79)	(89)
35-39	4.81	6.57	11.10	15.30	20.10
	(18)	(21)	(54)	(79)	(128)
40-44	6.47	7.84	12.01	20.65	21.01
	(25)	(29)	(64)	(101)	(108)
45-49	3.81	10.45	12.59	21.64	23.87
	(14)	(40)	(77)	(114)	(116)
50-54	4.36	6.07	10.17	18.23	22.30
	(15)	(22)	(64)	(112)	(118)
55-59	4.38	7.13	11.22	17.04	23.30
	(14)	(24)	(66)	(104)	(141)
60-64	4.48	8.74	8.85	15.18	21.52
	(13)	(27)	(48)	(86)	(127)
65-69	5.89	8.83	8.69	15.45	24.44
	(14)	(24)	(42)	(79)	(132)
70-74	10.39	7.97	12.86	15.83	24.90
	(19)	(17)	(52)	(69)	(116)
WTR ([b])	5.27	7.52	10.75	15.35	21.93

([a]) Rates per 100 000 person-years. Number of observed cases in brackets.
([b]) Rates standardized to the truncated world population 30 to 74 years.

birth. If risk increases with time, incidence increases more rapidly with age if risk is measured longitudinally (intra-cohort); conversely, if incidence decreases, the cross-sectional incidence (intra-period) will have a steeper slope. The two curves differ by the quantity βx, a linear function of age (Figure 3.18), and serve to remind us that the real increase in risk of a given cancer with age cannot be determined when its incidence changes over time. Unless it is specified *a priori*, based on other observations, that the changes are due to either cohort or period effects, the increase in risk can only be measured up to a term βx.

Table 3.20 gives cross-sectional incidence estimated for the year 1975 based on model (3.77) and longitudinal incidence for the cohort born around 1925, calcu-

Table 3.20   Incidence of malignant melanoma by age for women in Norway ([a])

	30-34	35-39	40-44	45-49	50-54	55-59	60-64	65-69	70-74
Cross-sectional 1975 ([b])	9.76	13.96	16.54	17.11	16.31	15.11	14.35	14.73	17.25
Longitudinal 1925 ([c])	2.80	5.72	9.68	14.32	19.50	25.80	35.01	51.34	85.89

([a]) Rate per 100 000 person-years.
([b]) Incidence estimated for the year 1975 from model 3.77.
([c]) Incidence estimated for the cohort born in 1925 from the model 3.78.

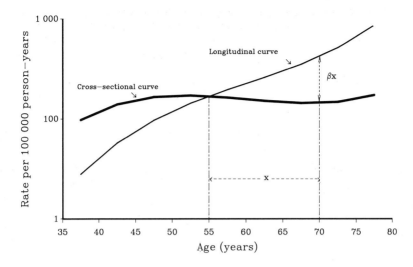

**Figure 3.18 Skin melanoma incidence in Norway, women; 1975
(cross-sectional curve), and for the generation born in 1925 (longitudinal curve)**

lated from the cohort version of the model given in formula (3.78). Here, the increase in risk with age is *a priori* better described by the longitudinal curve, insofar as sun exposure practices tend to change over generations. Furthermore, the cross-sectional curve gives a rather implausible description of the increase in risk with age. If this interpretation is correct, the cumulative risk of malignant melanoma for women aged between 30 and 74 years born in 1925 based on Table 3.20 is 1.25%. This risk has therefore increased from $(1.25/(1.077)^{25}) = 0.2\%$ for the generation born in 1900 to $(1.25 \times (1.077)^{15}) = 3.8\%$ for the generation of women born in 1940.

Table 3.19 can be reconstructed very accurately from the age-drift model using the data of Table 3.20 and a drift of 7.4%, except for the incidence over the first period in the age group 70-74 years, which is abnormally high. The estimated rate is in fact $17.25 \times e^{[0.074(1960 - 1975)]} = 5.68$.

Figure 3.19 shows rates estimated by cohort, under the longitudinal hypothesis. The change in shape observed between the oldest and youngest generations is quite likely to be mostly an artefact. This phenomenon once again shows how hard it is to model changes in risk with age: fitting a third-degree polynomial, which on average describes the data well in the observation period, undoubtedly leads to somewhat pessimistic estimates when extrapolated to young generations. Unfortunately, this uncertainty in the calculation of lifetime risk is inevitable, given that each cohort can only be observed over a limited age range.

Description of trend by cohort

Just as non-linear changes in risk with time leads to an age-period model, non-linear progression of risk with date of birth points to an age-cohort model. This model is satisfactory if the corresponding portions of the longitudinal incidence

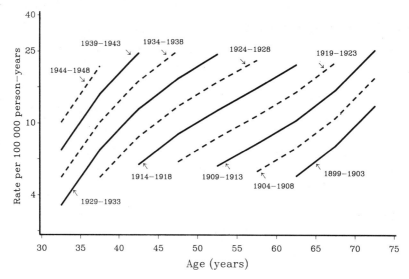

**Figure 3.19   Skin melanoma incidence in Norway;
estimated age-specific rate by birth cohort, women**

curves are parallel. In certain situations, a graphical representation can often show to what extent this condition is fulfilled [72]. Thus, Figure 3.20 shows the time trend of lung cancer incidence in Scotland by age group according to calendar period (Figure 3.20a) and date of birth (Figure 3.20b). Diverging curves in Figure 3.20a clearly show the inadequacy of an age-period model. On the other hand, the parallel segments in the corresponding parts of the curves seen in Figure 3.20b suggest that an age-cohort model fits well.

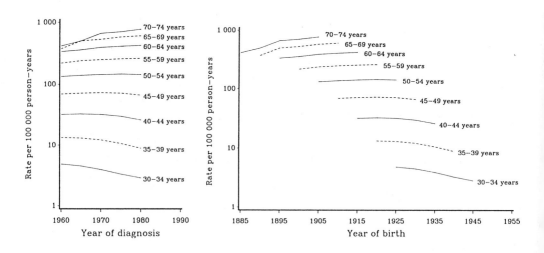

Figure 3.20   Trend in the age-specific incidence of lung cancer in Scotland; men

The age-cohort model is written:

$$\text{Log}\,(\lambda_{xu}) = \alpha'_x + \gamma_u \qquad \begin{array}{l} x_1 \le x \le x_g \\ u_1 \le u \le u_\ell \end{array} \qquad (3.79)$$

or, by writing explicitly the drift in the equation, as before (see formula 3.78):

$$\text{Log}\,(\lambda_{xu}) = \alpha'_x + \beta u + \text{non-linear terms in } u \qquad (3.80)$$

As already mentioned, the use of this model is illustrated with data on lung cancer incidence in Scotland between 1964 and 1980 among men aged between 30 and 74 years (see Table 3.21).

Table 3.21 **Incidence rates ([a]) of lung cancer in men in Scotland**

Age	Registration period				Estimated rate ([b])
	1963-66	1970-72	1973-77	1978-82	u = 1925
30-34	4.07	4.29	3.68	3.08	4.80
	(25)	(19)	(29)	(28)	
35-39	<u>15.14</u>	9.55	11.00	7.12	<u>13.09</u>
	(94)	(42)	(80)	(55)	
40-44	<u>29.94</u>	<u>29.21</u>	26.41	21.97	<u>32.22</u>
	(197)	(131)	(191)	(158)	
45-49	73.38	<u>73.40</u>	<u>69.52</u>	59.71	<u>71.59</u>
	(432)	(343)	(512)	(424)	
50-54	143.91	140.38	<u>143.31</u>	146.48	143.54
	(885)	(596)	(1070)	(1048)	
55-59	245.12	257.27	265.39	<u>268.85</u>	<u>259.72</u>
	(1483)	(1080)	(1729)	(1875)	
60-64	372.42	407.19	410.38	417.76	424.10
	(1923)	(1639)	(2618)	(2493)	
65-69	448.37	556.80	589.29	611.25	624.92
	(1654)	(1817)	(3305)	(3344)	
70-74	407.39	621.84	743.46	782.61	831.00
	(1015)	(1332)	(2969)	(3382)	
WTR ([c])	5.27	7.52	10.75	15.35	21.93

([a]) Observed rate per 100 000 person-years ; observed number in brackets.
([b]) Age-specific rate estimated for the generation born in 1925. Rates underlined correspond approximately. to the ages for which this cohort is actually observed.
([c]) Rates standardized to the truncated world population 30 to 74 years.

Note that the data used are not available at equidistant dates; it has therefore been necessary to reconstruct the cohorts, by dividing up the observation periods according to the cohorts that they include, and interpolating the corresponding person-years [73]. When there are three cohorts, the expectation of the observation k_{xt} for age x and time t can be written

$$E(k_{xt}) = \lambda_{x_1 u_1} M_1 + \lambda_{x_2 u_2} M_2 + \lambda_{x_3 u_3} M_3$$

where:

• u_1, u_2, u_3 and x_1, x_2, x_3 are respectively the average birth dates and average ages in this period-time interval of the three cohorts spanning this observation period at age x;

• M_1, M_2, M_3 are the estimated person-years of observation in the corresponding sub-regions of the lexis diagram; and

• λ_{xu} is the incidence rate from the chosen model.

Estimation of the model is then straightforward using maximum likelihood as before. The likelihood based on the Poisson distribution is, apart from a constant term,

$$L = -\sum_{xt} \hat{k}_{xt} + \sum_{xt} k_{xt} \, \text{Log}(\hat{k}_{xt}) \tag{3.81}$$

where $\hat{k}_{xt}$ is the value of k_{xt} estimated from the model.

For the data of table 3.21, the model:

$$\text{Log}(\lambda_{xu}) = \alpha(x) + \gamma(u) \tag{3.82}$$

where $\alpha(x)$ is a second-degree polynomial in x and $\gamma(u)$ a fifth-degree polynomial in u, provides a satisfactory fit ($\chi^2 = 24.8$ on 28 degrees of freedom).

Incidence rates and observed numbers are given in Table 3.21, as well as age-specific rates estimated for the cohort born in 1925. Relative risks for other

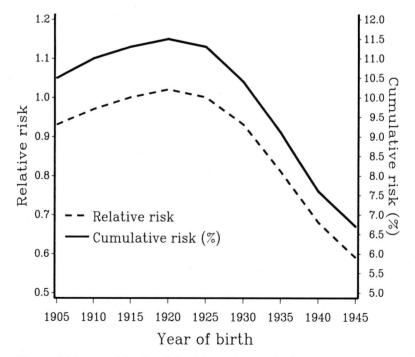

Figure 3.21 Trend in the risk of lung cancer in Scottish men born
between 1905 and 1945

**Table 3.22 Lung cancer risk ([a]) in Scotland by cohort,
for men born between 1905 and 1945**

	Year of birth								
	1905	1910	1915	1920	1925	1930	1935	1940	1945
Relative risk	0,93	0.97	1.00	1.02	1.00	0.93	0.81	0.68	0.59
Cumulative risk 30-74 years	10.50	11.00	11.30	11.50	11.30	10.40	9.10	7.60	6.70

([a]) Relative risk (reference 1925) and cumulative risk (%) are estimated from the age-cohort model

cohorts and corresponding cumulative risks from 30 to 74 years are given in Table 3.22 and Figure 3.21. Estimated rates corresponding to the observations are shown in Figure 3.22. This Figure shows the extent and the nature of the extrapolations carried out to obtain the cumulative risk for a given cohort.

In this example, a knowledge of the epidemiology of lung cancer would strongly suggest that risk has changed over successive cohorts. The fact remains that the fitting of a model, regardless of how good it is, does not prove whether an observed

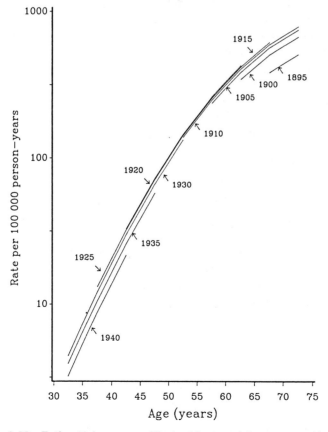

**Figure 3.22 Estimated age-specific incidence of lung cancer in Scotland
by birth cohort in men**

effect is due to period or cohort. For instance, in this example, the absence of non-linear effects associated with period implies that the *a priori* hypothesis of a multiplicative age-cohort model (equation 3.82) can be accepted. Taken in isolation, the quality of the fit tells little about the validity of this last model.

Often, however, non-linear changes occur over time in factors related to period and cohort, necessitating their simultaneous introduction into the model; we are then led to consider age-period-cohort models.

Age-period-cohort models

We saw that when an age-period or age-cohort model describes the data well, it is possible to summarize the data simply, either by cross-sectional mortality or incidence rate and a series of standardized rates for each period, or by a longitudinal mortality or incidence rate and a series of cumulative risks for each cohort. Even if there is no ultimate proof of the models' validity, they provide a more or less full reconstruction of the information present in the data, and an accurate representation of the time trend. We have also seen that when the nature of the model is known *a priori,* estimates of the corresponding parameters can be obtained.

On the other hand, when neither of the two models is adequate, parameterization according to one or another of the time scales is no longer justified. Furthermore, even when it is known that an age-period-cohort model underlies the data, it is impossible to estimate all the parameters, because of the algebraic relationship between the three study factors ($t = u + x$). It has been proposed that the linear term, the drift, be partitioned according to the goodness of fit of the age-period and age-cohort models (74). Unfortunately, as has already been stated, goodness of fit only indicates the size of the contribution of the non-linear terms characterizing period or cohort changes, not their respective absolute size. Note, for example, that a perfectly linear cohort effect combined with a purely quadratic period effect leads to an age-period model with perfect fit.

To show its various forms, we write the age-period-cohort model in the form :

$$\text{Log}\,(\lambda_{xtu}) = \alpha_0 + \alpha x + a(x) + \beta t + p(t) + \gamma u + c(u) \tag{3.83}$$

where $a(x)$, $p(t)$ and $c(u)$ are the non-linear effects associated with age, period and cohort respectively. Thus written, this model is not identifiable, because $t = u + x$. It can be shown that two versions of this model are:

• the age-cohort model corrected for non-linear period effects, which, using the relationship $\beta t = \beta x + \beta u$, can be written:

$$\text{Log}\,(\lambda_{xtu}) = \alpha_0 + (\alpha + \beta)x + a(x) + (\gamma + \beta)u + c(u) + p(t) \tag{3.84}$$

The linear coefficients of age and cohort are thus biased by β.

• the age-period model corrected for non-linear cohort effects, which, using the relationship $\gamma u = \gamma t - \gamma x$, can be written:

$$\text{Log}\,(\lambda_{xtu}) = \alpha_0 + (\alpha - \gamma)x + a(x) + (\beta + \gamma)t + p(t) + c(u) \tag{3.85}$$

where the coefficient of the linear term in age is now biased by $-\gamma$. The coefficient of the linear term in period, $\beta + \gamma$, is the same as the coefficient corresponding to cohort in model (3.84). This coefficient (the drift) is the sum of the rates of change according to period and cohort: it is the linear approximation of the trend in the neighbourhood of the reference year of observation ($t = 0$) and year of birth ($u = 0$) respectively, when a, c and p are modelled by polynomials of degree greater than 1.

We illustrate the use of the age-period-cohort model with data on cervical cancer in Birmingham, UK between 1960 and 1982 (see Table 3.23). Figure 3.23, which shows that the trends in each age group are very different, shows that an age-period model is certainly not appropriate. Fitting the age-cohort model gives a deviance of 51.9 on 30 degrees of freedom, which becomes 38.0 on 27 degrees of freedom when period is added as a factor, a significant reduction ($p = 0.003$). Estimates from models (3.84) and (3.85) are given in Table 3.24. Following Holford [75], effects of each factor are presented by separating the overall linear trend from the 'non-linear' effects which correspond here to departures from linearity. This approach differs from the polynomial modelling used here in the age-cohort model, particularly

Table 3.23   Cervical cancer incidence ([a]) in women in Birmingham, UK, between 1960 and 1982

Age	Registration period					Estimated rate ([b]) u = 1920
	1960-62	1963-66	1968-72	1973-76	1979-82	
25-29	1.58	2.80	3.56	7.03	13.50	4.24
	(7)	(17)	(31)	(55)	(91)	
30-34	8.44	8.67	10.80	13.86	19.95	14.76
	(40)	(51)	(82)	(90)	(149)	
35-39	22.58	24.57	16.11	16.29	22.79	27.57
	(117)	(153)	(118)	(98)	(151)	
40-44	<u>31.45</u>	38.48	27.47	21.52	21.68	<u>36.70</u>
	(154)	(263)	(214)	(126)	(128)	
45-49	30.21	<u>41.68</u>	40.72	29.83	22.17	<u>39.85</u>
	(150)	(265)	(338)	(183)	(125)	
50-54	28.46	37.70	<u>39.92</u>	35.96	22.72	<u>37.69</u>
	(136)	(243)	(312)	(239)	(134)	
55-59	34.20	33.10	36.38	<u>37.38</u>	36.59	<u>39.75</u>
	(148)	(202)	(277)	(209)	(225)	
60-64	34.27	27.13	32.40	36.39	<u>34.25</u>	<u>37.81</u>
	(130)	(146)	(231)	(208)	(189)	
65-69	34.12	30.48	23.72	24.60	33.45	33.06
	(106)	(137)	(146)	(127)	(173)	
70-74	41.59	32.55	30.08	27.78	25.62	33.54
	(101)	(111)	(148)	(118)	(114)	
75-79	37.45	27.82	26.02	21.97	20.88	24.64
	(65)	(67)	(89)	(66)	(70)	

([a]) Observed rates for 100 000 person-years; observed numbers in brackets.
([b]) Age-specific rates estimated for the cohort born in 1920. Underlined rates correspond to the age intervals for which the cohort is actually observed.

with regard to the interpretation of the drift. In this case, it should be considered to be the best approximation to the linear change in incidence over the whole observation period. The drift is small ($\beta + \gamma = 0.01070$), because the decrease observed in some age groups is balanced by a substantial increase in other age groups. A polynomial model with cohorts centred around 1920 and periods around 1970 would give a much larger drift, given that the increase at these dates was already quite marked and that this version of the drift estimates local increases. It is important to note that, although it is identifiable, the drift depends essentially on the model selected, and it must be interpreted with care.

Fortunately, these subtleties are often irrelevant. In most situations, the structure of the time trend is much simpler and the different parameterizations are more or less equivalent. In the complex example considered here, change in risk across cohorts after correcting for linear effects of period (Table 3.25) still provides quite a satisfactory picture of the underlying epidemiological situation.

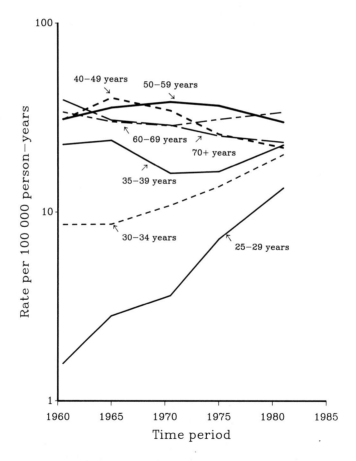

Figure 3.23 Trend in the age-specific incidence of cervical cancer in Birmingham, UK, between 1960 and 1982

**Table 3.24 Cervical cancer in Birmingham, UK.
Estimation of the age-period-cohort model**

Factor	Coding [b]	Deviation from linearity	Total [a]	
			Age-period	Age-cohort
Age	**x**	**a(x)**		
25	−5	−1.242	−1.765	−1.818
30	−4	−0.111	−0.529	−0.572
35	−3	0.399	0.085	0.053
40	−2	0.569	0.360	0.339
45	−1	0.537	0.432	0.422
50	0	0.366	0.366	0.366
55	1	0.304	0.409	0.419
60	2	0.138	0.347	0.368
65	3	−0.111	0.203	0.235
70	4	−0.212	0.206	0.249
75	5	−0.636	−0.113	−0.060
Linear effect			$\alpha - \gamma = 0.1046$	$\alpha + \beta = 0.1152$
Cohort	**u**	**c(u)**		
1885	−7	0.556		0.481
1890	−6	0.253		0.189
1895	−5	0.057		0.003
1900	−4	−0.070		−0.113
1905	−3	−0.224		−0.256
1910	−2	−0.211		−0.232
1915	−1	−0.071		−0.082
1920	0	−0.034		−0.034
1925	1	−0.052		−0.041
1930	2	−0.350		−0.329
1935	3	−0.599		−0.567
1940	4	−0.512		−0.469
1945	5	−0.186		−0.133
1950	6	0.317		0.381
1955	7	1.124		1.199
Period	**t**	**p(t)**		
1960-62	−2	−0.063	0.084	
1963-66	−1	0.054	0.043	
1968-72	0	0.040	0.040	
1973-76	1	0.012	0.023	
1979-82	2	−0.042	−0.021	

$$\alpha_0 = -8.249$$

| **Drift** | | | | $\beta + \gamma = 0.0107$ |

[a] The effect of the factor is obtained by summing the deviation from linearity and the linear effect corresponding to each of the models. Thus, the age effect at age 65 years (x = 3) in an age-cohort model corrected for nonlinear period effects is : $0.1152 \times 3 - 0.111 = 0.235$.
[b] Age, cohort and period variables are coded by corresponding integers, ignoring irregularities created by the observation periods. Age, cohort and period factors are centred around the categories 50-54, 1968-72 and 1920-25 respectively.

Table 3.25   Cervical cancer risk ([a]) in Birmingham, UK, by year of birth

	Year of birth												
	1890	1895	1900	1905	1910	1915	1920	1925	1930	1935	1940	1945	1950
Relative risk	1.20	1.00	0.89	0.77	0.79	0.92	0.97	0.96	0.72	0.57	0.63	0.87	1.46
Cumulative risk 25-79 years	1.99	1.66	1.47	1.28	1.31	1.52	1.59	1.58	1.19	0.94	1.03	1.44	2.41

([a]) Relative risk and cumulative risk (%) are estimated from the age-period-cohort model. Relative risks are normalized by the requirement that the sum of their logarithms is zero over the years considered.

Specific techniques and examples

Epidemiological evaluation of a secondary prevention campaign

The incidence of skin melanoma and associated mortality have shown a marked increase since the 1960s in most countries [73,76]. Some of this increase is most likely due to exposure to ultraviolet radiation, and another part can be attributed to improved diagnosis of these cancers. In theory, earlier detection of cases should limit the increase in mortality over time, or even reverse the trend. Accordingly, many countries or regions have developed intervention programmes, which in turn require evaluation. Even though secondary prevention programmes must ultimately be assessed on the basis of changes in mortality, the observation of larger increases in early-stage cases can also provide information on the effectiveness of the method of implementation of the programme.

A campaign conducted in Switzerland at the beginning of May 1988 had the twin objectives of primary prevention, aimed at educating the population about the dangers of prolonged exposure to the sun, and secondary prevention, through informing the public and the medical profession about the advantages of rapid and systematic examination (clinical and, if necessary, histological) of suspicious skin lesions. A year after this campaign was launched [77], only the second objective could be assessed. The ensuing analysis provides an example of the use of log-linear models to evaluate this type of chronological evolution.

The immediate objective of the campaign was to increase the number of cases diagnosed at an early stage, but it might also be expected that the number of advanced cases could also increase as a result of the intervention. The evaluation thus consisted of checking the assumption that the time trend prevailing before the campaign changed immediately after the launch of the campaign (that is, after June 1988), and that any increase was greater in early cases than in advanced cases.

For practical reasons, mainly related to the quality of cancer registration, data from before 1985 were not used to estimate the pre-campaign trend in incidence. Analysis was restricted to cases registered between 1 January 1985 and 30 April 1988 (three years and four months) and the campaign was assessed over the eight

Table 3.26   Skin melanomas by stage and calendar period in four Swiss registries

	Geneva		Neuchâtel		Vaud		St-Gall/Appenzell	
	Stage 1-2	Other ([a])	Stage 1-2	Other ([a])	Stage 1-2	Other ([a])	Stage 1-2	Other ([a])
1985								
Jan-Apr	6	6	–	3	12	7	7	5
May-Aug	9	3	3	–	14	17	7	4
Sep-Dec	9	4	3	1	13	8	8	5
1986								
Jan-Apr	9	4	1	1	13	14	5	5
May-Aug	11	5	–	–	10	13	12	9
Sep-Dec	7	7	4	2	14	13	10	7
1987								
Jan-Apr	8	5	3	1	15	12	4	6
May-Aug	17	7	1	4	22	10	6	12
Sep-Dec	5	4	3	–	7	16	7	6
1988								
Jan-Apr	5	3	4	3	9	8	4	4
May-Aug	20	12	9	3	23	12	17	12
Sep-Dec	12	4	4	4	24	17	5	5

([a]) Includes cases of unknown stage.

remaining months of 1988, when the effects of the intervention should have been apparent. In total, 734 skin melanomas were reported from January 1985 to December 1988 in the four participating regional registries (Geneva, Neuchâtel, St-Gall/Appenzell and Vaud). Given the short duration of the study period, it was not considered necessary to take denominators into account. On the other hand, monthly counts of cases were used, to allow for the effects of seasonal fluctuations.

In Switzerland, the melanoma incidence tends to increase markedly from the beginning of summer, and reach its lowest level during winter. It was decided *a priori* that a division of the year into three periods of four months (January to April, May to August and September to December) would provide a satisfactory description of the seasonal variation. Grouping into four-monthly periods also corresponded to the interval during which the effects of the campaign should have been noticeable, that is, the second and third periods of 1988. This grouping did not result in a significant loss of information compared to an analysis based on monthly data (χ^2 = 12.4 on nine degrees of freedom). All analyses were therefore carried out from data grouped in this way. For both practical and theoretical reasons, disease stages were also grouped. 'Early' cases were Breslow's stage 1 and 2 (up to and including 1.5 mm), while 'advanced' cases comprised those of stages 3 and 4 and unknown stage (7.9% of the total). Table 3.26 provides the data on which the analysis was based (see Table 3.27).

Table 3.27 Modelling of data from Table 3.26

Model	Estimate	Deviance	d.f.
Model A = Registry + Campaign + Year (continuous) + Four-month period			
• Four-month period ([a])			
Jan-Apr	1.00		
May-Aug	1.42 [1.16 ; 1.73]		
Sep-Dec	1.11 [0.90 ; 1.37]		
• Year ([b])	2.30 [–6.60 ; 12.1]		
• Campaign		114.9	88
Before campaign	1.00		
After campaign ([c])	1.46 [1.13 ; 1.89]		
Model B = Model A + registry x campaign		111.0	85
Model C = Model A + stage		99.0	87
Model D = Model C + stage x campaign			
Before campaign	1.00		
After campaign ([c])			
– early stages	1.63 [1.22 ; 2.19]		
– autres stages	1.24 [0.90 ; 1.71]	96.5	86

([a]) Relative risk.
([b]) Annual rate of increase (%).
([c]) Relative increase in number of cases.

The first step in the analysis was to assess whether there had indeed been additional increase in incidence from the start of the campaign, taking into account the prior trend and seasonal variation. Trend was modelled using year of incidence as a continuous variable, with the four-monthly periods to represent seasonal changes. Region of registration was also introduced into this model as a factor to take into account both the differences between the size of the populations (denominators) and possible differences in the prevalence of the risk factors in the populations covered by the four registries (model A). The model expresses the logarithm of the expected number of cases as a linear function of the various factors:

$$\text{Log}\,[\mu_{r\,q\,c}(t)] = \alpha_r + \beta_q + \gamma_c + \delta t$$

where r, q, c are the indices of the region, the four-monthly periods and the campaign respectively, and where t is the year of incidence. The model was fitted by maximum likelihood assuming that the number of cases follows a Poisson distribution of mean $\mu_{r\,q\,c}(t)$. The result is an estimate of the overall effect of the campaign equal to 1.46 [1.13 ; 1.89], which means that incidence was 46% higher than expected on the basis of the pre-campaign trend and seasonal variation.

The second step was a comparison of the effectiveness of the prevention campaign in the four registry regions, by adding an interaction term (registry x campaign)

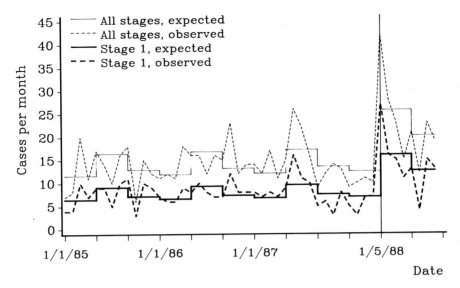

Figure 3.24 Observed and expected cases of skin melanoma before and after the start of a screening programme in Switzerland; both sexes combined; 1985–1988

to the above model, to allow for a possible different effect in each region (model B). The reduction in the deviance of 3.9 on three degrees of freedom led to the conclusion that there was no difference between the four regions with respect to the effect from the campaign.

The third step was to address the fundamental question as to whether the increase in incidence had been more marked for early stages. To test the hypothesis that the increase was identical for all stages, a model which included stage in addition to the other four factors included initially (registry, year, four-monthly period and campaign (model C)) was compared with a model augmented by an interactive term representing a campaign effect which differed for each stage (model D). The reduction in the deviance was 2.5 on one degree of freedom (p = 0.10). Despite the absence of a formal statistical significance at the 0.05 conventional level, the authors were convinced that the effect of the prevention campaign differed with respect to stage. The relative increase was estimated to be 1.63 [1.22 ; 2.19] in early cases and 1.24 [0.90 ; 1.71] in advanced cases, or 63% and 24% respectively. The campaign was therefore judged to be doubly effective on the basis of its first expected outcomes: (i) increased total incidence and (ii) a more marked increase in early cases.

The estimates obtained from fitting the final model (model D) provide the basis for calculating estimates which make up a smoothed curve (Figure 3.24). The number of expected cases can be calculated for any combination of values of the terms. For example, the number of cases over a whole year can be calculated by stage under the assumption that the prevention campaign either worked, or did not work.

In other words we can estimate the additional cases that were diagnosed during 1988, due to the effect of the screening campaign:

	Early stage	Other	Total
No screening	97	77	174
Screening	159	96	255
Additional cases	62	19	81
(% increase)	+ 64	+ 25	+ 47

Trends in cancer of the uterine cervix

In most western countries, the frequency of invasive cervical cancer has been decreasing for many years, almost certainly at least partly as a result of screening. However, a rise in incidence has recently been noted among young women in some countries. Various explanations have been offered, including an increase in sexual activity and the consequent increase in risk of infection by the human papilloma virus, an increase in the prevalence of smoking and decreased participation in screening programmes. Whatever the reasons for this phenomenon, it is of interest to examine the divergence by age of the time trend in different populations.

In Geneva, reliable incidence data are available from 1970. A study of time trends was first carried out on all invasive and microinvasive cases [78]. The time trend over the 18 years from 1970 to 1987 was analysed by modelling the logarithm of annual incidence rates by a linear function of year of diagnosis and estimating the parameters by maximum likelihood. Fitting the model

$$Log\,(\lambda_{xt}) = \alpha + \beta t$$

gave a rate of change of $\beta = -4.3\%$ per year [−6.0 ; −2.6], indicating a significant decrease in the crude incidence rate (Table 3.28, model B). The next step was to estimate the rate of change in the age-adjusted incidence from model (3.75):

$$Log\,(\lambda_{xt}) = \alpha_x + \beta t$$

which led to $\beta = -4.6\%$ [−6.3 ; −2.6] (model C).

The null hypothesis that the trends did not differ across age groups was tested by introducing a term for interaction between age group and year of diagnosis, which is equivalent to a different slope for each age group (model D) (see formula 3.74). Because of the significant improvement in the model's fit ($\chi^2 = 18.3$ on six degrees of freedom, $p < 0.05$), it was concluded that there was a real difference in trends between age groups, justifying different estimates of annual rates of change for each age group. These estimated rates of change are shown in Figure 3.25; estimates obtained by applying these rates of change to the incidence by age observed in 1970 are shown in Figure 3.26.

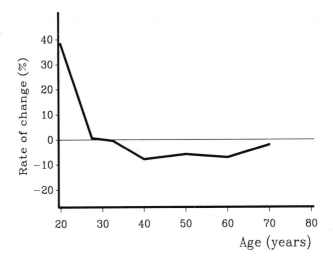

Figure 3.25   Age-specific rate of change in cervical cancer incidence in Geneva between 1970 and 1987

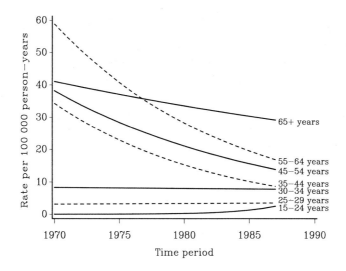

Figure 3.26   Trend in the age-specific incidence of cervical cancer in Geneva between 1970 and 1987

Although the numbers are small (480 cases observed in seven age groups over 18 years) and, consequently, the standard errors associated with the rates of change for each age group are high, the preceding analysis and data from Figures 3.25 and 3.26 suggest that there are three different types of time trend. The apparently increasing incidence for women less than 35 years could be a result of exposure to risk factors linked to sexual behaviour. In contrast, women aged 65 years and over, in whom incidence has only slightly decreased, might not have

Table 3.28 Modelling time trends by age group from annual rates of cancer of the uterine cervix in the canton of Geneva from 1970 to 1987 (all incident invasive and microinvasive cases)

Model	Rate of change %	95% CI	Deviance	d.f.
Model A = Constant			462.9	125
Log $(\lambda_{xt}) = \alpha$				
Model B = Year	−4.3	[− 6.0 ; −2.6]	438.3	124
Log $(\lambda_{xt}) = \alpha + \beta t$				
Model C = Year + Age	−4.6	[− 6.3 ; −2.6]	150.9	118
Log $(\lambda_{xt}) = \alpha_x + \beta t$				
Model D = Age ∗ Year				
Log $(\lambda_{xt}) = \alpha_x + \beta_x t$				
15-24 (4 cases)	38.3	[− 2.0 ; 95.1]		
25-29 (9 cases)	0.7	[−11.2 ; 14.2]		
30-34 (22 cases)	−0.4	[− 8.4 ; 8.3]		
35-44 (84 cases)	−7.8	[−11.8 ; −3.8]		
45-54 (92 cases)	−5.8	[− 9.7 ; −1.9]		
55-64 (101 cases)	−7.1	[−10.7 ; −3.5]		
65+ (168 cases)	−2.0	[− 4.9 ; 1.0]	132.6	112

benefited from screening as much as younger women either because screening for this cohort was not yet routine or, more likely, because they stopped being screened after menopause. Incidence decreases substantially and relatively uniformly only in women aged between 35 and 65 years. Most of this change can reasonably be attributed to screening.

Bibliographical notes

A more detailed discussion of the concepts and methods of graphs and spatial analysis can be obtained from Cliff and Haggett's *Atlas of disease distributions : analytical approaches to epidemiological data* [79], effectively a manual of statistical ecology. While mainly using examples from the field of transmissible diseases, including the historical data of John Snow, the book also deals with problems relevant to cancer epidemiology, such as nasopharyngeal cancer in China, clusters of mesothelioma cases in the USA and monitoring risk around nuclear power plants or in the region of Chernobyl. The book reviews the principal techniques used to define regions and to smooth data, and also considers the problem of detecting outliers and clusters, both spatial and spatio-temporal. Also discussed are methods for detecting autocorrelation, estimating spatial patterns and regression involving exposure factors in ecological analyses.

Another text brings together a series of papers on cancer mapping, including presentations of the principal mortality atlases published at the time [80]. Several articles of this latter monograph discuss the various problems raised in the geographical representation of epidemiological data on cancer, or comment on methodological issues, such as the choice of colour.

The recent article by Walter and Birnie [81] provides a survey of the 49 atlases which appear during the fifteen-year period ending in 1989. The atlases are examined and classified by population and disease, and by the mapping and statistical techniques adopted. The authors emphasize the diversity of methods used and the consequent difficulty in making comparisons across atlases.

Research into the analysis of the spatial distribution of cancer, and in particular on the detection of clusters, has been published recently; two publications of note are the proceedings of the meetings organized by the Royal Statistical Society of the UK, on cancer incidence near nuclear installations [82], and the review of Marshall [83].

Applications of the empirical Bayes and grouping methods proposed by Huel [43] are presented in a thesis by Colonna on geographical studies in the situation where incidence is low [21]. This paper also deals with autocorrelation and its measurement. The thesis by Mollie includes a detailed mathematical discussion of smoothing based on the Bayesian approach, with an application to cancer mortality in France [48]. On the same subject, articles by Clayton and Bernardinelli [84] and Bernardinelli and Montomoli [85] provide an original point of view and practical examples.

The epidemiological literature includes many studies which have tried to link risk and exposure at the level of groups, mainly defined geographically. These studies provide examples of the methods dealt with on page 141 of this chapter. Of particular note are three studies on dietary factors which appeared at the time when ecological correlation analysis first became widely used, and which clearly illustrate the methodological problems raised by measurement of exposure at the group level. The first study relates to the geographical correlation observed in the USA (across states) and in Europe (across countries) between alcohol and tobacco consumption on one hand and various cancer sites on the other [86]. The second study examines the relationship between dietary factors and the various types of cancer, using national statistics from 32 countries [87]. The third article also considers dietary factors, but includes diseases other than cancer [88].

A thesis by Viel compares the results of published case-control and cohort studies on the effect of pesticides with those that he obtained from ecological analysis of French data from the departements. These analyses are carried out using the method proposed by Gardner [51], a Poisson regression adjusting for latitude and longitude, and a correlation test modified to take into account autocorrelation, proposed by Clifford and coworkers [90]. The work provides a good example of geographical correlation methods applied to the study of an association involving an exposure which is difficult to quantify at the individual level.

There have been a number of studies published on cancer risk in migrants. Recent monographs published by the International Agency for Research on Cancer have considered Jewish migrants to Israel [91] and Italian migrant populations [60]. The first of these monographs is an excellent example of the use of information on the country of birth and time since arrival, in a country characterized by immigration from many countries. The second only considers one country of origin, Italy, but studies their outcome in a range of host countries.

Data on time trends in cancer incidence and mortality are essential for the development of public health policy. For this reason, it is surprising that the literature in this area is relatively poor. There has been little research on the simultaneous estimation of rates of change having variable precision. There is however a need for methods to allow data of this type to be presented in a more convincing manner. The only work in this area has been based on empirical Bayes methods, particularly in the estimation of cohort effects in the youngest and oldest cohorts. Breslow and Clayton have proposed the estimation of random effects based on autoregressive models, in which the estimate for each cohort is based on some information from earlier and later cohorts [92]. In contrast, Desouza has used data on the trend in several geographical areas, to estimate cohort effects in each area by making use of information from other study areas [93]. These methods have nonetheless been used very little, and their value in practice is still unknown. The current rate of progress in the analysis of longitudinal data suggests that there will be a rapid improvement in this situation [94].

The majority of research on time trends has involved relatively simple methods. This lack of sophistication is undoubtedly justified both by the lack of suitable computer software, and by the desire to publish observed data with only a minimum of smoothing compatible with the needs of graphical presentation. Research in this area has been published by Hakulinen and coworkers, on trends in cancer incidence in Nordic countries [95]; by Osmond and coworkers for trends in cancer mortality in England and Wales during 1951-80 [96], by Devesa and coworkers who carried out a fairly complete survey of trends of cancer incidence and mortality in the USA [97], by Lee and coworkers for trends in cancer incidence in Singapore [98], Hill and coworkers for those in France [64], La Vecchia and coworkers for Europe [99] and, finally, Coleman and coworkers who reviewed trends in cancer incidence and mortality using the data available from all five continents [73].

For a general discussion of methodological problems in the study of time trends, in particular those which are not statistical, two meeting reports may be of value [100,101].

REFERENCES

[1] Atlas graphique et statistique de la suisse. Berne, Bureau de statistique du Département fédéral de l'intérieur, 1914. (Statistique de la Suisse ; 191e livraison)

[2] CISLAGHI C, DECARLI A, LA VECCHIA C, LAVERDA N, MEZZANOTTE G, SMANS M. *Dati. Indicatori e mape di mortalita tumorale : Italia 1975/1977.* Bologna, Pitagora Editrice,1986

[3] SMANS M, MUIR CS, BOYLE P. *Atlas of cancer mortality in the European Community.* (IARC Scientific Publications, No 107), Lyon, IARC, 1992

[4] MASON TJ, McKAY FW, HOOVER R, et al. *Atlas of cancer mortality for US counties : 1950-1969.* Bethesda, US Department of Health, Education and Welfare, National Cancer Institute, 1975, (DHEW Publication ; No (NIH)75-780)

[5] *In* CLIFF AD, ORD JK, (eds). *Spatial processes : models & applications.* London, Pion, 1981, pp. 1-6

[6] TEPPO L, PUKKALA M, HAKAMA M *et al. Way of life and cancer incidence in Finland.* Helsinki, Finnish Cancer Registry, 1980, p. 18 ; pp. 40-44

[7] CARSTAIRS V, LOWE M. Small area analysis : creating an area base for environmental monitoring and epidemiological analysis. *Community Med* 1986, **8** :15-28

[8] DIRICHLET GL. Über die Preduction der positiven quadritschen Formen mit drei unbestimmten ganzen Zahlen. *J Reine Angew Math* 1850, **40** : 209-34

[9] CISLAGHI C, DECARLI A, LA VECCHIA C, MEZZANOTTE G, VIGOTTI MA. Trends surface and models applied to the analysis of geographical variations in cancer mortality. *Rev Epidémiol Santé Publ* 1990, **38** : 57-69

[10] Atlas of cancer mortality in the People's Republic of China : China map press n° 1358. Shanghai, Yan'an Xilu, 1979

[11] KEMP I, BOYLE P, SMANS M, MUIR C. *Atlas of cancer in Scotland 1975-1980 : incidence and epidemiological perspectives.* (IARC Scientific Publications, No 72), Lyon, IARC, 1985

[12] SMANS M, ESTÈVE J. Practical approaches to disease mapping. *In* P Elliott, J Cuzick, D English, R Stern (eds) : *Geographical and environmental epidemiology : methods for small area studies.* Oxford, Oxford University Press, 1992, pp. 141-150

[13] REZVANI A, DOYON F, FLAMANT R. *Atlas de la mortalité par cancer en France.* Paris, Les Éditions INSERM, 1986

[14] RYCKERBOER R, JANSSENS G, THIERS G. *Atlas de la mortalité par cancer en Belgique (1969-1976).* Brussels, Ministère de la santé publique et de la famille, Institut d'hygiène et d'épidémiologie, 1983

[15] GARDNER MJ, WINTER PD, TAYLOR CP, ACHESON ED. *Atlas of cancer mortality in England and Wales 1968-1978.* New York, John Wiley, 1983

[16] MORAN PAP. The interpretation of statistical maps. *J R Statist Soc B* 1948, **10** : 243-51

[17] GEARY RC. The contiguity ratio and statistical mapping. *Incorpor Statist* 1954, **5** : 115-45

[18] OHNO Y, AOKI K. Cancer deaths by city and county in Japan 1959-1971 : a test of significance for geographic clusters of disease. *Soc Sci Med* 1981, **15** : 251 : 8

[19] SMANS M. Analysis of spatial aggregation. *In* P Boyle, CS Muir, E Grundmann (eds) : *Cancer mapping.* Berlin, Springer, 1989, pp. 83-6. (*Recent Results in Cancer Research,* **114**)

[20] KNOX G. Epidemiology of childhood leukaemia in Northumberland and Durham. *Br J Prev Soc Med* 1964, **18** : 17-24

[21] COLONNA M. *Analyse de la distribution spatiale du cancer : problème posé par l'étude de faibles incidences* (Dissertation). Grenoble, Université des sciences sociales de Grenoble, Département informatique et mathématiques en sciences sociales, Laboratoire de statistique et analyse de données, 1991, 224 p.

[22] GARDNER MJ. Review of reported increases of childhood cancer rates in the vicinity of nuclear installations in the UK. *J R Statist Soc A* 1989, **152** : 307-25

[23] POCOCK SJ, COOK DG, BERESFORD SAA. Regression of area mortality rates on explanatory variables : what weighting is appropriate ? *Appl Statist* 1981, **30** : 286-95

[24] SCHULMAN J, SELVIN S, MERRILL DW. Density equalized map projections : a method for analysing clustering around a fixed point. *Stat Med* 1988, **7** : 491-505

[25] STONE RA. Investigations of excess environmental risks around putative sources : statistical problems and a proposed test. *Stat Med* 1988, **7** : 649-60

[26] Cook-Mozaffari PJ, Darby SC, Doll R, et al. Geographical variation in mortality from leukaemia and other cancers in England and Wales in relation to proximity to nuclear installations : 1969-78. *Br J Cancer* 1989, **59** : 476-85

[27] Jablon S, Hrubec Z, Boice JD. Cancer in populations living near nuclear facilities. *J Am Med Ass* 1991, **265** : 1403-8

[28] Kinlen LJ. Evidence for an infective cause of childhood leukaemia : comparison of a Scottish new town with nuclear reprocessing sites in Britain. *Lancet* 1988, **2** : 1323-27

[29] Kinlen LJ. The relevance of population mixing to the aetiology of childhood leukaemia. *In* WA Crosbie, JH Gittus (eds) : *Medical response to effects of ionising radiation.* London, Elsevier, 1989, pp. 272-8

[30] Potthoff RF, Whittinghill M. Testing for homogeneity. I. The binomial and multinomial distributions. *Biometrika* 1966, **53** : 167-82

[31] Potthoff RF, Whittinghill M. Testing for homogeneity. II. The Poisson distribution. *Biometrika* 1966, **53** : 183-90

[32] Muirhead CR, Ball AM. Contribution to the discussion of the Royal Statistical Society meeting on cancer near nuclear installations. *J R Statist Soc A* 1989, **152** : 376-77

[33] Muirhead CR, Butland BK. Testing for over-dispersion using an adapted form of the Potthoff-Wittinghill method. *In* FE Alexander, P Boyle (eds) : *Detecting localized clusters of disease.* Lyon : IARC. (IARC Scientific Publications, in preparation)

[34] *In* Cliff AD, Ord JK (eds). *Spatial processes : models & applications.* London, Pion, 1981 : p. 97

[35] Urquhart J, Black R, Buist E. Exploring small area methods. *In Methodology of enquiries into disease clustering.* London, London School of Hygiene and Tropical Medicine, 1989 : pp. 41-52

[36] Cuzick J, Edwards R. Spatial clustering for inhomogeneous populations. *J R Statist Soc B* 1990, **52** : 73-104

[37] Besag J, Newell J. The detection of clusters in rare diseases. *J R Statist Soc A* 1991, **154** : 143-55

[38] David FN, Barton DE. Two space-time interaction tests for epidemicity. *Br J Prev Soc Med* 1966, **20** : 44-8

[39] Mantel N. The detection of disease clustering and a generalized regression approach. *Cancer Res* 1967, **27** : 209-20

[40] *In* Cliff AD, Ord JK (eds). *Spatial processes : models & applications.* London, Pion, 1981 : 22-4

[41] Suomen Syöpäkartasto. *Atlas of cancer incidence in Finland : 1953-82.* Helsinki, Finnish Cancer Registry, 1987

[42] Ménégoz F, Colonna M, Lutz JM, Schaerer R. *Atlas du cancer dans le département de l'Isère.* Grenoble, Registre des cancers de l'Isère, 1989

[43] Huel G, Petiot JF, Lazar P. Algorithm for the grouping of contiguous geographical zones. *Stat Med* 1986, **5** : 171-81

[44] Clayton D, Kaldor J. Empirical Bayes estimates of age-standardized relative risks for use in disease mapping. *Biometrics* 1987, **43** : 671-81

[45] Besag J. Spatial interaction and the statistical analysis of lattice systems. *J R Statist Soc B* 1974, **36** : 192-936

[46] Mollie A, Richardson S. Empirical Bayes estimates of cancer mortality rates using spatial models. *Stat Med* 1991, 10 : 95-112

[47] Besag J, Kempton R. Statistical analysis of field experiments using neighbouring plots. Biometrics 1986, 42 : 231-51

[48] Mollié A. Représentation géographique des taux de mortalité : modélisation spatiale et méthodes bayesiennes [Dissertation]. Paris, Université Paris 6, 1990

[49] Morgenstern H. Uses of ecologic analysis in epidemiologic research. *Am J Public Health* 1982, **72** : 1336-44

[50] Durkheim E. *Suicide: a study in sociology.* New York, Free Press, 1951, pp. 153-80

[51] Gardner MJ, Winter PD. Extensions to a technique for relating mortality and environment – exemplified by nasal cancer and industry. *Scand J Work Environ Health* 1984, **10** : 219-23

[52] Hakama M, Hakulinen T, Pukkala E, Saxén E, Teppo L. Risk indicators of breast and cervical cancer on ecologic and individual levels. *Am J Epidemiol* 1982, **116** : 990-1000

[53] Blot WJ, Fraumeni JF. Geographic patterns of lung cancer : industrial correlations. *Am J Epidemiol* 1976, **103** : 539-50

[54] Richardson S. A method for testing the significance of geographical correlations with application to industrial lung cancer in France. *Stat Med* 1990, **9** : 515-28

[55] Cook DG, Pocock SJ. Multiple regression in geographical mortality studies with allowance for spatially correlated errors. *Biometrics* 1983, **39** : 361-71

[56] Mardia KV, Marshall RJ. Maximum likelihood estimation of models for residual covariance in spatial regression. *Biometrica* 1984, **71** : 135-46

[57] Buell P, Dunn JE. Cancer mortality among Japanese Issei and Nisei of California. *Cancer* 1965, **8** : 656-64

[58] Cairns J. The cancer problem. *Sci Am* 1975, 233 : 64-72 and 77-8

[59] Philips RL. Role of lifestyle on dietary habits in risk of cancer among seventh days adventists. *Cancer Res* 1975, **35** : 3513-22

[60] Geddes M, Parkin DM, Khlat M, Balzi D, Buiatti E. *Cancer in Italian migrant populations.* (IARC Scientific Publications, No 123), Lyon, IARC, 1992

[61] Buiatti E, Palli D, Decarli A et al. A case-control study of gastric cancer and diet in Italy. *Int J Cancer* 1989, 44 : 611-6

[62] Devesa SS, Schneiderman MA. Increase in the number of cancer deaths in the United States. *Am J Epidemiol* 1977, **106** : 1-5

[63] Yale University. Connecticut Cancer Epidemiology Unit. Forty-five years of cancer incidence in Connecticut : 1935-79. Bethesda, US Department of Health and Human Services, National Cancer Institute, 1986 (National Cancer Institute monograph, 70)

[64] Hill C, Benhamou E, Doyon F, Flamant R. *Évolution de la mortalité par cancer en France : 1950-1985.* Paris, Les Editions INSERM, 1989

[65] Cuzick J, Velez R, Doll R. International variations and temporal trends in mortality from multiple myeloma. *Int J Cancer* 1983, **32** : 13-9

[66] Kupper LL, Janis JM, Karmous A. Statistical age-period-cohort analysis : a review and critique. *J Chron Dis* 1985, **38** : 811-30

[67] Hinde J. Compound Poisson regression models. *In* : R Gilchrist, (ed) : *GLIM 82 : Proceedings of the international conference on generalised linear models.* New York , Springer Verlag, 1982, pp. 109-21

[68] Breslow N. Extra-Poisson variations in log-linear models. *Appl Statist* 1984, **33** : 38-44

[69] Breslow N. Score tests in overdispersed GLM's. *In* : M Decarli et al. (eds) : *Proceedings of GLIM 89 and the Fourth international workshop on statistical modelling.* New York, Springer, 1989, pp. 64-74

[70] Clayton D, Schifflers E. Models for temporal variation in cancer rates. I. Age-period and age-cohort models. *Stat Med* 1987, **6** : 449-67

[71] Clayton D, Schifflers E. Models for temporal variation in cancer rates. II. Age-period-cohort models. *Stat Med* 1987, **6** : 469-81

[72] Roush GC, Schymura MJ, Holford TR, White C, Flannery JT. Time period compared to birth cohort in Connecticut incidence rates for twenty-five malignant neoplasms. *J Nat Cancer Inst* 1985, **74** : 779-88

[73] Coleman M, Esteve J, Damiecki P. et al. Time trends in cancer incidence and mortality. (IARC Scientific Publications, No 121) Lyon : IARC, 1993

[74] Osmond C, Gardner MJ. Age-period and cohort models applied to cancer mortality rates. *Stat Med* 1982, **1** : 245-59

[75] Holford TR. The estimation of age, period and cohort effects for vital rates. *Biometrics* 1983, **39** : 311-24

[76] Muir CS, Nectoux J. Time trends : malignant melanoma of skin. *In* K Magnus (ed) : *Trends in cancer incidence : causes and practical implications.* Washington, Hemisphere Publ., 1982 : pp. 365-85

[77] Bulliard JL, Raymond L, Levi F et al. Évaluation épidémiologique préliminaire de la campagne suisse pour la prévention du mélanome malin. *Med Hyg* 1990, **48** : 370-4

[78] Bouchardy C, Fioretta G, Raymond L, Vassilakos P. Age differentials in trends of uterine cervical cancer incidence from 1970 to 1987 in Geneva. *Rev Epidémiol Santé Publ* 1990, **38** : 261-2

[79] Cliff AD, Haggett P. *Atlas of disease distributions : analytic approaches to epidemiological data.* Oxford : Basil Blackwell, 1988

[80] Boyle P, Muir, CS, Grundmann E (eds) *Cancer Mapping.* Berlin, Springer, 1989. (*Recents results in cancer research,* **114**)

[81] Walter SD, Birnie SE. Mapping mortality and morbidity patterns. *Int J Epidemiol* 1991, **20** : 678-689

[82] Royal Statistical Society meeting on cancer near nuclear installations. *J R Statist Soc A* 1989, **152** : 305-89

[83] Marshall RJ. A review of methods for the statistical analysis of spatial patterns of diseases. *J R Statist Soc A* 1991, **154** : 421-41

[84] Clayton D, Bernardinelli L. Bayesian methods for mapping disease risk. *In* P Elliott, J Cuzick, D English, R Stern (eds) : *Geographical and environmental epidemiology : methods for small area studies.* Oxford, Oxford University Press, 1992

[85] Bernardinelli L, Montomoli C. Empirical Bayes versus fully Bayes analysis of geographical variation in disease risk. *Stat Med* 1992, **11** : 983-1007

[86] Breslow NE, Enstrom JE. Geographic correlations between cancer mortality rates and alcohol-tobacco consumption in the United States. *J Natl Cancer Inst* 1974, **53** : 631-9

[87] Armstrong B, Doll R. Environmental factors and cancer incidence and mortality in different countries, with special reference to dietary practices. *Int J Cancer* 1975, 15 : 617-31

[88] Knox EG. Foods and diseases. *Br J Prev Soc Med* 1977, 31 : 71-80

[89] Viel JF. Étude des associations géographiques entre mortalité par cancers en milieu agricole et exposition aux pesticides. [Dissertation]. Paris : Université Paris XI, Faculté de Médecine Paris Sud, 1992

[90] Clifford P, Richardson S, Hémon D. Assessing the significance of the correlation between two spatial processes. *Biometrics* 1989, 45 : 123-34

[91] Steinitz R, Parkin DM, Young JL, Bieber CA, Katz L. *Cancer incidence in Jewish migrants to Israel, 1961-1981.* (IARC Scientific Publications, No 98), Lyon, IARC, 1989

[92] Breslow NE, Clayton DG. Approximate inference in generalized linear mixed models. Technical Report n° 106. Seattle WA : Department of Biostatistics School of Public Health, 1991 (Technical report; n° 106)

[93] Desouza CM. An empirical Bayes formulation of cohort models in cancer epidemiology. *Stat Med* 1991, 10 : 1241-56

[94] Zeger SL, Karim MR, Generalized linear models with random effects – A Gibbs sampling approach. *J Am Stat Assoc* 1991, **86** : 79-86

[95] Hakulinen T, Andersen AA, Malker B et al. *Trends in cancer incidence in the Nordic countries.* Helsinki : The Nordic Cancer Registries, 1986

[96] Osmond C, Gardner MJ, Acheson ED. Analysis of trends in cancer mortality in England and Wales during 1951-80 separating changes associated with period of birth and period of death. *Br Med J* 1982, **284** : 1005-8

[97] Devesa S, Silverman D, Young JL et al. Cancer incidence and mortality trends among whites in the United States, 1947-84. *J Natl Cancer Inst* 1987, **79** : 701-70

[98] Lee HP, Day NE, Shanmugaratnam K. Trends in cancer incidence in Singapore 1968-82. (IARC Scientific Publications, No 91), Lyon, IARC, 1988

[99] La Vecchia C, Lucchini F, Negri E, Boyle P, Maisonneuve P, Levi F. Trends of cancer mortality in Europe, 1955-1989. I. Digestive sites. *Eur J Cancer* 1992, **28** : 132-235

[100] Magnus K, ed. *Trends in cancer incidence. Causes and practical implications.* Washington DC : Hemisphere Publishing Corp, 1982

[101] Davis DL, Hoel D. Trends in cancer mortality in industrial countries. *Ann NY Acad Sci* 1990, **609**, New York

Chapter 4

Techniques for survival analysis

Survival analysis in descriptive epidemiology

The need for the estimation of survival rates[1] is twofold: the first objective is to describe the outcome, with time, of a given disease in a group of patients. The mortality associated with the disease can then be assessed in terms of setting public health priorities or providing prognostic information for a patient newly diagnosed with the disease. The second objective is to compare mortality between various groups of patients or to study survival according to individual characteristics such as sex, age, diagnosis or type of treatment in order to identify prognostic factors. Cancer registries are primarily concerned with the first, descriptive objective.

From this point of view, it is important to remember that survival rates routinely calculated from incident cases in a population should be distinguished from data of the same kind established from a series of hospital patients or from patients included in clinical trials.

Although the methods used in the two situations are identical, the groups studied in treatment evaluation are submitted to numerous selection criteria (recognized or unrecognized) and only rarely represent the full epidemiological diversity of the patient population. Survival rates estimated from incident cases (from which it is standard practice to remove cases discovered at death) can thus be noticeably different from hospital results, with the extent of difference depending on the selection process which affects the hospital population under study (see page 268). Conversely, survival rates established in an epidemiological context can only be used to estimate the overall efficiency of the health system, which depends not only on the quality of care but also on the accessibility of the system and the consequent likelihood of early diagnosis. For this reason, these rates do not lend themselves to retrospective evaluation of treatment even if the necessary information is available for some or all of the incident cases.

The analysis of survival data, like all epidemiological analysis, requires standardization of the case definitions. In particular, the diagnostic classification, including

---

[1] The expression "survival rates" will be used in this chapter as meaning survival probability, as it is current practice among clinicians, despite the fact that rate and probability are different concepts in theory.

site, subsite and histological type, may give rise to heterogeneity in the groups being studied. This issue will not be considered here.

We must also acknowledge the fundamental role of the stage of disease at the time of diagnosis. The apparent benefit of an early diagnosis, as measured by an increase in survival time, may be misleading if it only reflects the addition to the survival time of the *lead time* which separates early detection time from the time at which diagnosis is usually made clinically. Thus, screening and early detection may in reality be prolonging the period of morbidity while having no effect whatsoever on the natural history of the disease [1]. In fact, such arguments are not always easy to challenge in the absence of good information on the distribution of the time spent in the preclinical phase of the disease. However, if such were the situation, the survival curve would have about the same shape after the lead time for patients diagnosed early, and their age at death would not be changed [2]. In any case, the standardization of criteria defining date of incidence remains a fundamental objective.

The problems associated with data collection must not be ignored. In the study of survival, as in the study of disease incidence, it is essential to question the reliability of the data. In order to avoid bias, data collection systems should allow not only for the routine registration of death but also for the active verification of the status of cases for which no information on death has been received.

The primary objective of this chapter is to provide the means to calculate as precisely as possible the survival probability as a function of the time elapsed since the occurrence of the event marking the beginning of follow-up. This function of time defines the survival curve of the group under study. The necessary material is covered from page 216 to 222.

Survival data, like incidence data, are subject to sampling variation, that is, they can provide only an estimate of an unknown, underlying reality. For this reason, the degree of confidence to be attached to the results is also considered (confidence interval).

We will then examine (see page 231) methods that have been proposed to take account of the effect of competing causes of death, in order to provide a better understanding of the phenomenon under study: a cancer patient is not protected from other risks of death and adjustment for these is needed for assessing the specific effect of the cancer on the risk of death. Some authors calculate *cause-specific survival*, which only takes into account death due to the disease being studied. Among alternative methods that have been proposed, the most widely used is that of *relative survival*, based on the use of the *life table*, the principal concepts of which have been presented in Chapter 1. The reader will find the methods to overcome the possible lack of published life tables on page 236.

Methods to compare survival in two or more groups are dealt with in the second part of this chapter. These problems are very similar to those which were considered under the comparison of age incidence curves. Just as one might prefer the comparison of incidence curves as a whole to the comparison of cumulative risks alone, comparison involving whole survival curves is preferable to a comparison which only concerns survival probabilities at a given time point. However, one is often restricted to this latter comparison in the absence of appropriate data, resulting in the need for methods described briefly on page 246; unfortunately, routinely published data do not always provide all the details needed for making this point comparison.

When comparison is carried out over entire survival curves, the assumption is often made that the instantaneous mortality rates are proportional. In this situation, the optimal test, known as the log rank test, is effectively identical to the Mantel-Haenszel test discussed in Chapter 2. We will re-examine it in the context of survival distribution (see page 247).

Populations that are being compared sometimes experience different mortality patterns after the time of diagnosis: some are subject to a very high initial mortality followed by a long remission; others, in contrast, experience a more regular occurrence of deaths. In the former case, the Gehan-Breslow test, also presented in this section, is in principle more appropriate.

In certain situations, if the necessary information is available, survival comparisons can be made taking confounding factors into account. A further section discusses methods of adjustment or stratification which allow us to take account of confounding factors (see page 255).

When individual characteristics which might affect survival ('prognostic factors') are available for each case under follow-up, it is usual to assess the specific role played by each factor in the prediction of survival time. The stratification approach is however rapidly limited by sample size while it is still possible in some situations to use a modelling approach, despite the small number of subjects available. Cox's multiplicative model provides the necessary tool in this context and is discussed from page .

Calculation of long-term survival raises particular problems: because of ageing, the group is subject to an increasing risk of mortality from causes other than the disease under study. In this situation it becomes important to base comparisons on net survival, requiring the application of specific methods (see page 272).

A number of data sets obtained from cancer registries will be used to illustrate methods that have been mentioned: the first set of data refers to survival of incident cases of colon cancer in the French department of Côte-d'Or. This example illustrates the mathematical calculations required to establish survival probabilities by the actuarial method and their confidence limits. Survival of incident cases of skin melanoma in Geneva (Switzerland) will provide an example of the use of the Kaplan-Meier method. Data on colon cancer in Geneva will serve to illustrate the computation of relative survival rates and similar data from the canton of Vaud (Switzerland) will be considered with those from Côte-d'Or and Geneva to show how to carry out a comparative analysis.

Finally, we will use data from the Geneva cancer registry on various cancer sites to compare the results obtained by the relative survival method and those obtained by the cause-specific survival method where deaths not attributable to the disease are taken as censored observations.

Stratification methods will be illustrated by the comparison of survival distribution for men and women with melanoma, taking subsite as the confounding factor.

The more general modelling approach will be illustrated by the analysis of breast cancer survival in Geneva according to the type of health care system providing the treatment.

Estimation of survival distribution

When concepts associated with the study and interpretation of individual follow-up were discussed in Chapter 1, we presented the notion of *censored observations*, that is, observations which are incomplete and which require a specific methodology. In this section, we will illustrate different techniques proposed for the analysis of survival data. Although some of these techniques have been developed for clinical trials, they can be used in the present context with minor adjustments. Nevertheless, the choice of an analytical method and the interpretation of the results require a specific approach, because of the way the data are obtained, the size of the groups under study and the absence of randomization.

When there are no censored observations, survival probability after a given time is estimated simply by the ratio between the number of survivors at a specific date and the number in the group at the beginning of the study. This probability, called by some authors the direct survival rate, obviously cannot be calculated for individuals in the group for whom the period of follow-up is less than the time interval being considered. The group under study is therefore subdivided into subgroups in which the subjects have the same potential follow-up time and the survival probability calculated in each subgroup is assumed to be an estimate of the survival rate for the corresponding length of time. However, as the resulting probabilities have been obtained from different groups of patients, they will not in general provide a consistent survival curve, that is, the survival probability will not necessarily decrease with time.

In fact, observations with incomplete follow-up can still contribute to the estimation of survival for time intervals greater than the duration of their follow-up. This idea is being used in the following two methods which are also described in a more formal context in Chapter 1.

Estimation of crude survival

Actuarial method

The aim of this method is to study the survival of a group of subjects for whom a common event has occurred; for each subject the date of occurrences marks the beginning of follow-up. In the present context the common event which characterizes the group will be the diagnosis of cancer.

Follow-up of individuals comes to an end either at death, or on the date at which the individual is lost to follow-up, or on the date at which the individual is withdrawn from follow-up, for example for the purpose of analysis of the survival data. In fact, the date of withdrawal may be specific to each individual if assessment of status (living, deceased or lost to follow-up) is only carried out at regular intervals following the date of diagnosis; there may also be a single date of withdrawal if this assessment is carried out on the same date for all individuals (see page 227). The time between the date of diagnosis and the end of follow-up is called the *follow-up time*. Figure 4.1 illustrates the two follow-up procedures discussed above. Note that the recruitment period is generally less than the study period, for example, when we only want to consider cases which have a minimum follow-up time. On the graph, e_1, e_2 and e_3 represent the entry dates of new cases, f_1, f_2 and f_3 the end of individual observation periods, and the solid circles represent dates of assessment of status.

Theoretically, the method is applicable when new cases are recruited who have been diagnosed before their inclusion in the study group. These cases are only included in the calculation from the time when they are actually under observation and not from the date of their diagnosis. If such a precaution is not taken, mortality

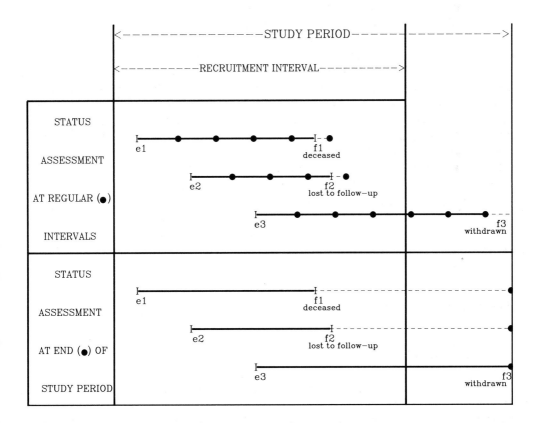

Figure 4.1 Principles of follow-up of cases in a survival study

during the period prior to their inclusion would be underestimated. Apart from the increased complexity in the calculations, it is generally preferable not to take these cases into consideration because of the selection biases to which they may be subject.

The first step of the actuarial method is the subdivision of the maximum observed survival time into intervals; the length of the intervals is set *a priori* taking into account the distribution of deaths over time, so that each interval, on average, has at least some deaths. If necessary, the intervals can be of unequal size.

The second step is the computation of the conditional probabilities in each interval which are defined by the proportion of those living at the start of the interval who were still living at the end of it. However, in order to account for subjects with shorter follow-up time, the number at risk at the beginning of the interval is reduced by half the number of subjects who were withdrawn or lost to follow-up during the interval. The total thus obtained is known as the corrected number of subjects at risk or the *effective number at risk*.

The probability of surviving to the end of a given interval is obtained by multiplying together the conditional probabilities over all the intervals preceding this time point. Survival is obtained by linear interpolation for all other time.

Table 4.1   Calculation of survival probabilities by the actuarial method (incidence of colon cancer in males in Côte-d'Or, France, between 1976 and 1982)

Interval (months) t_i, t_{i+1} (1)	Number at risk in t_i n_i (2)	Number censored r_i (3)	Death d_i (4)	Effective number at risk N_i (5)	Conditional probability of death q_i (6)	Conditional probability of survival s_i (7)	Survival rate S_{i+1} (8)
0-6	411	1	145	410.5	0.353	0.647	0.647
6-12	265	1	40	264.5	0.151	0.849	0.549
12-18	224	0	32	224.0	0.143	0.857	0.471
18-24	192	2	16	191.0	0.084	0.916	0.431
24-30	174	15	15	166.5	0.090	0.910	0.392
30-36	144	15	4	136.5	0.029	0.971	0.381
36-42	125	15	13	117.5	0.111	0.889	0.339
42-48	97	10	4	92.0	0.044	0.956	0.324
48-54	83	11	0	77.5	0.000	1.000	0.324
54-60	72	13	1	65.5	0.015	0.985	0.319

Columns (1) to (4) give observed data; data in columns (5) to (8) have been calculated.

Let:

- t_i, t_{i+1} be the interval end-points ($0 \leq i \leq I - 1$),
- n_i be the number of subjects surviving and followed up at date t_i (number at risk),
- r_i be the number of subjects withdrawn or lost to follow-up in the interval $]t_i, t_{i+1}]$,
- d_i be the number of deaths in the interval $]t_i, t_{i+1}]$,
- $N_i = n_i - (r_i / 2)$ be the corrected number at risk,

- $q_i = d_i / N_i$ be the estimates of the conditional probability of dying in the interval $]t_i, t_{i+1}]$,
- $s_i = 1 - q_i$ be the conditional probability of being alive at t_{i+1} given that the subject was at risk at t_i, and

- $S_{i+1} = \prod_{j=0}^{i} s_j$, the survival probability at t_{i+1}.

The method has the advantage of using all available information, as opposed to the direct survival method, which is based only on cases which have a follow-up time at least equal to the time for which survival probability is being calculated. On the other hand, the method relies on the assumption, sometimes debatable, that those for whom observations are censored are subject to the same force of mortality as cases for whom follow-up is complete.

Table 4.1 shows the details of this calculation using data from the Côte-d'Or on colon cancer in males. Figure 4.2 shows the corresponding survival curve. An interval of six months has been used. Cases lost to follow-up and cases withdrawn from follow-up are treated in the same way and considered to be censored observations.

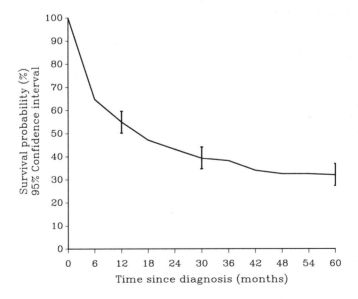

Figure 4.2 Survival of male colon cancer patients in Côte-d'Or, diagnosed between 1976 and 1982

Kaplan-Meier Method

This procedure relies on the same principles as the actuarial method. However, the time intervals are not set *a priori* but are determined by the occurrence of death:

the conditional probabilities of surviving between two dates of death are estimated every time a death occurs. As in the actuarial method, the probability of survival, from the start of follow-up, is obtained by the product of probabilities calculated for each successive interval.

Intervals are usually defined in days. The method requires the calculation of as many survival probabilities as there are deaths, except if several deaths occur on the same day. It is particularly suited to analysing data from small groups. An observation which is censored between two deaths does not affect the cumulative probability of survival, which remains constant in this interval; in principle, it is not necessary to know the exact dates when such observations are censored. However, it is necessary to know the number of censored observations between two deaths which is subtracted from the number at risk at the start of the next interval.

Let:

- t_i be the ith observed time of deaths $1 \leq i \leq I$,
- d_i be the number of observed deaths at t_i,
- r_i be the number of censored observations in interval $[t_i, t_{i+1}[$,
- $n_i = n_{i-1} - d_{i-1} - r_{i-1}$ be the number at risk just before time of deaths occurring in t_i: to obtain n_i, subtract from n_{i-1} the deaths which took place at t_{i-1} and all other cases for which follow-up ended in the interval $[t_{i-1}, t_i[$
- $s_i = 1 - (d_i/n_i)$ be the conditional probability of being alive in $]t_i, t_{i+1}]$ given the subject was at risk at t_i, and
- $S_i = \prod_{j=1}^{i} s_j$ be the probability of surviving after t_i. This probability is constant up to date t_{i+1} inclusive.

The details of the computation are shown in Table 4.2 which refers to data from Geneva for skin melanoma in males. The corresponding survival curve is graphed in Figure 4.3.

We can see that the successive conditional probabilities are calculated here from the true number at risk at the moment when death takes place and not from a number obtained by subtracting half those censored in the interval, as is done in the actuarial method. Furthermore, the latter method assumes a constant force of mortality by interval, while the Kaplan-Meier method makes no assumption about the underlying instantaneous rate.

In practice, both methods give very similar results when they are applied to large groups, which is one of the reasons why most registries traditionally use the actuarial method, the application of which in medicine goes back to J. Graunt [4]. The fixed intervals of the actuarial method are perfectly suited to the classic presentation of survival probability for a given number of years after diagnosis, for example, 1, 3 or 5 year survival. However, the existence of modern computer software makes the application of the Kaplan-Meier method much easier than in the past, and it may be better to consider using it more widely, even for large groups,

Table 4.2   Calculation of the probabilities of survival by the Kaplan-Meier method (incidence of skin melanoma for males, Geneva, Switzerland, 1970)

Day of death	Day (number) of censored observations	Number of deaths	Number of censored observations	Number at risk	Conditional survival at t_i	Survival probability between t_i and t_{i+1}
t_i (1)	(2)	d_i (3)	r_{i-1} (4)	n_i (5)	s_i (6)	S_i (7)
373		1		13	0.923	0.923
643		1		12	0.917	0.846
672		1		11	0.909	0.769
975		1		10	0.900	0.692
1173		1		9	0.889	0.615
	1542(1)					
1645		1	1	7	0.857	0.527
	1891(1)					
	1920(1)					
	2055(1)					
	2148(1)					
	2167(1)					
2481		1	5	1	0.000	0.000

Columns 1 to 3 as well as the first line of column 5 (actual size of the group) give observed data; other values are calculated.

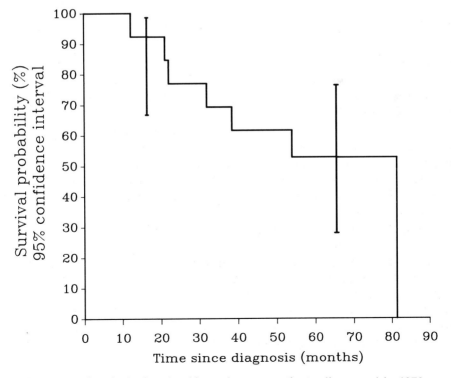

Figure 4.3   Survival of male skin melanoma patients diagnosed in 1970 in Geneva, Switzerland

both for its greater precision and because it is more appealing than the actuarial method in the context of modern tools of survival data analysis.

Confidence interval for a survival rate

The estimation of variability of a survival rate becomes essential when its calculation is carried out on small groups of patients. The computation of confidence limits is usually undertaken for estimating the cumulative survival rates at a given time point. Determining several successive intervals gives an approximate idea of the 'confidence band' within which the real survival curve is taken to be, although, strictly speaking, it does not define the 95% confidence interval of the curve. It is sometimes useful to estimate the confidence intervals of the conditional probabilities of survival, cumulative not from the date of origin but from a given time. For example, one might focus on subjects who have survived for at least two years after diagnosis. The calculations are based on the same methodology.

The estimation of a confidence interval for a cumulative rate S_i is based on the estimation of its variance, which depends in turn on whether the group is *open* or *closed*[2].

In a closed group, survival at time t_i is the proportion of those surviving: $S_i = n_i/n_0$, where n_0 is the initial number and n_i is the number of survivors at time t_i. In this situation, the variance of S_i is simply:

$$V_i = \frac{S_i (1 - S_i)}{n_0} \qquad (4.1)$$

that is, the variance of the estimated probability from n_0 trials among which there are n_i successes (Binomial law).

In the usual situation where the group is open, the number of subjects at risk is decreased over time by censoring; the variance is thus larger than if the entire group had been followed up. Nevertheless, it is smaller than it would be in a closed group which would also have counted n_i survivors and which would have produced the same estimate of survival. In this situation, the initial size of the group would have been

$$n'_0 = \frac{n_i}{S_i} \qquad (4.2)$$

Peto [5] suggests using this theoretical number to determine an upper bound for the variance. Thus, the corresponding standard error is

$$E_i = \sqrt{\frac{S_i (1 - S_i)}{n'_0}} = S_i \sqrt{\frac{1 - S_i}{n_i}} \qquad (4.3)$$

---

[2] See the definition of these terms in Chapter I, page 22

Greenwood [6] based an estimate of the variance of S_i on the estimated variance of the conditional probabilities s_j, which are directly derived as variances of a proportion, since at each time t_j, s_j is the proportion of survivors in the group of subjects at risk of death just before t_j.

Thus:

$$Var\ (s_j) = \frac{s_j\ (1 - s_j)}{n_j} \tag{4.4}$$

Furthermore, since:

$$Log\ (S_i) = \sum_{j=1}^{i} Log\ (s_j) \tag{4.5}$$

the standard method [7] of calculating the variance of Log (s_j) based on the variance of s_j (4.4) can be used to show that

$$Var\ [Log\ (S_i)] = \sum_{j=1}^{i} \frac{Var\ (s_j)}{s_j^2} = \sum_{j=1}^{i} \frac{1 - s_j}{n_j\ s_j} \tag{4.6}$$

and, consequently, that

$$V_i = Var(S_i) = S_i^2 \sum_{j=1}^{i} \frac{1 - s_j}{n_j\ s_j} \tag{4.7}$$

which is the formula that Greenwood established for the actuarial method by replacing n_j, the number at risk at the beginning of the interval, by the effective number at risk N_j. Insofar as this result depends on the estimate of the variance (4.6) being valid for large samples only, this formula can lead to an under-estimation of the variance for long time intervals when the group size is not sufficiently large [8]. This estimate and that proposed by Peto are shown in Table 4.3, in which calculations of variance are made from the data in Table 4.1.

Column 5 of Table 4.3 is obtained by induction:

$$V_0 = 0$$

$$V_{i+1} = V_i\ s_i^2 + S_{i+1}^2\ \frac{(1 - s_i)}{n_i\ s_i} \tag{4.8}$$

The number calculated in column 6 and the standard error in column 7 are obtained from (4.2) and (4.3).

In general, the confidence interval of size α for a survival rate θ can be calculated by

$$\frac{|\ S_i - \theta\ |}{SE\ (S_i)} < Z_{\alpha/2} \tag{4.9}$$

Table 4.3   Calculation of standard errors by Greenwood's and Peto's methods

i (1)	n_i (2)	S_i (3)	S_{i+1} (4)	Greenwood $\sqrt{V_{i+1}}$ (5)	Peto n'_0 (6)	Peto E_{i+1} (7)
0	411	0.647	0.647	0.0236	409.7	0.0236
1	265	0.849	0.549	0.0246	408.0	0.0246
2	224	0.857	0.471	0.0247	408.0	0.0247
3	192	0.916	0.431	0.0245	403.6	0.0246
4	174	0.910	0.392	0.0242	367.1	0.0255
5	144	0.971	0.381	0.0242	328.3	0.0268
6	125	0.899	0.339	0.0242	286.4	0.0280
7	97	0.956	0.324	0.0242	256.2	0.0292
8	83	1.000	0.324	0.0242	222.3	0.0314
9	72	0.985	0.319	0.0244	181.8	0.0346

The numbers in columns 1 to 4 are from Table 4.1 and those in the remaining columns have been derived from formulae 4.8, 4.2 and 4.3.

where θ is the probability of survival to be estimated at t_i and $SE(S_i)$ is the standard error of its estimator S_i. If $SE(S_i)$ is replaced by one or another of the standard errors in Table 4.3 (columns 5 and 7), a symmetric interval is obtained as:

$$[S_i' , S_i''] = S_i \pm Z_{\alpha/2} SE (S_i) \qquad (4.10)$$

since when time t is fixed, the estimate of the survival rate at time t is approximately normally distributed.

As Rothman suggests [9], it is also possible to calculate an interval whose

limits always lie between 0 and 1, by substituting the quantity $\sqrt{\dfrac{\theta(1-\theta)}{n''_0}}$ for $SE(S_i)$ in equation (4.9) with

$$n''_0 = \frac{S_i (1 - S_i)}{V_i} \qquad (4.11)$$

where V_i is either Greenwood's variance or the maximum variance postulated by Peto. The confidence interval is then obtained by solving equation (4.9) for θ:

$$[S'_i, S''_i] = \frac{n''_0}{n''_0 + Z_{\alpha/2}^2} \left[S_i + \frac{Z_{\alpha/2}^2}{2n''_0} \pm Z_{\alpha/2} \sqrt{\frac{S_i(1 - S_i)}{n''_0} + \frac{Z_{\alpha/2}^2}{4n''^2_0}} \right] \qquad (4.12)$$

The choice between the many different ways of calculating the confidence interval depends on practical considerations and on how conservative an estimate is required. For routine calculations, most scientists in cancer registries use the wider symmetric confidence interval (4.10) with the Greenwood standard error. We prefer to use (4.12) with the theoretical number n''_0 derived from Greenwood's variance (4.11). In fact it has been shown that this method on average provides the most satisfactory result [10]. Note however that the symmetric confidence interval derived by Peto is an easily-obtained estimate of the magnitude of the variability of the survival probability estimate.

Table 4.4 shows survival probability at 12, 30 and 60 months for cancer of the colon in men in Côte-d'Or between January 1976 and December 1982, and confidence intervals obtained using the three methods discussed. The differences are only noteworthy after 60 months, when Peto's interval is substantially wider.

Table 4.4   Confidence intervals for survival; data from Table 4.1.

Time since diagnosis (months) t_i	Survival probability S_i	Greenwood Rothman	Greenwood symmetric	Peto symmetric
12	0.549	0.501 ; 0.596	0.501 ; 0.597	0.501 ; 0.597
18	0.471	0.423 ; 0.519	0.422 ; 0.519	0.422 ; 0.519
24	0.431	0.384 ; 0.480	0.383 ; 0.479	0.383 ; 0.479
30	0.392	0.346 ; 0.441	0.345 ; 0.440	0.342 ; 0.442
60	0.319	0.273 ; 0.368	0.271 ; 0.367	0.251 ; 0.387

Median survival time

With the preceding methods, the distribution of survival times can be correctly estimated in the presence of censoring without making assumptions about the analytical shape of this distribution. However, by not adopting parametric models, we cannot use the method of maximum likelihood, which is an effective tool for estimating parameters such as life expectancy and its confidence interval. In all the methods previously described, it is accepted practice to estimate quantiles of the distribution of survival. In particular, the median survival time is the time at which the survival rate is equal to 50%. This value can be estimated from the curve calculated using one of the methods previously described. The median survival time is a readily calculated location parameter which provides an easily interpretable summary of the data.

In the actuarial method, a unique value of this median is usually obtained because the survival curve is continuous and, more often than not, strictly decreasing. If S_i and S_{i+1} are respectively the survival rates at the end points of the intervals which include the value 0.5, then the median of the observed distribution is obtained by linear interpolation:

$$m = t_i + \frac{S_i - 0,5}{S_i - S_{i+1}} (t_{i+1} - t_i) \qquad (4.13)$$

for data relating to cancer of the colon in Côte-d'Or (Table 4.1), the observed median is

$$m = 12 + \frac{0.549 - 0.500}{0.549 - 0.471}(18 - 12) = 15.77 \, \text{months} \tag{4.14}$$

If the survival probability is estimated by the Kaplan-Meier method, there is in general no time for which the observed survival rate is exactly equal to 0.5. The observed median can be taken as the date of the first death corresponding to a survival rate less than or equal to 0.50. For the data on melanoma (Table 4.2), the survival rate is not less than 0.5 before the last observed event, which is a death at 2481 days. Strictly speaking, the median survival is thus 2481 days, or six years and nine months. In fact, in this example, it is clear that the estimate is imprecise because of the small number of observed cases. As a general rule, the variability of this parameter can be substantial. Therefore, it is important that it be accompanied by its confidence interval.

Figure 4.4, based on hypothetical data, shows that a confidence interval for the median can be obtained by simply inverting the functions representing the lower and upper confidence limits of the survival probability. The confidence region R_α for the median is thus contructed from the confidence interval of the survival probability defined as in the previous paragraph. A time point t is included in the confidence region of the median if the confidence interval for S_t includes 0.50:

$$R_\alpha = \left[t \mid \left(S_t - \frac{1}{2} \right)^2 < Z^2_{\alpha/2} \, V_t \right] \tag{4.15}$$

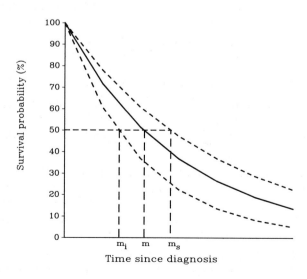

Figure 4.4 **Confidence interval of median survival**

When the actuarial method is used, the upper and lower confidence limits of the median are determined by interpolation. For example, survival following cancer of the colon in Côte-d'Or is greater than 0.501 at 12 months and greater than 0.423 at 18 months (lower bound of the confidence interval) (Table 4.4); the survival time for which the lower bound of the confidence interval is exactly equal to 0.5 is thus found between 12 and 18 months. This time is obtained by linear interpolation:

$$12 + \frac{0.501 - 0.500}{0.501 - 0.423} \times 6 = 12.08\,\text{months} \qquad (4.16)$$

Similarly, survival is less than 0.519 at 18 months and less than 0.480 at 24 months (upper bound of the confidence interval) (Table 4.4). Survival will thus be less than 0.50 at 20.85 months. Therefore the confidence interval of the median is [12.08 ; 20.85].

When the Kaplan-Meier method is used, the upper and lower confidence limits of the median are obtained by determining respectively the first and last date of death for which the confidence interval of survival includes the value 0.50 [11,12]. When this method is applied to the data in Table 4.2, it is seen that the confidence interval of S_t includes 0.50 from t = 975 days and that all the subsequent time points are those which correspond to survival probabilities for which the confidence interval includes 0.5. As a result, the confidence interval of the median extends from two years and eight months to infinity, illustrating the imprecision obtained with a small number of cases.

Collecting data for survival analysis

In the usual situation of an open group, we have just seen that the calculation of survival rates requires specific variables for each member of the group:

- date at which follow-up started (date of incidence)
- date when follow-up ended
- status of the subject at this date (dead, living, lost to follow-up).

we have also seen that the date at which follow-up ended for each individual is either the date of death, the last date at which the subject was known to be alive for those who were lost to follow-up, or the date at which follow-up is ended for all subjects as a result of the study being concluded.

This information can be obtained either on an ongoing basis or retrospectively. It comes in general from a variety of sources. These sources are rarely perfect and can give rise to selection biases of different kinds, especially when they involve routine forms of data reporting. For example, failure to notify certain deaths results in the overestimation of survival. The same effect occurs indirectly when the number of individuals lost to follow-up is underestimated, since these cases are then wrongly counted in the numerator and denominator of the survival probabilities. More subtle biases can arise when the amount of information obtained on an individual depends on his or her status. For example, the status of a patient may be better known simply because of a regular presentation to an oncology department or, conversely, because a death has been recorded. Consequently, no matter how good routine reporting sources may be, it is advisable to carry out a regular update to check the status of all subjects not known to have died, probably using reporting sources independent of those already employed routinely. In other words, for these cases, *passive* follow-up should be complemented by *active* follow-up which may involve searches of official records, direct contact with the patient or the patient's family or other sources.

From an administrative point of view, it is sensible to carry out these updates individually at regular intervals from the date at which follow-up started, for example at every fifth anniversary of the date of incidence. This procedure ensures that the tasks required for active follow-up are ongoing throughout the year rather than all being carried out at once when it is time to analyse the data. Whatever procedure is used, the duration of follow-up should be ended at the date of the last update which ends the follow-up period for the subject.

When the survival probability is calculated for all incident cases, follow-up of subjects who are officially recorded as having left the geographic area covered by registration should be censored at the date of departure, and should be treated as lost to follow-up. Following subjects outside this area can introduce a bias if it is routinely easier to obtain information on death or, conversely, on the surviving patients. A death which occurs outside the registration area obviously should not be counted even if it is known to have occurred. Updates should be organised in such a way that cases lost to follow-up in the literal sense of the term, that is, those cases for which it is not known whether they have left the area or not, are the exception.

Calculating survival probability solely from cases residing in an area for the whole follow-up period has the apparent advantage of characterising the effectiveness of regional medical care. However, when departure from the area is linked to stage of disease (and to the survival probability which follows from it), this way of proceeding might plausibly introduce a bias in the results. For example, suppose that foreign workers with cancer routinely return home, as soon as their condition worsens, to die in their own country. There is unfortunately no ideal solution to resolve this difficulty; only the appraisal of each individual situation ensures that resulting biases are appropriately evaluated.

The mode of follow-up can have a considerable effect on the reliability of results obtained in survival analysis. It is instructive to compare the follow-up procedures used in Côte-d'Or, Geneva and the Swiss canton of Vaud (from where the data used as examples in this chapter have been drawn). Following accepted practice, incident cases in the three regions which are known only from death certificates are excluded from calculation.

In Côte-d'Or, follow-up of patients is based on routine registration of deaths and on an annual update at a fixed time to check the status of all cases. Routine registration identifies approximately 75% of deaths occurring in patients with cancer of the colon. This percentage varies with age, treatment and survival time. The status of patients for whom there is no report of death is obtained on a fixed date, partially from government registry offices at the place of birth (except for foreign-born subjects) and partially from clinicians (gastroenterologists, surgeons and general medical practitioners). Alltogether, in 98% of cases it is thus known whether the patient is living or dead.

In Geneva, follow-up is carried out from two sources of information, one being the updating of the database from routine notification of death, the second resulting from a regular check-up at five-yearly intervals from the date at which follow-up started, for subjects believed to be alive. There are multiple sources of information on deaths: the cancer registry has the right to obtain from the health authority a copy of all death certificates which mention cancer as a cause of death. The registry can be incidentally informed of death when collecting missing data from the hospital records. Finally, information on death is obtained annually by merging records of incident cases with death records at a national level. This link-up of data is based on the date and place of birth. The five-year update is done by manually consulting population records, allowing the registry to note dates of any definite departures and to stop follow-up accordingly. Deaths which might otherwise have escaped detection can also be detected by this manual consultation. It is important to emphasise that cases are only included in the calculation of survival for the period covered by the five-year update. Events which follow this update are not taken into consideration even if they are already registered. In particular, deaths occurring after the time when the update takes place must not be included in the analysis.

In the canton of Vaud, follow-up is based principally on the regular linkage between mortality files held by the Federal Swiss Office of Statistics, and the registry of incident cases. Linkage is achieved by a series of computer processes accompanied by manual verification. The routine update also involves an investigation of cases presumed living, through the municipal population registries in order to determine status and dates of any departures from the canton. Active follow-up is organized and status is determined at a single fixed date for all cases (31 December).

Estimation of net survival

The study of survival in a population subgroup is often motivated by the supposition that the subgroup is subject to a risk of death different from that experienced by other individuals in the population. For example, people with cancer generally experience a much higher mortality than the general population in the years immediately following diagnosis. Insofar as the increase in risk due to the disease being studied tends to diminish, mortality progressively returns to 'normal'. Overall survival probability should therefore be considered as the result of two components, corresponding respectively to the disease being studied and to all other causes taken together.

Thus a *net survival* can be defined as that which might occur if the risks of death other than the cancer were removed. Its complement is none other than the *net probability* of death (see Chapter 1, page 34). Analysing the net survival probability is thus equivalent to the analysis of the excess mortality in the group under study.

To the extent that it is accurately estimated, net survival probability tends to become constant as deaths due to cancer decrease. It then represents the percentage of subjects who can be considered to be cured of the cancer under study. The time period corresponding to the point when net survival probability becomes constant can thus be interpreted as a recovery period. As for all estimates, this value is only valid as an average for the group; it does not exclude the possibility of a fatal recurrence for certain individuals outside this time period.

The justification for calculating the additional risk due to the cancer under study is particularly clear when considering an older age group, because the force of mortality from other causes increases with age. As a group ages over time, net survival probability tends to be decreasingly well represented by observed survival probability, which is increasingly determined by death from other causes. The estimation of net survival probability also responds to the need to make comparisons between subpopulations from the same region or between populations from different regions where the mortality due to other causes may differ such that the comparison of overall survival probabilities might lead to biased conclusions.

The determination of net survival probabilities implicitly assumes that the risk of death from the cancer being studied and the risk of death from other causes are independent, that is, *not interactive* (see Chapter 1, page 34 for the definition of this term). In fact, with cancer, the two risks seem to be positively correlated: the presence of cancer and its treatment cause an increase in the force of mortality from other causes. The inverse situation cannot however be excluded. When survival time increases, the survivors of the group might benefit from a reduction in the risk of death from other causes, because of better medical care or a decrease of risk-related behaviour. It will be seen later that such interactions cannot be totally ignored when deciding which method to use in estimating net survival or when interpreting the results.

There are two classical methods available to estimate the probability of surviving a given disease: the method of *cause-specific survival* and that of *relative survival*.

Cause-specific survival

The principle of this method is simple: the cause of each death is assessed and only those deaths that can be attributed to the disease under study are counted. Other deaths are considered as simply termination of follow-up (in the same way as cases lost to follow-up and observations which are censored at the end of the study). Calculation of cause-specific survival can also be carried out by the actuarial method or by the Kaplan-Meier method. Under both methods, survival rates are obtained disregarding deaths from other causes. However, if these methods are used, note that it is assumed that the process leading to death from cancer is independent of the process leading to death from other causes, an assumption which is often only approximately true (for example, when a suicide occurs following the diagnosis of advanced cancer).

The method of cause-specific survival is sometimes used in a clinical setting if follow-up is of sufficient quality to distinguish between deaths due to the disease under study and other deaths. The method can only be applied to epidemiological data when the cause of death is routinely recorded, a situation which does not generally hold in population registries. Whatever the situation, the method of cause-specific survival comes up against the difficulties of determining cause of death such as the doubtful reliability of information supplied by the certifying doctor and the arbitrary choice of the primary cause of death when there are multiple or associated pathologies. Moreover, it would seem practically impossible, as much as it would be appropriate, to take into consideration deaths caused by secondary effects of treatment.

Relative survival

The method of relative survival [13] does not require knowledge of the cause of death and thus avoids the difficulties associated with its determination. The method involves calculating, at each time period t, the *relative survival probabilities* defined by the relationship

$$S_c(t) = \frac{S_o(t)}{S_e(t)} \tag{4.17}$$

where $S_o(t)$ and $S_e(t)$ are respectively observed survival and expected survival at time t.

Expected survival corresponds to the mortality of the general population, taking into account the initial distribution in the group of prognostic factors which one wishes to control for. If only age (the effects of which should always be accounted for) is considered, the expected survival $S_e(t)$ is provided by the proportion of survivors that would be predicted at time t in a group having the same initial age structure as the group under study, but subject only to the force of mortality of the general population. The adjustment is thus a standardisation of the indirect type. The calculation of the expected number of survivors is firstly done for each subgroup defined by age at diagnosis in single years or by larger age groups according to the available life tables. Expected deaths are then summed. If n_x is the number of subjects of age x at the beginning of follow-up and $S_{ex}(t)$ is the probability of survival at time t for a subject with initial age x, then the number of survivors at time t for this age group is

$$e_x(t) = n_x S_{ex}(t) \tag{4.18}$$

The total number of survivors at this time is thus:

$$\sum_x e_x(t) = \sum_x n_x S_{ex}(t) \tag{4.19}$$

Consequently, the overall expected survival is

$$S_e(t) = \frac{\sum_x n_x S_{ex}(t)}{\sum_x n_x} \tag{4.20}$$

that is, the average survival probability at time point t, weighted by the initial number.

Remember that survival after t years of a group of individuals aged x at diagnosis whose follow-up can only terminate only with the death of the subjects (ie, a closed group) is equal to the ratio of the number of survivors of age x+t to the number of survivors of age x. Thus

$$S_{ex}(t) = \frac{\ell_{x+0.5+t}}{\ell_{x+0.5}} \tag{4.21}$$

by using the data and expressions of the life table (see page   in this chapter and Chapter 1). The half year results from the fact that the table is related to the birthday, while in fact an individual considered to be aged x is, on average, aged x + 0.5. The number of survivors at age x + 0.5 is obtained by linear interpolation of the values given in the table:

$$\ell_{x+0.5} = \frac{\ell_x + \ell_{x+1}}{2} \tag{4.22}$$

Even if the calculation of expected survival does not have to be very precise (in particular concerning relatively short survival times, for which observed survival is generally substantially less than expected survival), the simplest method is to use a table which gives the number of survivors at each birthday. When the computation is carried out from a table in which the age groups are of a duration Δx greater than one year (known as an abridged life table, for example, by five-yearly age groups), the correction is made in the same way and the value will correspond to the number of survivors at age x + Δx/2.

The life table which is used should reflect the general mortality of the region at the appropriate time. If the rate of mortality does not change too quickly and if follow-up is over a long time, adopting a life table which relates to the middle of this time period will be adequate. For example, a table based on a population census carried out in 1980 can be suitable for a cohort recruited in 1975 and followed up for ten years. If the time for which survival probability is calculated increases, it might be necessary to adopt mortality rates derived from several successive tables. If the survival of the general population improves, the use of only one table could produce an artificial improvement in the relative survival by underestimating the expected survival of more recent cohorts. Furthermore, it will be seen in the following section that the construction of a life table does not present any special difficulties when complete data on the population and deaths are available, and that large numbers guarantee precise results.

When prognostic factors other than age and sex are identified, it is preferable to calculate expected survival by taking them into account. Examples of such factors are marital status, ethnicity and socioeconomic status. Their incorporation in the analysis can be achieved if the data necessary to construct the life tables are available as a function of these variables.

As an example, Table 4.5 shows some of the calculations used to establish expected survival for cancer of the colon for males in Geneva between 1970 and 1979.

Table 4.5   Calculation of the expected number of survivors[a] for cancer of the colon for males in Geneva, Switzerland; incident cases 1970-1979

Age (years)	Survivor function	Number at risk	Expected proportion of survivors [b] after:					Expected number of survivors [b] after:				
x,x+1	ℓ_x	N_x	1 year	2 years	3 years	4 years	5 years	1 year	2 years	3 years	4 years	5 years
1	2	3	4	5	6	7	8	9	10	11	12	13
15-19	9831	4	0.9989	0.9978	0.9963	0.9945	0.9926	4.00	3.99	3.99	3.98	3.97
20-24	9777	1	0.9982	0.9963	0.9947	0.9932	0.9918	1.00	1.00	0.99	0.99	0.99
25-29	9686	5	0.9985	0.9971	0.9958	0.9945	0.9933	4.99	4.99	4.98	4.97	4.97
30-34	9616	3	0.9987	0.9975	0.9960	0.9943	0.9926	3.00	2.99	2.99	2.98	2.98
35-39	9556	1	0.9983	0.9966	0.9943	0.9915	0.9886	1.00	1.00	0.99	0.99	0.99
40-44	9474	19	0.9972	0.9943	0.9907	0.9864	0.9820	18.95	18.89	18.82	18.74	18.66
45-49	9340	22	0.9956	0.9912	0.9854	0.9783	0.9712	21.90	21.81	21.68	21.52	21.37
50-54	9136	29	0.9927	0.9854	0.9764	0.9658	0.9552	28.79	28.58	28.32	28.01	27.70
55-59	8807	34	0.9889	0.9778	0.9634	0.9459	0.9283	33.62	33.24	32.76	32.16	31.56
60-64	8331	60	0.9811	0.9622	0.9393	0.9124	0.8855	58.87	57.73	56.36	54.74	53.13
65-69	7579	75	0.9696	0.9392	0.9041	0.8642	0.8243	72.72	70.44	67.81	64.82	61.82
70-74	6509	72	0.9517	0.9033	0.8515	0.7963	0.7410	68.52	65.04	61.31	57.33	53.36
75-79	5104	61	0.9256	0.8511	0.7766	0.7022	0.6277	56.46	51.92	47.37	42.83	38.29
80-84	3501	47	0.8816	0.7630	0.6468	0.5329	0.4191	41.43	35.86	30.40	25.05	19.70
85-89	1900	16	0.7286	0.4569	0.2905	0.2297	0.1689	11.66	7.31	4.65	3.68	2.70
90-94	363	5	0.6398	0.2796	0.0895	0.0696	0.0497	3.20	1.40	0.45	0.35	0.25
Total		454	0.9474	0.8947	0.8455	0.7999	0.7543	430.10	406.18	383.86	363.14	342.43

[a] Life table for Geneva 1976-80 (Table 4.9).
[b] Columns 4 to 8 are derived from column 2; columns 9 to 13 are derived from the preceding columns. For example, the expected proportion of survivors after three years for the age group 50 to 54 years is:

$$\frac{\ell_{50+3+2.5}}{\ell_{50+2.5}} = \frac{\ell_{55.5}}{\ell_{52.5}} = \frac{(4.5 \times 8807 + 0.5 \times 8331)/5}{(9136 + 8807)/2} = 0.9764$$

The number of expected survivors is therefore $29 \times 0.9764 = 28.32$. Columns 4 to 8 of the last line are obtained from the last five columns. Expected survival at five years for the whole group is $342.43/454 = 0.7543$.

The above calculations have been obtained from the life table based on five-yearly age intervals shown in Table 4.9. This table has been constructed using the method described below (see page 236). When a life table by single years of age is available, the calculations are based on annual and not five-yearly interpolations and are slightly more accurate. As an example, the expected survival of the same group has also been estimated from the Swiss life table (1978-1983) by single years of age in Annex 1. Initially, the survivors at regular yearly intervals are used and then those at five-yearly anniversaries as if the life table had been abridged. Table 4.6 shows the results using these different methods.

Table 4.6 Expected number of survivors from two life tables for cancer of the colon in men in Geneva, Switzerland (incident cases 1970-1979)

Time since diagnosis (years)	Expected number of survivors		
	Geneva table 1976-1980	Swiss table [a] 1978-1983	
	Quinquennial	Annual	Quinquennial
1	430.1	433.1	432.3
2	406.2	412.3	410.6
3	383.9	391.9	389.8
4	363.1	371.8	369.9
5	342.4	352.0	349.9

[a] See Annex 1.

The results obtained from the Swiss life table show that the use of a five-yearly table hardly changes the estimate of the expected number of survivors obtained from the annual life table. On the other hand, the earlier Geneva life table (1976-1980) gives estimates which are noticeably less than those obtained from the Swiss life table (1978-1983). The observed differences probably reflect real differences in mortality both between Switzerland as a whole and Geneva, and between time periods. However, Table 4.7 shows that the differences between the relative survival probabilities are no more than 2%, which is certainly smaller than the differences between the results obtained with this method and alternative methods described below.

The confidence interval of the relative survival probability is proportional to that of the observed survival if the random variation in expected survival can be assumed to be negligible. The standard error for S_c is thus

$$SE(S_c) = \frac{SE(S_o)}{S_e} \tag{4.23}$$

Table 4.8 gives cause-specific and relative survival for various cancer sites at five years estimated from data from Geneva. For cause-specific survival, deaths have been attributed to the cancer concerned when the first three numbers of the

Table 4.7 Expected and relative survival probabilities from two life tables for cancer of the colon in men in Geneva, Switzerland (incident cases 1970-1979)

Time since diagnosis (years)	Observed survival[a]	Expected survival		Relative survival	
		1976-1980[b]	1978-1983[c]	1976-1980[b]	1978-1983[c]
1	0.601	0.947	0.954	0.634	0.630
2	0.479	0.895	0.908	0.535	0.528
3	0.402	0.846	0.863	0.475	0.466
4	0.352	0.800	0.819	0.440	0.430
5	0.324	0.754	0.775	0.429	0.418

[a] Actuarial survival probability calculated from three-monthly intervals.
[b] Geneva life table (Table 4.9).
[c] Annual Swiss life table (Annex 1).

Table 4.8 Cause-specific and relative survival probabilities; Geneva, Switzerland (incident cases 1970-1977)

Site (sex)	Survival probabilities at 5 years	
	Relative	Cause-specific
Stomach (M)	0.16	0.19
Colon (M)	0.35	0.37
Colon (F)	0.37	0.36
Lung (M)	0.09	0.11
Breast (F)	0.69	0.71
Prostate	0.40	0.46
Ovary	0.29	0.30
Bladder (F)	0.38	0.45

ICD 8 code for the primary cause of death (coded by the Registry according to the WHO rules) correspond to the code for the site. Note that under this procedure, carried out in a registry where the causes of death are systematically verified and corrected if necessary, the specific rates for most sites are more optimistic than those obtained by the method of relative survival. This difference can be explained by the fact that, in contrast to cause-specific survival, the method of relative survival attributes to the cancer any deaths resulting from the secondary effects of treatment or from diseases caused by the same risk factors as the cancer.

The method of relative survival is also based on the assumption that the general mortality, as it is described by the life table of the population adequately takes account of all causes of mortality, except for the specific cause under study. This cause is considered to be negligible in comparison to all other causes of death. Only on this condition can relative survival provide an acceptable approximation to net survival. If this assumption does not hold, net survival will be overestimated as a result of the overestimation of the mortality due to other causes. For example, it is known that in women aged 50 to 54 years mortality from breast cancer is responsible for approximately one death in six. If the method of relative survival is applied to this cause in this age group, net survival will be markedly overestimated. If death rates by cause are available for the general population, it is possible to calculate probabilities of death and then of survival by subtracting the risk of death due to the cancer under study. However, this precaution is rarely taken in practice. Indeed, it has been suggested that this correction is excessive, because the group under follow-up is still at risk of developing a second malignancy at the same site [13]. In addition, the life expectancy of a group of patients may in fact be less than that in the general population, as a result of the factors to which the patients have been exposed. These factors can lead to an increase in the risk of dying from other causes (for example, other diseases related to tobacco in people with lung cancer). In this case, the relative survival could be less favourable because of factors associated with the disease rather than because of the disease itself. The cause-specific survival, on the other hand, would not be affected by the occurrence of these deaths, since they would be attributed to other causes.

As we have indicated above, the determination of the time point t at which relative survival becomes constant leads to an estimate of the percentage $S_c(t)$ of people cured, because t corresponds to the moment at which deaths due to the cause under study are no longer recorded. Graphically, from t onwards the observed and expected survival curves become parallel on a logarithmic scale. In practice, a plateau of this kind in the relative survival is not uncommon even when deaths due to the cancer under study continue to be recorded. Furthermore, the relative survival may even start rising from a certain point onwards. Some authors have attributed this increase to the fact that mortality in surviving patients, who are receiving good medical care, can in the long term be less that that in the general population. This explanation is nonetheless incompatible with the interpretation of relative survival as an estimate of net survival. We will see (page 242) that this effect is more frequently due to a methodological bias [14].

Constructing a life table

Life tables established by national statistical services are usually available to calculate expected survival in the absence of cancer. However, it can happen that there is no life table suitable for the population being studied, either because the last official table is out of date or because the population being followed is too selected for its mortality to be described by the official table available. In this situation, a table can be built from available mortality rates (or calculated specifically for the purpose) provided they are sufficiently reliable and statistically accurate. Frequently, these conditions can only be fulfilled by using a table abridged in five-year age groups, and a long period of follow-up to calculate the mortality rates.

The method described below provides approximate results but sufficient accuracy for the objective. The results differ by definition from those which official statistical services would calculate from similar data; national tables are in fact made by using various methods to smooth the data and, especially in older age groups, are based on mathematical models of mortality. These procedures are not discussed here.

We saw in Chapter 1 that the life table was defined entirely by the probabilities of dying in the different age groups and that these probabilities could be directly estimated from mortality rates (Chapter 1, formula 1.31):

$$q_x = \frac{2\lambda_x \Delta_x}{2 + \lambda_x \Delta_x}$$ (4.24)

where λ_x is the annual mortality rate for the age group x and Δ_x the length in years of the age interval. In a five-yearly table, the probability of dying for each age group is obtained by

$$q_x = \frac{10\lambda_x}{2 + 5\lambda_x}$$

It is usual however to break down the first five-year interval by estimating the probability of dying in the first year of life separately. Thus, for the first age group (x = 0), and taking into account the concentration of deaths in the first days of life, it may be accepted that

$$q_0 = \lambda_0$$ (4.25)

and, from the formula above, the probability of dying during the four following years is estimated as

$$q_1 = \frac{8\lambda_1}{2 + 4\lambda_1}$$ (4.26)

Up until the age group 70-74 years, this formula provides sufficient accuracy. For older age groups, Reed and Merrel's formula is recommended [15]. For $\Delta_x = 5$ this formula gives:

$$q'_x = 1 - e^{(-5\lambda_x - \lambda_x^2)}$$ (4.27)

The number of survivors at the beginning of each five-year period can then be calculated by applying the successive probabilities of death starting with the initial number (root of the table), equal for example to 10 000:

$$\ell_{x+5} = \ell_x (1 - q_x)$$ (4.28)

As an example, Table 4.9 shows the results obtained from mortality rates observed in Geneva between 1976 and 1980. The calculation of the probability of death q_x is based on formula (4.24) up to q_{75} and on formula (4.27) after that.

Alternative methods

As we have seen, the method described previously for calculating cause-specific and relative survival probabilities raise problems of interpretation which have led many authors to look for alternative solutions to the estimation of net survival.

**Table 4.9   Calculations of the probability of death and of survivors by age from morta-
lity rates observed in men in Geneva, Switzerland, between 1976 and 1980**

Age x	Mortality rate λ_x	Probability of death q_x	Survivor function[a] ℓ_x
0	0.010605	0.010605	10 000
1	0.000623	0.00249	9 894
5	0.003610	0.00180	9 869
10	0.000427	0.00213	9 852
15	0.001100	0.00548	9 831
20	0.001861	0.00926	9 777
25	0.001456	0.00725	9 686
30	0.001250	0.00623	9 616
35	0.001725	0.00859	9 556
40	0.002855	0.01417	9 474
45	0.004409	0.02180	9 340
50	0.007342	0.03605	9 136
55	0.011103	0.05402	8 807
60	0.018901	0.09024	8 331
65	0.030487	0.14116	7 579
70	0.048424	0.21597	6 509
75	0.074263	0.31397	5 104
80	0.119394	0.45731	3 501
85	0.174174	0.59392	1 900
90	0.311673	0.80900	363
95+	0.532710	0.94752	19

[a] The number of survivors at a given age is obtained by linear interpolation from these numbers. For
example, the number of survivors at 33 years is given by:

$$\ell_{33} = \frac{(2 \times 9616 + 3 \times 9556)}{5}$$

Results obtained by the method of cause-specific survival depend closely upon the
quality of information available on causes of death. Systematic national differences
in the coding of causes of death make this method unsuited to comparisons between
registries. Relative survival, derived from expected survival as in the previous section, is equally subject to methodological biases which will be briefly discussed
before presenting other methods.

The group being followed is often heterogeneous with respect to factors influencing both net survival and survival from competing causes, and hence observed
survival. Observed survival is consequently an average value which depends not
only on the initial structure of the group but also on the changes that the group
experiences over time with respect to these different factors. For obvious reasons,
the force of mortality acting on the group in the long term is generally closest to
the mortality in the group with the longest lifespan [14,16]. The calculation of expected survival as described above does not take into account changes in the group
over time, consequently the ratio between observed and expected survival will generally lead to overestimation of net survival over long time periods.

When age is the factor being considered, the consequences of this phenomenon can be easily demonstrated. Individuals in the group under study may end follow-up for one of three reasons, all of which are dependent on age: death from the disease under study, death from other causes and withdrawal from follow-up for reasons other than death. If $\lambda_x(t)$, $\mu_x(t)$ and $\gamma_x(t)$ are the corresponding instantaneous rates for each age x, then the force of mortality to which the group is subject at time t is a weighted average for which the weight $w_x(t)$ changes over time. This can be written

$$v(t) = \sum_{x=1}^{g} w_x(t) \, [\lambda_x(t) + \mu_x(t)] \qquad (4.29)$$

where $w_x(t)$ is the proportion of individuals aged x years present in the population at time t. Using the notation of formula (4.17), this proportion is equal to

$$w_x(t) = \frac{w_x(0) \, S_{cx}(t) \, S_{ex}(t) \, \Gamma_x(t)}{\sum\limits_{x=1}^{g} w_x(0) \, S_{cx}(t) \, S_{ex}(t) \, \Gamma_x(t)} \qquad (4.30)$$

where $\Gamma_x(t)$ is the probability that an individual aged x years has a potential follow-up time greater than t.

$$\Gamma_x(t) = e^{\left[-\int_0^t \gamma_x(t)\right]}$$

If the net survival and the potential follow-up time are independent of age, the weighting becomes proportional to the expected number of survivors:

$$w_x(t) = \frac{w_x(0) \, S_{ex}(t)}{\sum\limits_{x=1}^{g} w_x(0) \, S_{ex}(t)}$$

and the net mortality rate comes out from the summation over age:

$$v(t) = \lambda(t) + \sum_{x=1}^{g} w_x(t) \, \mu_x(t)$$

Therefore, the observable survival probability can be written

$$S_o(t) = e^{-\int_0^t v(u)\,du}$$

$$= e^{-\int_0^t \lambda(u)\,du} \, e^{-\int_0^t \frac{\sum\limits_{x=1}^{g} w_x(0) \, S_{ex}(u) \, \mu_x(u)}{\sum\limits_{x=1}^{g} w_x(0) \, S_{ex}(u)}\,du}$$

Furthermore, since

$$\mu_x(t) = -\frac{S'_{ex}(t)}{S_{ex}(t)}$$

it follows that

$$S_o(t) = S_c(t)\, e^{\displaystyle\int_0^t \frac{\sum_{x=1}^{g} w_x(0)\, S'_{ex}(t)}{\sum_{x=1}^{g} w_x(0)\, S_{ex}(t)}\, dt}$$

Since the term to be integrated is equal to the derivative of the logarithm of $\Sigma\, w_x(0)\, S_{ex}(u)$,

$$S_o(t) = S_c(t) \sum_{x=1}^{g} w_x(0)\, S_{ex}(t) \tag{4.31}$$

This formula implies that the observed survival is the result of two independent forces of mortality and that in this case relative survival correctly estimates net survival.

When the net survival or potential follow-up time depend on age, this relationship no longer holds true. In the long term, relative survival then tends to estimate the net survival of age groups which have the greatest life expectancy. In particular, if the potential follow-up time depends on age when the net survival is constant, the estimate of net survival by relative survival is biased.

In principle, the changes in the group over time can be accounted for in the calculation of expected survival, as in the method proposed by Ederer and Heise [17] and programmed by Rothman and Boice [18]. Instead of calculating expected survival from the initial number in each age group ($N_x(0)$), it is estimated at time $t + \Delta t$ for subjects still living at time t. Conditional expected survival $\bar{s}_e(t + \Delta t)$ is then the average of expected survival probabilities at different ages, weighted by the proportion of subjects still subject to the risk of dying at time t:

$$\bar{s}_e(t + \Delta t) = \sum_{x=1}^{g} w_x(t)\, s_{ex}(\Delta t) \tag{4.32}$$

The probability $s_{ex}(\Delta t)$ that an individual aged x years living at time t will still be living at the end of the time period ($t + \Delta t$) is obtained from the life table. For example, if a five-yearly table is used

$$s_{ex}(\Delta t) = \frac{\ell_{x+0.5+\Delta t}}{\ell_{x+0.5}}$$

Expected survival of the group is then given by the cumulative product of the average survival over each five-year interval:

$$S_e(t_i) = \prod_{j=1}^{i} \bar{s}_e(t_j) \tag{4.33}$$

This method will be termed Ederer II, as opposed to Ederer's method previously described (Ederer I, see page 231).

It can be seen that if the net mortality rate $\lambda_x(t)$ does not depend on age, $S_c(t)$ is factorised as before:

$$S_o(t) = e^{-\int_0^t \sum_{x=1}^{g} [w_x(u)(\lambda(u) + \mu_x(u))]\,du}$$

$$= S_c(t)\, e^{-\int_0^t \sum_{x=1}^{g} [w_x(u)\,\mu_x(u)]\,du}$$

$$= S_c(t) \cdot S_e(t) \tag{4.34}$$

where $S_e(t)$ now denotes expected survival after taking into account the group structure at each time point t. This last formula holds whether or not the follow-up time depends on age. This characteristic was noted by Hakulinen [16] who proposed replacing $w_x(t)$ by $w_x^*(t)$ in the calculation of expected survival where

$$w_x^*(t) = \frac{w_x(0)\,S_{ex}(t)\,\Gamma_x(t)}{\sum_{i=1}^{g} w_x(0)\,S_{ex}(t)\,\Gamma_x(t)} \tag{4.35}$$

that is, by a weight which corrects for the distortion of age structure caused by censoring but in which net survival no longer plays a role. This expression gives the same result as (4.33) if net survival does not depend on age. It also provides an expected survival which is not affected by the value of net survival when it depends on age. In contrast, the Ederer II estimate derived in (4.32) and (4.33) provides an expected survival which depends on net survival and thus on the cancer being studied.

When $S_{cx}(t)$ does not depend on x but $\Gamma_x(t)$ does, for example when the population ages and increasingly older patients enter the study, Ederer II and the method of Hakulinen are preferable to Ederer I, which can lead to biases of the order of 10% [16].

When $S_{cx}(t)$ depends on x, Ederer II will systematically give results which are less than those of Hakulinen's method if net survival decreases with age. In fact, because they experience a larger number of deaths from cancer, the oldest subjects will be withdrawn more quickly from the calculation of expected survival, which will consequently be overestimated.

The original proponent of relative survival [19] clearly intended to calculate the net survival of a group of patients and not simply to provide an indicator of relative risk of dying. However, the parameter being estimated when net survival depends on age has never been clearly defined. Implicitly, most authors are in favour of estimating the net survival of the group by the ratio of observed and expected survival. Explicitly taking age into account, this ratio can be written

$$\overline{S}_c(t) = \frac{\sum_{i=1}^{g} n_x S_{ex}(t) S_{cx}(t)}{\sum_{i=1}^{g} n_x S_{ex}(t)} \tag{4.36}$$

and thus corresponds to the average of net survival probabilities weighted by the expected number of survivors.

As stated before and shown by formula (4.36), the estimate of $\overline{S}_c(t)$ will always be closest to the net survival of the subgroup that has the greatest life expectancy. Considering the goal of this type of calculation, it would seem preferable to calculate the average of net survival probabilities, weighted by the initial numbers of subjects followed up and not by the expected number of survivors at time t:

$$\tilde{S}_c(t) = \frac{\sum_{i=1}^{g} n_x S_{cx}(t)}{\sum_{i=1}^{g} n_x} \tag{4.37}$$

A relative survival estimate based on direct standardisation of relative survival calculated separately for each age group can in theory be obtained in this way. However, it is less likely that this calculation can be made in practice, because of the statistical instability of the estimates for the older age groups. In addition, it can be questioned whether subjects who are diagnosed with cancer at 80 years should play the same role in the calculation of survival in the long term as those who were diagnosed with cancer at 40 years. The expected survival of elderly patients is moreover difficult to estimate from available data.

This discussion shows that the calculation of relative survival should be placed in the context of the classical methods for estimating the parameters of a survival model. This would have the two-fold advantage of providing both a better definition of the concept and a standard method for calculation. It seems natural in this context to estimate the net probability rate using a proportional hazards model (see page 260) where baseline hazard is a step function:

$$\lambda(t,\mathbf{z}) = e^{\beta \mathbf{z}} \sum_{k=1}^{m} \tau_k I_k(t) \tag{4.38}$$

where $\mathbf{z}$ is a vector of covariates including age which might influence net survival, $I_k(t)$ is the indicator function of the kth interval ($I_k(t) = 1$ if t is in the interval, $I_k(t) = 0$

if it is not), and m the number of intervals being considered in the whole period under study.

Estimating such a model from individual observations (for subject i, t_i is survival time, δ_i the status living or dead in t_i, z_i the vector of covariates and x_i the initial age) is easily achieved by the maximum likelihood method. The logarithm of the likelihood can be written (see Chapter 1, page 19):

$$L(\beta,\tau) = -\sum_{i=1}^{n} \Lambda\,(t_i\,,\,z_i) + \sum_{i=1}^{n} \delta_i \log\,[\lambda(t_i\,,\,z_i) + \mu\,(t_i + x_i\,,\,z_{1i})] \qquad (4.39)$$

where $\mu(t_i + x_i,\,z_{1i})$ is the mortality rate at age $t_i + x_i$ for a subject in the general population characterized by z_{1i}, the value of the covariate z_1, subvector of the covariate z for which these data are available (e.g., sex and ethnic group).

After substituting (4.38) for λ in (4.39), the first and second derivatives of $L(\beta,\tau)$ are obtained. Then, using the Newton Raphson method, the values $\hat{\beta}, \hat{\tau}$, which maximize $L(\beta,\tau)$ are derived. The confidence intervals of these parameters are obtained simultaneously by inversion of the matrix of second derivatives with respect to β and τ at the maximum. It can be shown that in practice this method amounts to describing observed deaths in each interval by the sum of expected deaths based on the risk of overall mortality (μT_k) and of deaths resulting from the disease under study (λT_k), where T_k is the time spent in this interval by patients in the cohort who have respectively rates μ and λ [20].

Applying this method to the survival data for cancer of the colon in Geneva (1970-1979) shows that net survival does not depend on sex but strongly depends on age (appropriate significance tests are given below, see page 274). The mortality rate for age group 65 to 74 years is $e^{0.59} = 1.8$ times bigger than that for age group 0 to 64 years and for age group 75 to 99 years is $e^{0.91} = 2.5$ times bigger (Table 4.10).

The cumulative mortality rate, the corresponding net survival and their confidence intervals are obtained from $\lambda(t,z)$ and from the standard errors of β and τ by using the formulae already described in Chapter 1 (see for example formula 1.36) as well as the standard procedures for calculating asymptotic variances [7].

If $u_1, u_2 \ldots u_m$ are the limits of the intervals used to define the baseline hazard step function and if $t \in [u_\ell, u_{\ell+1}]$

$$\Lambda\,(t,z) = e^{\hat{\beta}z} \sum_{k=1}^{\ell-1} \hat{\tau}_k\,(u_{k+1} - u_k) + \hat{\tau}_\ell\,(t - u_\ell) \qquad (4.40)$$

$$S_c\,(t,z) = e^{-\Lambda\,(t,z)} \qquad (4.41)$$

Table 4.10 gives values calculated for five and ten years and survival probabilities obtained by other methods. It will be seen in the present case that relative

Table 4.10 Survival probability([a]) of patients with cancer of the colon in Geneva, both sexes, 1970-1979

	Age at time 0 (years)			Total
	< 65	65-74	≥ 75	
Numbers				
At risk	322	292	326	940
expected at 10 years([b])	287.1	182.5	84.8	554.3
Crude survival([c])				
5 years	0.51 (0.03)	0.31 (0.03)	0.18 (0.02)	0.33
10 years	0.45 (0.04)	0.19 (0.03)	0.08 (0.02)	0.24
Net survival				
Ederer I([c])				
5 years	0.54 (0.03)	0.37 (0.03)	0.32 (0.03)	0.42
10 years	0.50 (0.04)	0.30 (0.05)	0.30 (0.09)	0.40
Likelihood method([d])				
$\hat{\beta}$	0	0.59 (0.12)	0.91 (0.12)	–
5 years	0.56 (0.03)	0.35 (0.03)	0.24 (0.03)	0.40
10 years	0.51 (0.04)	0.30 (0.04)	0.19 (0.03)	0.36
Cause-specific survival				
5 years	0.57 (0.03)	0.38 (0.03)	0.25 (0.03)	0.40
10 years	0.55 (0.03)	0.31 (0.04)	0.21 (0.03)	0.36

([a]) The standard error of each estimate is given in brackets.
([b]) Calculations from the Swiss life table (1978-83).
([c]) Crude survival is calculated by the actuarial method with intervals of three months. Relative survival is obtained by the Ederer I method (4.17).
([d]) Estimation of β is obtained by the maximum likelihood method and survival analysis is deduced from these values and from that of τ (not reproduced here) by using (4.39) and (4.40).

survival is more optimistic than net survival obtained by the maximum likelihood method (Figure 4.5). The difference is particularly noticeable for older age groups. In this situation, the cause-specific survival can be calculated from the same data using causes of death as assessed by nosologists at the Geneva registry. Specific survival is slightly higher for the younger age groups than the estimate obtained by the maximum likelihood method but it is the same for the group as a whole. For the oldest age group, cause-specific survival is closer to the maximum likelihood estimate than the relative survival calculated by the Ederer I method.

Calculations not given here show that in this case the Hakulinen method provides results which are close to those of the Ederer I method (0.42 to 5 years and 0.42 to 10 years for the whole group). The last two methods would suggest that the time at which cancer of the colon can be considered to be cured is five years, because relative survival is then no longer decreasing. The maximum likelihood method is in fact stricter and would reject this assumption. The estimate of the average rate of mortality τ in the interval 5 to 10 years is 0.019 with a standard error equal to 0.008. In fact, the Ederer method overestimates relative survival for

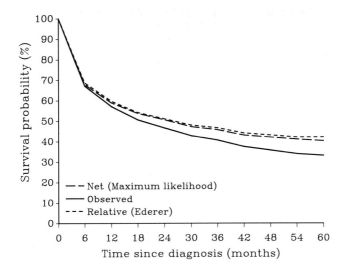

Figure 4.5   Observed and relative survival of colon cancer patients diagnosed between 1970 and 1979 in Geneva, Switzerland; both sexes

the oldest age group on the one hand and overall relative survival on the other hand by weighting each age group with expected survivors

$$(0.5 \times 287.1 + 0.3 \times 182.5 + 0.3 \times 84.8) / 554.3 = 0.40$$

(while the average weighted by the initial numbers would be 0.37).

Other alternatives to the Ederer method have been proposed. Breslow [21], Andersen and coworkers [22], and Hill and coworkers [23] proposed a model in which the presence of the disease multiplies the risk in the general population by a constant. Pocock and coworkers [24] have suggested a model similar to that described in this section, in which the risk added by the disease decreases exponentially with time. We would also suggest that the additive model is more natural in this context. However, the multiplicative model has certain advantages which have already been explained in detail [22].

Methods of comparison

Introduction

In some situations, comparison of survival between two groups can only be made at one time point on the survival curve, for example at five years. The method used in this situation is described below. Generalization from this comparison to the whole survival curve can nonetheless lead to incorrect results : survival probabilities at five years in the two groups might be the same even though the two survival curves are different as a whole. This is a common situation in clinical practice, especially when two groups are treated with different therapies (e.g., surgery versus radiography) having effects which may be unequally distributed over time. The choice of a specific time point to evaluate survival will thus be arbitrary. Furthermore, when the groups are small in size, a survival rate at a given time point is subject to a relatively large random error and observed differences may appear to be due to chance, while the more powerful overall comparison between survival curves might lead to a significant difference.

Except in particular situations, there is therefore a strong argument to comparing the whole of the two curves, provided that the necessary data are available. The problem is then to summarize all differences between the curves by a suitable indicator and then to use an appropriate test. The methods described below (see page 248) illustrated with data on cancer of the colon in Côte-d'Or, Geneva and the canton of Vaud provide a way to answer these questions.

Furthermore, it is not unusual for the groups being compared to be unequally distributed with regard to age, sex and stage of disease at diagnosis. The comparison should take these prognostic factors into account by a method based on an appropriate stratification, provided that the necessary information is available for each subject. This method will be illustrated by data from Geneva on the survival of subjects with malignant melanoma by site and sex (see page 255).

A substantial amount of research has been carried out over the last two decades in the area of semiparametric models of survival, which simultaneously take into account various prognostic factors defined on an individual basis [25, 26]. Among these, the proportional hazards model has been of particular interest because of its simplicity and effectiveness (see page 260). We will present this model using breast cancer data from the Geneva Cancer Registry to assess the influence of health care systems on survival.

Long-term survival cannot be compared between groups without considering competing causes of death. This consideration leads to the comparison of relative survival between groups, (see page 272). Despite the above-mentioned difficulties, it may be that a point comparison of two rates is appropriate or that, as is often the case, the basic data are not available to make an overall comparison. The method to be used in this situation will be presented briefly below.

Comparison of crude survival probabilities

Test to compare two survival rates

Observed survival probabilities are often only published in the form of an actuarial rate at a given time (e.g., survival rate at five years). Evaluating the statistical significance of the observed differences between two or more populations requires information on the variability of the rates, which unfortunately is rarely available. Knowledge of the number of cases initially entered in the study is not sufficient to correctly estimate the variability. If the observed number of survivors at a given time is known, the upper limit of the variance of the survival rate can be calculated (see page 222) and a slightly conservative comparison can be made. Implementation of the test is straightforward as soon as an estimate of the variability of the rates is available.

Let $S_1(t)$ and $S_2(t)$ be the survival rates at time t, estimated using one of the two methods described in the first part of this chapter (see pages 216 and 219) and let $V_1(t)$ and $V_2(t)$ be the estimates of their variance. For a given value t_0 of t, the quantity

$$\varepsilon = \frac{S_1(t_0) - S_2(t_0)}{\sqrt{V_1(t_0) + V_2(t_0)}} \qquad (4.42)$$

follows an approximately normal distribution and provides an appropriate statistic to test the hypothesis of equality of the rates in t_0. For example, the five-year survival rates in men following cancer of the colon are obtained using the actuarial method as 0.324 (Geneva) and 0.348 (canton of Vaud). As the standard errors obtained by Greenwood's method are 0.0228 and 0.0216, we have :

$$\varepsilon = \frac{0.324 - 0.348}{\sqrt{0.0228^2 + 0.0216^2}} = -0.76$$

It is therefore concluded from this value that five-year colon cancer survival for men does not differ significantly between the canton of Vaud and Geneva.

When standard errors are estimated from initial numbers (as if there were no censored observations), the standard error for Geneva is 0.0220. The proximity of this value to 0.0228 can be explained by the fact that the majority of subjects were followed up for five years. Conversely, the standard error in the canton of Vaud is 0.0187 instead of 0.0216 because the percentage of censored observations is high among the 650 cases. In this situation, it is particularly important to provide a correct estimate of variance. In fact, the upper limit of the variance calculated solely from the 114 survivors observed at 60 months would be 0.0263 which is a slight over-estimation.

In general, it is highly recommended that survival rates be presented with their standard errors to provide the basis for making more reliable comparisons.

Rank tests to compare survival curves

The objective of these tests is to compare two or more survival curves making optimum use of the available information about the survival of patients in the different groups. They are part of a family of tests which are the extensions to censored data of methods based on ranks [27]. Even if the data were not censored, it is inappropriate to make a simple comparison of average survival times of two populations, because survival times do not follow the normal distribution which is a prerequisite for the validity of classical tests. Non-parametric procedures (rank tests in particular) allow us to overcome this difficulty.

When observations are complete, the implementation of a rank test requires ordering all survival times within the two groups in ascending order, assigning a score c_i to the observation of rank i, then calculating the observed sum C of c_i for one of the samples and, finally, comparing C to its expected value E(C) under the assumption that ranks are randomly assigned between the two samples. If, in reality the survival times in one of the samples are on average greater than in the other, their ranks will be on average higher and C will be significantly greater than E(C). The scores c_i are chosen in such a way that the resulting tests are efficient against certain alternatives in the framework of the largest possible family of survival distributions. In the Mann-Whitney test, for example, the score c_i of an observation is simply its rank i in the classification. In the Savage test, the score c_i is equal to the expectation of the observation of rank i in a sample from a distribution with a constant mortality rate (that is, an exponential distribution). For n observations, this score is equal to:

$$c_i = \frac{1}{n} + \frac{1}{n-1} + \dots + \frac{1}{n-i+1}$$

The extension of these methods to censored data requires the assignment of a score to observations censored between the ith and the (i + 1)th survival time, for which it is only known that survival time exceeds t_i. When the Savage test is extended to censored data, it becomes very similar to the Mantel-Haenszel test described in Chapter II (see page 77). In the framework of survival comparisons it is known as the *logrank test* [28]. The generalization proposed by Gehan and Breslow [29, 30] of the Mann-Whitney test (or the Kruskal-Wallis test for more than two populations) is similar to the logrank test. Both tests are based on a comparison of observed deaths d_i with expected deaths e_i in a group, at each time point t_i where at least one death is observed. The two tests only differ in the weight given to the observed differences ($d_i - e_i$). Application of the logrank test to the comparison of three populations is given below.

Let:

- k = 1,2,3 be the three groups being compared,
- t_i be the dates at which at least one death occurred,
- d_{ki} be the number of observed deaths at t_i in group k,
- e_{ki} be the number of expected deaths at t_i in group k,
- D_i be the total number of deaths occurring at t_i,
- n_{ki} be the number of subjects at risk just before t_i in group k, and
- N_i be the total number of subjects at risk just before t_i.

The test is based on the comparison of the total number of observed deaths in each group k, $(O_k = \sum_i d_{ki})$, with the number of deaths $(E_k = \sum_i e_{ki})$ that might have been observed if the force of mortality was the same in the three groups. The number of expected deaths in each group should be calculated at each time point t_i when at least one death occurred. The comparison takes into account not only the total number of observed deaths in each group before a given date but also the date at which these deaths occurred. It is possible that the overall proportion of deaths is the same in the three groups over the entire time period under consideration, but that there is an unequal distribution of survival times in the groups due to differences between the instantaneous mortality rates. Figure 4.6 shows ten-year survival for men with colon cancer in Geneva, Côte-d'Or and the canton of Vaud. The observed rates are practically identical in the three registries after the fifth year, while survival is better in the canton of Vaud before this date.

Table 4.11 gives the breakdown of counts used in the test at a time point t_i when at least one death occurred.

Under the null hypothesis, the observed number of deaths in each of the three groups would be proportional to the respective numbers of subjects at risk in each group at this date. The numbers e_{ki} of expected deaths under this hypothesis are therefore:

$$e_{1i} = D_i \times \frac{n_{1i}}{N_i} \qquad e_{2i} = D_i \times \frac{n_{2i}}{N_i} \qquad e_{3i} = D_i \times \frac{n_{3i}}{N_i}$$

Table 4.11   Logrank test. Breakdown of counts at each time point t_i when one or more deaths occurred

	Group 1	Group 2	Group 3	Total
Deceased	d_{1i}	d_{2i}	d_{3i}	D_i
Alive	$n_{1i} - d_{1i}$	$n_{2i} - d_{2i}$	$n_{3i} - d_{3i}$	$N_i - D_i$
Total	n_{1i}	n_{2i}	n_{3i}	N_i

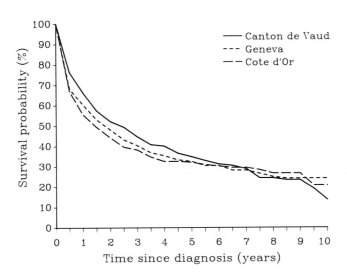

Figure 4.6   Survival of male colon cancer patients in the canton of Vaud, Switzerland (1974-1983), Geneva, Switzerland (1970-1979) and Côte-d'Or, France (1976-1982)

giving the total numbers of expected deaths:

$$E_1 = \sum_i e_{1i} \qquad E_2 = \sum_i e_{2i} \qquad E_3 = \sum_i e_{3i}$$

The objective of the test is to judge whether the sum of the differences between the observed and expected numbers in each group $(O_k - E_k)$ differs significantly from zero. The test is identical in principle to the Mantel-Haenszel test described in Chapter 2 (see page 77). However, the distribution of deaths in this case is multinomial leading to a three-dimensional hypergeometric distribution for d_{ki} when the total number of deaths D_i is fixed, rather than the multinomial distribution which results when the number of deaths follows a Poisson distribution. The variances and covariances of d_{ki} are thus :

$$\text{Var}\,(d_{ki}) = \frac{D_i n_{ki}\,(N_i - n_{ki})\,(N_i - D_i)}{N_i^2\,(N_i - 1)} \tag{4.43}$$

$$\text{Cov}\,(d_{hi},\,d_{ki}) = \frac{-\,D_i\,n_{hi}\,n_{ki}\,(N_i - D_i)}{N_i^2\,(N_i - 1)} \tag{4.44}$$

from this, we derive the symmetric variance-covariance matrix **V** of $(O_k - E_k)$ which, when comparing three groups, is of dimension 3×3; the diagonal elements are

$$v_{kk} = \sum_i \text{Var}\,(d_{ki}) \qquad 1 \leq k \leq 3 \tag{4.45}$$

and the remaining elements

$$v_{kh} = \sum_i \text{Cov}\,(d_{ki},\,d_{hi}) \qquad 1 \leq k \leq 3, \qquad 1 \leq h \leq k \tag{4.46}$$

The definition of the expected numbers implies that the sum of O_k is equal to the sum of E_k : it is therefore sufficient to know the deviations $(O_k - E_k)$ in two of the groups in order to know the deviation in the third. To assess the size of the deviation between all pairs of observed and expected values, it is therefore sufficient to retain two of the three groups. The significance is determined from the statistic:

$$T_1 = w_{11}(O_1 - E_1)^2 + w_{22}(O_2 - E_2)^2 + 2\,w_{12}(O_1 - E_1)\,(O_2 - E_2) \tag{4.47}$$

where w_{hk} are the elements of the inverse of the variance-covariance matrix of $(O_1 - E_1)$ and $(O_2 - E_2)$:

$$\mathbf{W} = \begin{bmatrix} w_{11} & w_{12} \\ w_{12} & w_{22} \end{bmatrix} = \mathbf{V}^{-1} = \frac{1}{v_{11} \times v_{22} - v_{12}^2} \begin{bmatrix} v_{22} & -v_{12} \\ -v_{12} & v_{11} \end{bmatrix} \tag{4.48}$$

under the null hypothesis of equal survival, the statistic T_1 follows a χ^2 law on two degrees of freedom. Formula (4.47) can be easily generalized to r groups and is expressed in matrix form as:

$$T_1 = (O - E)' \, W \, (O - E) \qquad (4.49)$$

where $(O - E)$ is the vector made up of the r − 1 differences between the observed and expected numbers in the first r − 1 groups, and W is the inverse of the variance-covariance matrix of the first r − 1 differences of $(O_k - E_k)$. When T_1 exceeds the critical value corresponding to χ^2 on r − 1 degrees of freedom, it can be concluded that the r survival curves are different. The test of a more specific alternative hypothesis is carried out in a way analogous to that in Chapter 2, page 90. For example, a trend test is based on the statistic :

$$T_1^* = \frac{\left[\sum_k x_k (O_k - E_k) \right]^2}{\mathrm{Var}\left[\sum_k x_k (O_k - E_k) \right]} = \frac{[X' (O - E)]^2}{X' V X} \qquad (4.50)$$

where $X' = (x_1, \ldots x_r)$ is the vector corresponding to the r levels of a quantitative variable such as disease stage or age group which may have an influence on survival. T_1^* follows a χ^2 distribution on one degree of freedom and provides a more powerful test than T_1 for specific alternative hypotheses defined *a priori*. Contrasts, particularly pairwise comparisons, between groups can be tested with the same statistic. It is worth noting however that if a large number of comparisons of this kind are made, the type one error associated with the final result could be seriously underestimated.

The homogeneity of survival rates in 2 groups can be evaluated by a conservative test, approximating formula (4.49) by

$$T_2 = \sum_{k=1}^{r} \frac{(O_k - E_k)^2}{E_k} \qquad (4.51)$$

under the assumption that T_2 is distributed as χ^2 on r − 1 degrees of freedom [31,32]. Because of its simplicity, the statistic T_2 is sometimes calculated first when a rapid result is needed; if it gives a non-significant result, more precise tests can still be carried out.

Table 4.12 shows some of the calculations involved in the comparison of five-year survival following cancer of the colon in males in Geneva (incident cases 1970-83), Côte-d'Or (incident cases 1976-80) and the canton of Vaud (incident cases 1974-83).

Table 4.12 Comparison of survival following cancer of the colon among males in the canton of Vaud, Switzerland (incident cases 1974-83), Geneva, Switzerland (incident cases 1970-83), and in Côte-d'Or, France (incident cases 1976-80)

t_i(month)	Vaud		Geneva		Côte-d'Or		Total		Expected		
	n_{vi}	d_{vi}	n_{gi}	d_{gi}	n_{ci}	d_{ci}	N_i	D_i	e_{vi}	e_{gi}	e_{ci}
1	650	80	454	80	411	80	1 515	251	107.7	75.2	68.1
2	568	18	349	18	331	25	1 248	61	27.8	17.1	16.2
3	546	18	329	15	306	15	1 181	48	22.2	13.4	12.4
4	520	15	314	13	291	10	1 125	38	17.6	10.6	9.8
5	501	21	300	5	281	6	1 082	32	14.8	8.9	8.3
6	476	14	295	5	275	9	1 046	28	12.7	7.9	7.4
7	460	9	289	12	265	6	1 014	27	12.2	7.7	7.1
.	.	.	.	.	.	.	.	.	.	.	.
.	.	.	.	.	.	.	.	.	.	.	.
.	.	.	.	.	.	.	.	.	.	.	.
57	125	3	128	0	66	0	319	3	1.2	1.2	0.6
58	118	0	128	1	66	0	312	1	0.4	0.4	0.2
59	118	1	127	0	63	0	308	1	0.4	0.4	0.2
60	116	2	127	1	61	0	304	3	1.1	1.3	0.6
Total	$O_v = 369$		$O_g = 292$		$O_c = 270$			931	E_v=406.6	E_g=279.6	E_c=244.8

The logrank test is calculated from the variance-covariance matrix of the observations:

$$V = \begin{bmatrix} 214.55 & -114.33 & -100.21 \\ -114.33 & 183.09 & -68.76 \\ -100.21 & -68.76 & 168.97 \end{bmatrix}$$

If the test is calculated from the first two groups, we obtain (cf formula 4.48):

$$W = \frac{1}{26\,210.6} \times \begin{bmatrix} 183.09 & 114.33 \\ 114.33 & 214.55 \end{bmatrix}$$

Applying formula (4.47) gives:

$$T_1 = \frac{1}{26\,210.6}[183.09 \times (-37.6)^2 + 214.55 \times (12.4)^2 + 2 \times 114.33 \times (-37.6) \times (12.4)]$$

$$T1 = 7.07$$

The simplified test (formula 4.51) gives:

$$T_2 = \frac{(369 - 406.6)^2}{406.6} + \frac{(292 - 279.6)^2}{279.6} + \frac{(270 - 244.8)^2}{244.8} = 6.62$$

which, as stated previously, is slightly less than the result of the exact test.

Overall, survival differs between the three groups (p = 0.029). The test T_1^* applied with values of **X'** equal to (1, −1, 0) and (0, 1, −1) shows that survival differs between the canton of Vaud and Geneva ($T_1^* = 3.99$, using the first value of **X'**, p < 0.05), but not between Geneva and Côte-d'Or ($T_1^* = 0.34$, using the second value of **X'**). Figure 4.6 showing ten-year survival demonstrates clearly the reason for this apparent contradiction: mortality is initially less in the canton of Vaud, while the five-year survival rate here is almost the same as in Geneva (see the test described above page 247).

The difference between survival curves is often characterized by a constant ratio R between instantaneous death rates. This ratio is a measure of the relative risk of death in one group compared to another. The quantity

$$\tilde{R}_{kh} = \frac{O_k/E_k}{O_h/E_h} \tag{4.52}$$

can be taken as an estimate of this ratio if it is between 0.5 and 2, but it has been shown to be an underestimate when it is too far from unity [21]. In this latter case, estimation of the relative rate by maximum likelihood in the context of the Cox model (see page 263) is preferable. The Mantel-Haenszel estimate can also be calculated from the series of contingency tables obtained for each date of death as in Table 4.11:

$$\hat{R}_{kh} = \frac{\left[\displaystyle\sum_i \frac{d_{ki}(n_{hi} - d_{hi})}{N_i'} \right]}{\left[\displaystyle\sum_i \frac{d_{hi}(n_{ki} - d_{ki})}{N_i'} \right]} \tag{4.53}$$

where $N_i' = n_{ki} + n_{hi}$

The force of mortality in group k is R_{kh} times higher than that to which group h is subjected. The logrank test evaluates the hypothesis $R_{kh} = 1$ against the alternative $R_{kh} \neq 1$. It is optimum in this situation.

When rates are not proportional and the ratio of the forces of mortality decreases over time as in the example above, the difference between curves will be more correctly determined by the Gehan-Breslow test, which only differs from the logrank test in the weighting of the differences between the observed and expected numbers. The principle of this test is based on the calculation of a score for each of the groups being compared. This score summarizes all possible pairwise comparisons of survival times: all follow-up times t_{kj} in group k are compared to all follow-up times t_{lh} in the other groups and:

• $\psi(k,j,l,h) = +1$ if the comparison of t_{kj} and t_{lh} indicates that subject j has a better survival probability, and

• $\psi(k,j,l,h) = -1$ if the comparison of t_{kj} and t_{lh} indicates that subject j has poorer survival;

the value 0 is given to ψ when the comparison is inconclusive, either because of equal survival times or censored observations. The score associated with group k $\sum_j \left[\sum_{l,h} \Psi(k,j,l,h) \right]$ is higher to the extent that survival times in the group are on average greater than those of all the other groups. It is easy enough to verify that, ignoring its sign, this score is equal to

$$C_k = \sum_i N_i\, d_{ki} - n_{ki}\, D_i = \sum_i N_i \left(d_{ki} - D_i\, \frac{n_{ki}}{N_i} \right) \tag{4.54}$$

where the summation extends over all the dates of death. In other words, C_k is again obtained as a sum of the differences between observed and expected numbers over all time points at which a death occurs. However, unlike the logrank test, this sum is weighted by the total number of subjects still at risk at this date. Any given difference will thus have a weight which is higher for short follow-up times, when N_i is still large, while its effect on the score will be negligible for long follow-up times if the number of subjects still under observation is small. Figure 4.6 suggests that this statistic will be particularly sensitive in the first years to large observed differences between the canton of Vaud, Geneva and Côte-d'Or.

The score C_k is calculated for each of the first $r-1$ groups, and the variance-covariance matrix of the C_k is constructed from:

$$v_{kk} = \sum_i N_i^2\, \mathrm{Var}\,(d_{ki}) \tag{4.55}$$

$$v_{kh} = \sum_i N_i^2\, \mathrm{Cov}\,(d_{ki}, d_{hi}) \tag{4.56}$$

where the variance and covariance are defined by formulas (4.43) and (4.44). When comparing three groups, the statistic T_3, analogous to T_1, is written:

$$T_3 = w_{11}\, C_1^2 + w_{22}\, C_2^2 + 2\, w_{12}\, C_1\, C_2$$

where, as previously described, W_{ij} denotes the terms of **W**, the inverse of the variance-covariance matrix of the parameter estimates for the two groups involved in the calculation.

As the value of C_k is generally very high, each score in the numerical application given below has been divided by the number of thousands of conclusive comparisons carried out (with score equal to either +1 or −1). This operation obviously does not change the proposed weighting and reduces the differences to an order comparable to that obtained for the logrank test. The calculations were carried out with data from the canton of Vaud, Geneva and Côte-d'Or; 1 156 446 conclusive comparisons were carried out and the modified score (per 1000) in each of the groups is:

$$C_1 = -50.04\ ;\ C_2 = 18.17\ ;\ C_3 = 31.87$$

which indicates that survival time is on average longer in the first group. To evaluate the significance of this difference, the variance and covariance of these scores are calculated using (4.55) and (4.56) modified by the weighting above. The result is the matrix

$$\begin{bmatrix} 184.74 & -96.85 & -87.89 \\ -96.85 & 155.60 & -58.75 \\ -87.89 & -58.75 & 146.64 \end{bmatrix}$$

W being the inverse of the matrix **V** defined by the first two rows and columns of the matrix above, we have:

$$\mathbf{W} = \frac{1}{19\,365.6} \begin{bmatrix} 155.60 & 96.85 \\ 96.85 & 184.74 \end{bmatrix}$$

and the value of the statistic:

$$T_3 = \frac{1}{19\,365.6} [155.60 \times (-50.04)^2 + 184.74 \times (18.17)^2 + 2 \times 96.85 \times (-50.04) \times (18.17)]$$

$$= 14.17$$

The three global tests thus lead to the conclusion that survival in the first five years is significantly different between the three registries. Gehan-Breslow's test provides a much larger value ($T_3 = 14.17$) than that obtained for T_1 ($T_1 = 7.07$) or T_2 ($T_2 = 6.62$) as it takes greater account of differences observed at the beginning of the curve and, as Figure 4.6 shows, differences between the Canton of Vaud and the other two registries are present mainly in the initial period. These results suggest that long-term survival is actually the same in the three registries but that artefacts linked to the definition of the date of incidence and to the mechanisms of follow-up may have led to the differences observed in the initial period.

Obviously not every test described in this section needs to be used for each data set under study, nor should a test be selected solely for its convenience. In fact, the choice of a test should, as always, be dictated by a hypothesis made prior to the examination of the survival curves. As Gehan-Breslow's test can behave unpredictably in certain circumstances [26], caution is recommended in its use. In particular, the result of this test should be ignored if it does not produce significance when the logrank test does, especially when there is a large number of censored observations.

Stratified comparison of crude survival

The survival of a group of patients is generally associated with many prognostic factors which are themselves related. When survival of two or more groups are compared, it is crucial to take into account known prognostic factors. Thus, the difference of colon cancer survival between Geneva and the canton of Vaud might be partially explained by differences in the distribution of clinical stages between the two regions: it would be preferable to compare the two geographic areas 'holding stage constant'. The opposite situation can also occur: a difference in survival between groups may go unrecognized if a major determinant of survival within groups is ignored.

Regardless of the distribution of the prognostic factors in the various groups, a comparison holding these factors constant will tend to increase the power of the test that is used by decreasing the within group variability. Accounting for these factors in the analysis is achieved through an adjustment based on an appropriate stratification as follows.

For each category (or stratum) of the factor under consideration, the approach described in the previous paragraph is used (see page). We calculate, for each group k and stratum j, the number of observed deaths (O_{kj}) and the number of deaths that would occur (E_{kj}) if, in each stratum, the force of mortality had been the same in each of the groups being compared. In other words, the expected number e_{kji} of deaths at date t_i in group k is calculated and summed separately for each stratum j. Evaluation of the difference between observed and expected numbers is based on the sum of results from all strata.

In order to simplify the notation, we first show how to carry out the adjustment for a two-group comparison in the presence of a two-category prognostic factor. Generalization to any number of groups and categories is immediate. The method is illustrated by comparing survival between patients with malignant melanoma of the legs and patients with melanoma at another site (using data from Geneva). As sex is known to be a prognostic factor for melanoma, it should be considered in the comparison.

In the case of two groups, only one needs to be considered. we take the group (k = 1) of patients with melanoma of the legs. Thus:

- for males (stratum j = 1)

$$O_{11} = \sum_i d_{11i}, \quad E_{11} = \sum_i e_{11i}$$

$$v_{11} = \sum_i Var(d_{11i})$$

- for females (stratum j = 2)

$$O_{12} = \sum_i d_{12i}, \quad E_{12} = \sum_i e_{12i}$$

$$v_{12} = \sum_i Var(d_{12i})$$

variances in each stratum being calculated using formula (4.43).

Observed and expected number of deaths in the group of patients with skin melanoma of the legs are added over the two strata:

$$O_{1.} = O_{11} + O_{12} \; ; \; E_{1.} = E_{11} + E_{12} \qquad (4.57)$$

similarly, the variance of $O_{1.}$ (the within-stratum variance) is obtained by addition of the variances of O_{11} and O_{12}

$$Var(O_{1.} - E_{1.}) = v_{11} + v_{12} \qquad (4.58)$$

then the quantity

$$T_1 = \frac{(O_{1.} - E_{1.})^2}{Var(O_{1.} - E_{1.})} \qquad (4.59)$$

is calculated; under the null hypothesis of equal survival, the statistic T_1 follows a χ^2 distribution with one degree of freedom. Comparison of T_1 with the critical value of the corresponding χ^2 distribution tells us if the two survival curves differ overall, after correcting for sex.

An appropriate formula similar to (4.51), based only on observed and expected data in the two groups can also be used:

$$T_2 = \frac{(O_{1.} - E_{1.})^2}{E_{1.}} + \frac{(O_{2.} - E_{2.})^2}{E_{2.}} \qquad (4.60)$$

T_2, under the null hypothesis, approaches (but is greater than) a χ^2 with one degree of freedom. The significance of T_2 is sufficient to conclude that the groups have different survival probabilities, but calculation of T_1 is necessary if T_2 is not significant.

When more than two groups are being studied, the calculation of the within-group covariance using formulae (4.44) and (4.46) and the generalization of (4.58) provides the basis for carrying out the adjusted global test and the associated tests on one degree of freedom given on page 251 In this case, the observed and expected numbers calculated from the obvious generalization of formula (4.57) to more than two groups are used in formulae (4.49) and (4.50).

Table 4.13 gives survival data by site for incident cases of malignant skin melanoma among males and females in Geneva between 1970 and 1982. Melanomas of the legs make up group 1; sites from the rest of the body form group 2. The data are illustrated in Figure 4.7.

The unadjusted comparison of group 1 (legs) and group 2 (other sites) using the logrank test shows significantly better survival in group 1:

$$\chi^2_{1df} = \frac{(20 - 31.7)^2}{21.3} = 6.4$$

If the comparison is made without taking into account the patients' sex, it could be concluded that the mortality rate is approximately twice as high ($p < 0.01$) in group 2 than in group 1 (4.52).

Table 4.13   Survival of patients with malignant skin melanoma([a]) in Geneva, Switzerland. Incident cases 1970-1982

Year	Group 1[b]				Group 2[b]			
	Number at risk	Observed deaths	Expected deaths[c]	Survival (standard error)	Number at risk	Observed deaths	Expected deaths[c]	Survival (standard error)
1	80	3	8.0 (5.6)	0.96 (0.021)	180	24	19.0 (5.6)	0.88 (0.023)
3	76	7	19.3 (13.2)	0.92 (0.031)	149	55	42.7 (13.2)	0.73 (0.031)
5	69	14	25.4 (17.2)	0.83 (0.041)	138	66	54.6 (17.2)	0.68 (0.033)
10	22	20	31.7 (21.3)	0.67 (0.068)	37	78	66.3 (21.3)	0.52 (0.048)

([a]) Number of patients living and still under follow-up, cumulative deaths and survival are given for the end of the year under consideration. These values are based on calculations using a month as the time unit.
([b]) Group 1: 83 patients with melanoma of the skin of the leg. Group 2: 204 patients with other skin melanomas.
([c]) Variance in brackets.

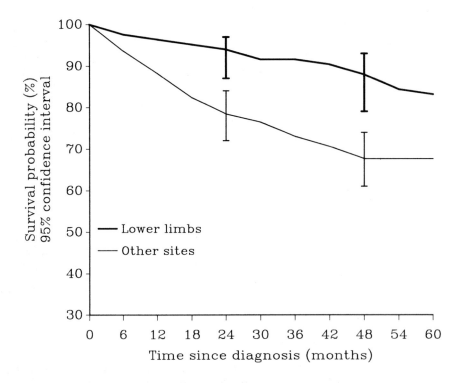

Figure 4.7   Survival of skin melanoma patients by site, Geneva, Switzerland (incident cases 1970-1982); both sexes

In fact, it is known that sex plays a strong prognostic role in the survival of melanoma patients: women have a better survival than men. As melanoma of the legs is much more frequent in women (64/146 = 43.8%) than in men (19/141 = 13.5%), the observed effect can partially be explained by sex.

Table 4.14 gives the same survival data for each sex separately. After adjustment (see formula 4.58), the comparison becomes:

$$T_1 = [(7+13) - (9.9+16.2)]^2 / (8.2+8.7) = 2.2 \quad (p = 0.14)$$

Thus, the hypothesis of equal survival for the two sites can no longer be rejected after taking sex into account. The relative mortality rate is now estimated to be 1.08/0.77 = 1.4, a value which no longer differs significantly from unity.

Figure 4.8 shows that these results should be examined even more closely since, survival for group 1 (legs) is better than that of group 2 (other sites) regardless of sex or follow-up time. We see that, in men, there are only 19 cases of melanoma of the legs. Thus estimation of survival rates in this stratum is imprecise : for this latter patients the confidence intervals of survival probability at five and ten years

Table 4.14   Comparison of survival of subjects with malignant skin melanoma by site and sex in Geneva, Switzerland. Incident cases between 1970 and 1982([a])

Year	Group 1				Group 2			
	Number at risk	Observed deaths	Expected deaths ([c])	Survival (standard error)	Number at risk	Observed deaths	Expected deaths ([c])	Survival (standard error)
Males								
1	18	1	2.9 (2.5)	0.95 (0.051)	102	20	18.1 (2.5)	0.84 (0.034)
3	16	3	6.4 (5.4)	0.84 (0.084)	82	40	36.6 (5.4)	0.67 (0.043)
5	14	5	7.8 (6.5)	0.74 (0.101)	75	47	44.2 (6.5)	0.62 (0.044)
10	5	7	9.9 (8.2)	0.56 (0.138)	20	56	53.1 (8.2)	0.43 (0.060)
Females								
1	62	2	2.6 (1.5)	0.97 (0.022)	78	4	3.4 (1.5)	0.95 (0.024)
3	60	4	8.6 (4.7)	0.94 (0.030)	67	15	10.4 (4.7)	0.82 (0.043)
5	55	9	12.9 (6.9)	0.86 (0.044)	63	19	15.1 (6.9)	0.77 (0.047)
10	17	13	16.2 (8.7)	0.71 (0.077)	17	22	18.8 (8.7)	0.66 (0.073)

([a]) Number of patients living and still under follow-up, cumulative deaths and survival are given for the end of the year under consideration. These values are based on calculations using a month as the time unit.
([b]) Group 1: melanoma of the skin of the leg (18 male and 64 female patients). Group 2 : other skin.
([c]) Variance in brakets.

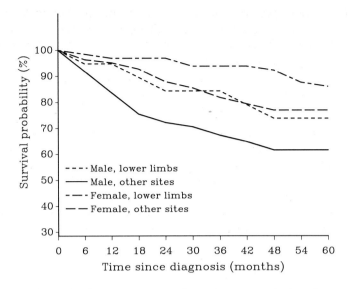

Figure 4.8   Survival of skin melanoma petients by sex and site, Geneva, Switzerland (incident cases, 1970-1982)

are respectively [0.54 ; 0.94] and [0.28 ; 0.84]. One might conclude that the role of site can not be definitely excluded, and that the problem requires further research.

Taking account of a prognostic factor in the comparison of survival between groups presumes that there is no interaction between this factor and the group. If, in the example above, survival of subjects with melanoma of the legs was better than that of other sites in men and worse in women, a single test based on summing the differences between the two strata would not have made sense. Only a separate analysis in men and in women would be acceptable. The value of this latter kind of analysis depends however on the number of subjects in each stratum (if the number is small the comparison has less power), the number of categories of the factor to be taken into account (when the number of tests carried out is large, there is a substantial increase in the probability of type one error) and the interpretability of the interaction.

The Cox model

The proportional hazards model

The limits of the stratification method described above are quickly reached as the number of patients under study decreases in relation to the number of strata particularly when the number of covariables or of their levels increase. In this case, there will inevitably be a large number of survival times for which one or more of the groups will no longer provide subjects at risk of dying, thus making the results from the test increasingly imprecise. In describing all the data by one model, the comparisons to be made are summarized by those between the few parameters which characterize the model itself. The information which was not available in the data is effectively replaced by information provided by the equation defining the distribution of the survival data under study. The benefit is however only real if the model is sufficiently valid.

The classical analytical models (exponential, Weibull; see Chapter 1, page 29) are often too rigid to take into account the diversity of situations which are encountered in practice. Methods with more general applicability, based on principles analogous to those used in linear regression, have therefore been developed. The most frequently used in survival analysis is the proportional hazards model [25], which states that the instantaneous mortality rate depends on covariables through a multiplicative parameter applied to an unspecified background or baseline rate $\lambda_0(t)$:

$$\lambda(t, \mathbf{z}) = \lambda_0(t) \, e^{\beta \mathbf{z}} \qquad (4.61)$$

where $\mathbf{z}$ is a vector of covariables and β a vector of coefficients measuring the intensity of the effect of the components of vector $\mathbf{z}$. Thus, when $\mathbf{z}$ is the indicator of membership in a subgroup, this model implies that, at each time point t, the mortality rate in the subgroup ($\mathbf{z} = 1$) is proportional to the mortality rate for the rest of the study sample ($\mathbf{z} = 0$):

$$\lambda(t, 1) = \lambda_0(t) \, e^{\beta} = \lambda(t, 0) \, e^{\beta} \qquad (4.62)$$

where $\theta = e^{\beta}$ is consequently the relative mortality rate of the subgroup with respect to the rest of the sample. θ is also a good approximation of the relative risk of dying at time t when the cumulative mortality rate is small.

As a rule, the ratio of hazard rates for any two values of $\mathbf{z}$:

$$\frac{\lambda(t, \mathbf{v})}{\lambda(t, \mathbf{u})} = e^{\beta(\mathbf{v} - \mathbf{u})} \qquad (4.63)$$

is independent of time, giving rise to the name, *proportional hazards model*. This model is often called semiparametric because the background rate $\lambda_0(t)$, unlike the relative rate, is not specified by a parametric model.

When the factor under study is defined by a qualitative variable with r categories, the variable $\mathbf{z} = (z_2...z_r)$, where the z_i are $r - 1$ indicator variables defining membership of the subgroups corresponding to $r - 1$ categories of the factor, is constructed: for $2 \leq i \leq r$, $z_i = 1$ if the subject falls into the ith category and $z_i = 0$ otherwise. The first category of the factor is characterized by $z_i = 0$, $2 \leq i \leq r$. The choice of the particular role played here by the first category is obviously arbitrary. Thus, if the covariable under study is stage at diagnosis, coded into three classes of increasing severity, two indicator variables are constructed. A subject in stage 1 is coded as $z_2 = 0$ and $z_3 = 0$, a subject in stage 2 as $z_2 = 1$ and $z_3 = 0$ and a subject in stage 3 is defined by $z_2 = 0$ and $z_3 = 1$.

The coefficient β_i corresponding to the indicator variable z_i allows the calculation of θ_i, the relative mortality rate for patients in the category compared to those in the first category. Thus, in the previous example, $\theta_2 = e^{\beta_2}$ is the relative rate of subjects in stage 2 with respect to subjects in stage 1. The relative rates of any two categories can then be derived from the previously described relative rates by simple division, the choice of standard categories being entirely arbitrary. Still using the example of disease stage, θ_3/θ_2 measures the relative rate of the subjects in stage 3 compared to those in stage 2, and similarly for all pairs of categories.

The proportional hazards model has already been discussed in the context of incidence data (Chapter 2). There, it was noted that the ratio of incidence rates in two populations with different cancer risks was frequently independent of age. This variable played the same role as time since diagnosis in the present situation. The constancy of the ratio implied that the age-incidence curves for the two populations were parallel when plotted on a logarithmic scale.

In survival analysis, the hazard rate itself is not usually calculated. Nevertheless, analogous graphical properties can be demonstrated from the estimation of survival probability itself. Since:

$$S(t , \mathbf{z}) = e^{- \Lambda_0(t) \, e^{\beta \mathbf{z}}} \tag{4.64}$$

we have:

$$\mathrm{Log} \, [- \mathrm{Log} \, (S(t , \mathbf{z}))] = \mathrm{Log} \, [\Lambda_0(t)] + \beta \mathbf{z} \tag{4.65}$$

an equation which shows that the proportional hazards model is also a generalized linear model in which the intercept with the Y-axis is the logarithm of the cumulative background rate at the specified time interval. This relationship also shows that, if the negative of the logarithm of survival probability is plotted on a logarithmic scale for two values $\mathbf{u}$ and $\mathbf{v}$ of $\mathbf{z}$, the two curves will differ from each other by a translation of value $\beta(\mathbf{v} - \mathbf{u})$. Drawing these two curves in practice helps to assess the validity of the model.

Just as the linear regression method is used in the context of normally-distributed observations to assess the specific effect of a risk factor (see Chapter 3, page 158), fitting the model $\lambda_0(t) \, e^{\alpha \mathbf{x} + \beta \mathbf{z}}$ to survival data allows the effect of a variable $\mathbf{z}$ to be evaluated after correcting for a confounding variable $\mathbf{x}$. The regression method is successful where a stratification method would have failed because it assumes that the effect of $\mathbf{z}$ is the same regardless of the value of $\mathbf{x}$. In contrast, the method of stratification evaluates the effect of $\mathbf{z}$ for all categories of variable $\mathbf{x}$, which means that a larger number of observations is required for the analysis. When the model is judged to be inadequate, it is obviously possible to construct a model which is slightly modified in each stratum by defining a baseline rate $\lambda_0(t)$ exclusive to it. Equivalently, interaction terms expressing that the effect of **z** is no longer the same for different categories of **x** can be introduced into the model. It should however be remembered that overly complicating the model risks sacrificing a large part of its value, as much in its interpretability as in its effectiveness.

Principle of the Cox model estimation

The estimation of the vector β in the model (4.61) has been described in detail in Chapter 1, page 30. In this section, the application of these principles to survival analysis is described for malignant melanoma of the lower limbs, already used to illustrate comparative methods. The covariable under study here is sex, defined by $z = 1$ for female subjects and $z = 0$ for male subjects. The model (4.61) implies that the instantaneous mortality rate for men is $\lambda_0(t)$ and that of women is $\theta\lambda_0(t)$ where $\theta = e^\beta$.

Since under the model, two subjects of the same sex have the same mortality rate, it is clear that there is one chance in two that one will survive longer than the other. Furthermore, since θ is the relative mortality rate for women with respect to men, a man has the probability $1/1+\theta$ of surviving longer than a woman. Similarly, the probability that a woman will survive longer than a man is $\theta/1+\theta$

If at the time point t_i, n_{1i} men and n_{2i} women are still under follow-up and if a subject characterized by the covariable z_i dies, the probability of this death occurring among the $n_{1i} + n_{2i}$ possible deaths is, by extension of the previous concept:

$$p_i(\beta) = \frac{e^{\beta z_i}}{n_{1i} + n_{2i}\, e^\beta} \tag{4.66}$$

When the mortality rate $\lambda_0(t)$ is not given by a parametric model, the likelihood can only be based on the order of the observations. In this case, it is equal to the probability that the m deaths occur in the observed order and that they had preceded the censored time that followed them. By repeated application of formula (4.66), the likelihood is obtained as:

$$V(\beta) = \prod_{i=1}^{m} p_i(\beta) \tag{4.67}$$

the estimate $\hat{\beta}$ of β is the value which maximizes the logarithm of $V(\beta)$:

$$L(\beta) = Log[\,V(\beta)\,] = \sum_{i=1}^{m} [\,\beta z_i - log(n_{1i} + n_{2i}\, e^\beta)\,] \tag{4.68}$$

To obtain $\hat{\beta}$, the derivative of this function with respect to β is set equal to zero:

$$C\,(\beta) = \sum_{i=1}^{m} \left[z_i - \frac{n_{2i}\,e^{\beta}}{n_{1i} + n_{2i}\,e^{\beta}} \right] \tag{4.69}$$

known as the *score*. Noting that $\hat{\theta} = e^{\hat{\beta}}$ and $d_{2.} = \sum_{i=1}^{m} z_i$ is the total number of deaths observed in women, the equation $C(\beta) = 0$ is equivalent to:

$$\sum_{i=1}^{m} z_i = d_{2.} = \sum_{i=1}^{m} \frac{n_{2i}\,\hat{\theta}}{n_{1i} + n_{2i}\,\hat{\theta}} \tag{4.70}$$

an expression which indicates that the total number of deaths observed in women is consistent with the proportions of female deaths predicted by the model at each observed date of death.

The variance of $\hat{\beta}$ is obtained from the second derivative of $L(\beta)$. Thus, in the context of this example, we have:

$$I(\beta) = -\frac{d^2 L(\beta)}{d\beta^2} = \sum_{i=1}^{m} \frac{n_{1i}\,n_{2i}\,e^{\beta}}{(n_{1i} + n_{2i}\,e^{\beta})^2} \tag{4.71}$$

Since the likelihood curve is concave around its maximum, its second derivative is negative (see Figure 4.9). The bigger the absolute value of its second derivative, the greater the curvature of $L(\beta)$ and the more precise is the estimate (see Chapter 1,

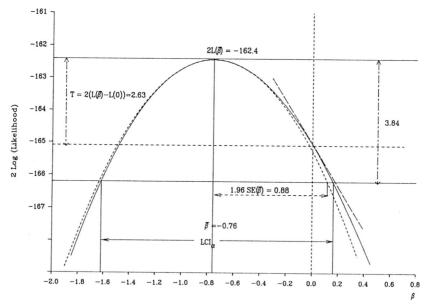

Figure 4.9 Likelihood and associated statistics. Cox model for survival of skin melanoma patients by sex, Geneva, Switzerland (incident cases 1970-1982)

page 17). Similarly, the greater the curvature is, the more $C(\beta)$ is variable in the vicinity of $\hat{\beta}$. It can be shown that the variance of $\hat{\beta}$ is closely approximated by the inverse of $I(\beta)$ and that $I(\beta)$ itself is a good approximation of the variance of $C(\beta)$.

Under the previous reasoning, we suppose that a single death occurs at each time t_i. In practice, this is rarely the case as the measurement of time is never precise enough to allow all deaths to be ordered. This situation is particularly true for data from registries when only the month of death is recorded. When D_i deaths have been observed at time t_i, the available information on survival time could have been generated by the observations defined by all possible orders of the identical survival times. There are therefore $D_i!$ possible configurations. it can be seen that a calculation based on the above principle becomes practically impossible as soon as D_i increases in size past a few units. In practice, the probability $p_i(\beta)$ is approximated by the quantity:

$$p_i^*(\beta) = \frac{\theta^{d_{2i}}}{(n_{1i} + n_{2i}\theta)^{D_i}}$$

(4.72)

which is proportional to the probability that d_{1i} male deaths and d_{2i} female deaths are observed out of a total of D_i deaths observed at time point t_i. The equations (4.68), (4.69), (4.70) and (4.71) in our example thus become:

$$L(\beta) = \sum_{i=1}^{m} [\, \beta d_{2i} - D_i \log (n_{1i} + n_{2i}e^{\beta}) \,]$$

(4.73)

$$C(\beta) = \sum_{i=1}^{m} \left[d_{2i} - D_i \left(\frac{n_{2i}\, e^{\beta}}{n_{1i} + n_{2i}\, e^{\beta}} \right) \right]$$

(4.74)

$$d_{2.} = \sum_{i=1}^{m} \left[D_i \left(\frac{n_{2i}\, \hat{\theta}}{n_{1i} + n_{2i}\hat{\theta}} \right) \right]$$

(4.75)

$$I(\beta) = \sum_{i=1}^{m} \left[D_i \, \frac{n_{1i}\, n_{2i}\, e^{\beta}}{(n_{1i} + n_{2i}\, e^{\beta})^2} \right]$$

(4.76)

The likelihood suggested by Cox is defined for each survival time by the probability that the D_i deaths have the observed configuration at this date:

$$p_i^c (\beta) = \frac{\theta^{d_{2i}}}{\sum_{\ell \subset C} \theta^{k(\ell)}}$$

(4.77)

where C is the totality of choices of d_{2i} deaths among the $n_{1i} + n_{2i}$ subjects present in the study at t_i, and $k(\ell)$ is the number of female subjects in the combination ℓ. The expression (4.72) is an approximation to (4.77), and is used in most computer software for survival analyses.

Table 4.15   Likelihood of the Cox model; prognostic value of sex on survival of subjects with melanoma of the legs in Geneva, Switzerland (Incident cases 1970-1982)

Date	Males		Females		Contribution to the likelihood[a]		
	death	at risk	death	at risk	$p_i^*(\beta)$	$\log p_i^*(0)$	$\log p_i^*(\hat{\beta})$
2	0	19	1	64	$\theta/(19+64\theta)$	-4.419	-4.650
4	1	19	0	63	$1/(19+63\theta)$	-4.408	-3.881
12	0	18	1	63	$\theta/(18+63\theta)$	-4.394	-4.620
18	1	18	0	62	$1/(18+62\theta)$	-4.382	-3.850
23	1	17	0	62	$1/(17+62\theta)$	-4.369	-3.829
28	0	16	2	62	$\theta^2/(16+62\theta)^2$	-8.713	-9.133
38	1	16	0	60	$1/(16+60\theta)$	-4.331	-3.786
43	0	15	1	60	$\theta/(15+60\theta)$	-4.317	-4.523
44	1	15	0	59	$1/(15+59\theta)$	-4.304	-3.752
52	0	14	1	59	$\theta/(14+59\theta)$	-4.290	-4.488
54	0	14	2	58	$\theta^2/(14+58\theta)^2$	-8.553	-8.953
55	0	14	1	56	$\theta/(14+56\theta)$	-4.248	-4.454
65	1	9	0	28	$1/(9+28\theta)$	-3.611	-3.095
66	0	7	1	26	$\theta/(7+26\theta)$	-3.497	-3.713
68	0	7	1	22	$\theta/(7+22\theta)$	-3.367	-3.610
81	0	6	1	19	$\theta/(6+19\theta)$	-3.219	-3.460
102	0	6	1	18	$\theta/(6+18\theta)$	-3.178	-3.428
110	1	6	0	17	$1/(6+17\theta)$	-3.135	-2.636
155	1	2	0	4	$1/(2+4\theta)$	-1.792	-1.353

$$2L(0) = -165.1 \quad 2L(\hat{\beta}) = -162.4$$

[a] See (4.67), (4.68), (4.72) ; $\theta = e^\beta$; $\hat{\beta} = 0.76$

Table 4.15 gives dates of observed death, number of subjects under follow-up at each date and the contribution of each death to the likelihood. The approximation (4.72) is used in case of identical survival times. Figure 4.9 shows the function $2L(\beta)$ in the vicinity of $\hat{\beta}$ which, in this case, is -0.76 ($\hat{\theta} = 0.47$). Here the test of the hypothesis $\beta = 0$ has as its objective the comparison of the survival between male and female subjects, and could be carried out by the logrank test. In the context of the maximum likelihood method, there are several classical tests available [33] (see Chapter 1); it is of note that one of them will again lead to the logrank test.

The likelihood ratio test

$$T1 = 2[L(\hat{\beta}) - L(0)] \tag{4.78}$$

has a χ^2 distribution under the null hypothesis. Its number of degrees of freedom is equal to the dimension of β. In the example given, the number of degrees of freedom is equal to unity and $T_1 = 2.63$ ($p = 0.11$).

Furthermore, $2[L(\hat{\beta}) - L(\beta_0)]$ has this distribution if $\beta = \beta_0$. We define around $\hat{\beta}$ all the values of β which, given the observations, are not rejected by the test T_1, that is, those for which

$$2[L(\hat{\beta}) - L(\beta)] < Z^2_{\alpha/2} \tag{4.79}$$

This interval is classically known as the likelihood-based confidence interval, and noted as LCI_α in Figure 4.9.

Wald's test is based on the variance of $\hat{\beta}$, obtained from the matrix of the second derivatives of L. In the example where β is of dimension 1,

$$T_2 = \frac{\hat{\beta}^2}{Var(\hat{\beta})} \tag{4.80}$$

is a χ^2 variable on one degree of freedom. Here, the standard error associated with the estimate β is calculated from $1/I(\beta)$ and is 0.451, therefore $T_2 = (-0.76)^2/(0.451)^2 = 2.84$. indicating that we can not exclude the possibility that β is null.

The variance of $\hat{\beta}$, allows a confidence interval for β to be constructed using the usual expression:

$$CI_\alpha = \hat{\beta} \pm \left[Z_{\alpha/2}\sqrt{Var(\hat{\beta})} \right]$$

This interval is derived in the same way as the interval LCI except that $2[L(\beta) - L(0)]$ is replaced by its quadratic approximation (see Figure 4.9 and Chapter 1, page 17).

The Score test is based on the vector of first derivatives of the likelihood which, in the example, reduces to the function $C(\beta)$. The statistic

$$T_3 = \frac{C(0)^2}{I(0)} \tag{4.81}$$

assess the magnitude of the slope of the tangent to the likelihood curve $2L(\beta)$ at the value of β being tested (here 0). If it is not possible to reject the hypothesis that this line is horizontal, then it should be concluded that 0 is acceptable as a value of β. In the example, $T_3 = 2.98$. Since, from formula (4.75)

$$C(0) = d_2 - \sum_{i=1}^{m} D_i \frac{n_{2i}}{n_{1i} + n_{2i}}$$

it can be seen that the score test is based on the same statistic as the logrank. The variance $I(0)$ is exactly that obtained in (4.43) if there are no ties ($D_i = 1$ for each t_i). It is slightly different if there are ties (since each term of the sum defining it is multiplied by $(N_i - 1)/(N_i - D_i)$). Using $p_i^c(\beta)$ (4.77) instead of the approximation $p_i*(\beta)$ to calculate the likelihood would give exactly the same variance as (4.43) and the score test will thus be identical to the logrank test in all cases.

The previous example illustrated the use of the Cox model to estimate the relative rate for a single dichotomous factor. The principles applicable when more than one categorical or continuous factor is studied (the case in fact for which the model was developed) have been described in Chapter 1. These principles are exactly the same: only the expression of the model is more complicated. In the construction of these models, the mortality rate $\lambda_0(t)$ has been considered to be a nuisance parameter. However, in practice, it is often desirable to estimate the survival curve corresponding to this background rate. The principle of the Kaplan-Meier method (see formula 1.22) is used here, but the number of deaths at time point t_i is related to a modified denominator to take account of the fact that not all individuals under follow-up at time point t_i are subject to the same risk of death. The estimate of $S_0(t)$ is therefore given by the formula:

$$\hat{S}_0(t) = \prod_{t_i \le t} \left(1 - \frac{D_i}{\sum_{j \subset R_i} \hat{\theta}_j} \right) \qquad (4.82)$$

in which each individual in group R_i of subjects at risk of death at time t_i is no longer counted as one but as a value equal to its relative rate.

Example of an adjustment using Cox's model

Survival data based on hospital records are often considered to be a biased representation of the overall situation. In particular, survival rates calculated from these data may be better than those obtained from the ensemble of incident cases. One explanation for this phenomenon is that cases not treated in hospital are often those that are very advanced or that have not been treated at all. Hospital statistics would therefore represent a selection of favourable cases, for which survival is overestimated in comparison to the general population.

The Geneva cancer registry routinely collects the place of treatment of all incident cases (public university hospital or other health care centre). The survival of patients treated in these two health centres can thus be compared. Breast cancer data are given as an example [34]. The 1105 women diagnosed between 1975 and 1982, were allocated to two groups depending on their place of treatment. The two groups were then compared using a Cox model with one covariable z, indicating group membership (z=1 corresponds to the group treated in a university hospital):

$$\lambda(t) = \lambda_0(t) \ e^{\beta z} \qquad (4.83)$$

The hypothesis of equal death rates in the two groups ($\beta = 0$) is evaluated by the score test (4.81) which, in this case, corresponds to the logrank test. The value obtained ($T_3 = 29.9$) corresponding to a χ^2 on one degree of freedom is very significant ($p < 10^{-5}$). The likelihood ratio test (4.78) obviously confirms this result ($T_1 = 33.2$).

The estimate of the relative rate obtained by maximizing the Cox likelihood is:

$$\hat{\theta} = e^{\hat{\beta}} = 2.04$$

indicating that the mortality rate is about twice as high for patients of the public university hospital as for those of other health care centres.

Since there is no reason to suspect that health care is inferior in university hospitals, it is important to take into account factors which might lead to the selection of cases with a poorer prognosis into public health care institutions. One possibility may be that the public hospital receives advanced cases which require complicated treatment and have poorer prognoses. There may also be selection by social class associated with the higher financial contribution required of patients in the private sector. Clinical stage, social class and age have therefore been examined in order to assess this assumption. It is known that these three variables have a prognostic role and Table 4.16 shows that they have a different distribution in the two health care systems. Consequently, they should be taken into account in the comparison (see page 255) otherwise all or part of their effect may be attributed to the type of hospital health care system.

Clinical stage, which has a fundamental importance in this context, is used to illustrate the model-fitting for a qualitative variable. This variable has four categories, with an associated vector of indicator variables $\mathbf{x} = (x_2, x_3, x_4)$ defined by:

- Localized only $(x_2 = 0, x_3 = 0, x_4 = 0)$
- Regional involvement $(x_2 = 1, x_3 = 0, x_4 = 0)$
- Metastases $(x_2 = 0, x_3 = 1, x_4 = 0)$
- Unknown $(x_2 = 0, x_3 = 0, x_4 = 1)$

These three variables are then included in the model which is written:

$$\lambda(t, \mathbf{x}, z) = \lambda_0(t) \, e^{(\alpha_2 x_2 + \alpha_3 x_3 + \alpha_4 x_4 + \beta z)} \qquad (4.84)$$

the variable z still being the variable of interest indicating the health care system as defined.

Table 4.16 : Distribution (%) of prognostic variables available by   health care system for breast cancer in Geneva, Switzerland (Incident cases 1975-1982)

Age (years)	< 50	50-64	65-74	75+
University hospital (N=808)	25	25	25	25
Other (N=297)	33	31	18	18

Stage	Local	Regional	Metastasis	Unknown
University hospital (N=808)	47	39	10	4
Other (N=297)	60	27	1	12

Social class	Manual workers	Office workers	Executives	Unknown
University hospital (N=808)	29	35	13	23
Other (N=297)	20	39	19	22

The estimate $\hat{\theta} = e^{\hat{\beta}}$ which maximizes the likelihood of observations for this model is the relative mortality rate 'adjusted for stage' for the university hospitals. Its value ($\hat{\theta}$ = 1.91) is only slightly less than the previous value, showing a small confounding effect due to the fact that the stage at diagnosis is on average more advanced in public hospitals.

The test of the hypothesis β = 0 from the likelihood ratio gives a value T_1 = 22.8. By the score test, the value obtained is T_3 = 21.0. These values are very significant in both cases, indicating that the effect of hospital type remains after taking stage into account.

The logrank test with stratification described earlier (see page 255) could have been used to solve this problem. In fact, it would have provided the same results as a Cox model with stratification specifying:

$$\lambda_{\mathbf{x}}(t) = \lambda_{\mathbf{x}0}(t) \, e^{(\beta z)} \tag{4.85}$$

This equation implies, as does (4.84), that there is the same relative rate between public hospitals and other health care systems for each stage $\mathbf{x}$. However, it allows for the possibility that the baseline hazard rates might differ for each stage. The maximum likelihood here is the product of the likelihoods of the proportional hazards model written separately for each stage. To obtain the score test for the hypothesis β = 0, scores calculated for each stage are first summed and the variance of this sum is calculated by addition of the within-stage information related to β. The test is then the ratio of the two sums and is identical, apart from the way in which ties are dealt with, to the logrank test with adjustment for the stage given page... Its value (T_3 = 19.4) is very close to that obtained above, (T_3 = 21.0), and the estimate of β ($\hat{\theta}$ = 1.85) is little different from that derived from the model (4.84), that is, $\hat{\theta}$ = 1.91. This result confirms that the stage at diagnosis is responsible for only a small part of the difference observed between the two types of hospitals.

The adjustment for all other available variables is summarized in Table 4.17. Although social class and age have some prognostic value, they do not qualitatively change the previous conclusion since the estimate of β, after adjusting for these variables, still corresponds to a relative rate of 1.56 which is significantly different from unity.

Figure 4.10 gives survival observed in the two groups. Survival predicted by the model for each of the hospital types is also given. The predicted survival for other health care system is given for a group of patients with an identical distribution of stage, age and social class to that of the patients treated in the public university hospitals. The difference between the curve predicted and observed for patients outside university hospitals is an estimate of the portion of the improvement in survival which can be explained by the most favourable distribution of the recorded prognostic factors in patients treated outside the public sector.

This result suggests that factors other than stage, age and social class as recorded by the registry may lead patients with worse prognoses to be treated in university hospitals. The presence of a large number of cases of unknown stage among patients treated in other health care systems could distort the comparison,

Table 4.17 Cox's model for breast cancer survival data from Geneva, Switzerland (Incident cases 1975-1982)

	$\hat{\beta}(^a)$	$SE(\hat{\beta})$	$\hat{\theta}(^b)$	Score test(^{c})
Health care system				
University hospital	0.445	0.14	1.56*	29.9
Other	0	–	1.00	
Stage				
Local involvement	0	–	1.00	21.0
Regional involvement	0.801	0.12	2.23*	
Metastases	2.482	0.16	11.97*	
Unknown	1.399	0.19	4.05*	
Age (years)				
< 50	0	–	1.00	11.6
50-64	0.247	0.16	1.28	
65-74	0.440	0.16	1.55*	
75+	1.424	0.16	4.16*	
Social class				
Manual workers	0	–	1.00	10.0
Office workers	− 0.135	0.13	0.87	
Executives	− 0.001	0.18	1.00	
Unknown	− 0.425	0.14	0.65*	

(^{a}) Estimate obtained when all variables (stage, age and class) are included in the model.
(^{b}) The asterisk indicates variables for which the 95% confidence interval excludes 1 ($\hat{\beta}/SE(\hat{\beta}) \geq 1.96$).
(^{c}) Test of effect of the health care system after inclusion of the corresponding variable in the model. The first model is the crude test of effect equivalent to the logrank test without adjustment.

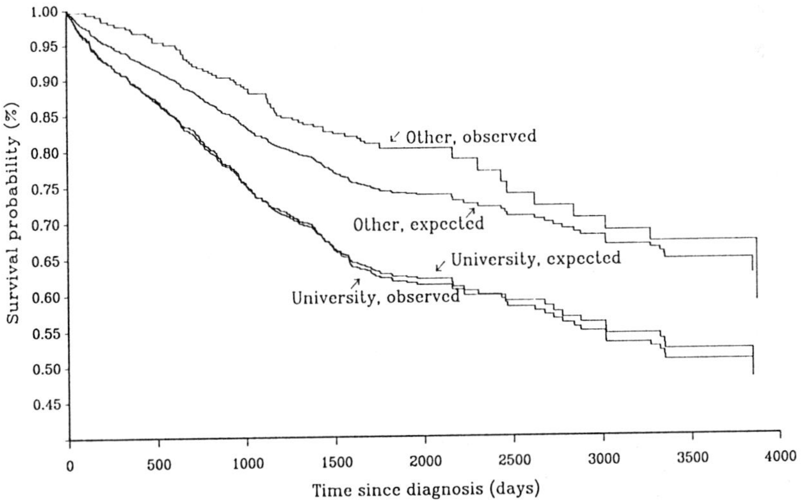

Figure 4.10 Observed and adjusted survival of breast cancer patients by type of hospital – Geneva – Cases diagnosed between 1978 and 1982

as could cases of advanced clinical stages which are almost all treated in university hospitals. It is therefore worth repeating the analysis, limiting the comparison to patients whose tumours were at an early stage, either being localized or only showing regional involvement. The results are not modified substantially although the estimate of $\hat{\theta} = 1.54$ is decreased as is the score test ($T_2 = 7.57$), showing that part of the difference observed for unknown stage was incorrectly attributed to an effect of the health care system.

These results do not correspond to the commonly held notion of better survival in leading hospitals; effects of selection other than those which have been controlled for are probably responsible for the findings. Furthermore, it is known that adjustment by class can leave residual differences with respect to confounding factors because of the phenomenon of within group variation. Classification into three clinical stages only partially accounts for the characteristics of the disease. Fitting stage categories more finely, even though impossible due to the lack of the necessary information, would have improved the results.

Phenomena of this kind have been described by Feinstein [35] to illustrate the paradox attributed to Will Rogers. Convinced of the mediocre intellectual level in California even among higher socio-economic classes, Rogers noted that the average cultural level in California improved even when underprivileged people from Oklahoma emigrated there. This emigration obviously caused a similar phenomenon in Oklahoma. A similar situation occurs with the retrospective reclassification of clinical diagnoses of cancer [35]. Reclassification effectively leads to the worst cases of localized cancer being categorized as regional stage, although these cases have on average a better prognosis than those of the category in which they are now classified. The result is a purely fictional improvement in the survival rate in both categories.

Comparison of net survival

Differences between the survival distributions in several groups are often difficult to interpret because the overall mortality observed is partially due to competing causes of death. These causes, however, are not the object of the comparison and the extent of their effect can vary from one group to another. These difficulties can be very pronounced when a comparison is to be made over a long time period, in particular when the groups being compared do not have the same age distribution or life expectancy. Comparison is then carried out using net survival.

The methods discussed in the previous sections for comparing survival between two or more groups apply without change if the net survival is estimated by the cause-specific survival method (see page 230). In effect, dates of death not caused by the cancer under study are considered as censored observations. However, as noted above, it is not generally advisable to use this method because of inaccuracies in the classification of the causes of death. Other methods such as relative survival should thus be considered to estimate net survival. Unfortunately, the analysis is then not as simple and should be adapted from principles used above to carry out the comparison of crude survival.

The comparison of two relative survival rates at a given time point (e.g., five years) can be easily carried out by calculating their variances, which are in turn obtained directly from the crude survival analyses. A test analogous to that given in formula (4.42) can then be easily carried out. This approach is however subject to the same criticism as for crude survival.

Note that the use of relative survival does not remove the need to account for age in the comparisons. In fact, as we have seen before (Table 4.10) and as we will confirm below, net survival, like crude survival, is often dependent on age. Relative survival should therefore also be adjusted for the effect of age before any interpretation of observed differences is made. Myers and Hankey [36] and Hakulinen [37] have resolved this problem by calculating relative survival in subgroups which are homogeneous for the main determinants of net survival and by calculating a relative survival rate for the whole group using the method of direct standardisation (see Chapter 2, page 56). Myers and Hankey compared relative survival for different cancer sites between Blacks and Whites after adjusting for age and stage. Hakulinen compared relative survival between Finland and Norway after adjusting for age. However, this method accounts rather imperfectly for the effect of age and depends to some extent on the choice of the standard population. Furthermore, as for crude survival, comparison of survival at specified time points is rarely the only problem of interest. Consequently, methods have been proposed for comparing entire net survival curves and adjusting for confounding variables. We will only describe here the principles underlying these methods and suggest further reading for the reader who wishes to apply them.

One possibility is to adopt a method analogous to the Mantel-Haenszel test, by considering the distribution of deaths in the groups for each interval appearing in the actuarial survival curve (Table 4.11). Brown [38] and Hakulinen [39,40] have constructed tests of this kind, based on the maximum likelihood method. The distribution of the number of deaths d_{ki} for time interval i among the n_{ki} subjects in group k is a binomial distribution:

$$d_{ki} \rightsquigarrow \text{binom}(n_{ki}, 1 - r_{ki} s_{ki}^*)$$

where r_{ki} is the relative survival of the n_{ki} individuals in group k who were living at the beginning of the interval and s_{ki}^* is their expected survival, calculated from the life table, and taking into account the competing forces of mortality. The test of the hypothesis that the r_{ki} are equal is however more complicated than the Mantel-Haenszel test: when n_{ki} and the number of deaths are fixed, d_{ki} has a noncentral hypergeometric distribution with variance and covariance depending on r_{ki}. Although identical in all groups for each interval i under the null hypothesis, the r_{ki} nevertheless remain unknown, and in order to carry out the test, they must be estimated.

Moreover, this method makes implicitly the unrealistic assumption that all individuals at risk of death at the beginning of the interval have the same expected survival s_{ki}^*. Its application would in principle require stratification of the variables influencing survival so that, for each level j of the stratification variable, the n_{kji} individuals at risk at the beginning of the interval would have the same expected survival s^*_{kji}. Stratification of this kind is always possible for age and sex, for which the existing life tables allow the calculation of expected survival probability s^*_{kji}.

When groups being compared have the same mortality hazard for other causes, this stratification will make expected survival identical for individuals in the different groups being compared within each stratum thus created. The logrank test with stratification then applies without change since, under the null hypothesis, the probabilities of dying are identical. In this special case, stratification by age avoids the need to adjust for competing causes. Adjusting for age using Cox's model is also possible. However, if age classes are included directly in the model equation, the effect of age is implicitly considered as being multiplicative; since a large part of this effect is created by the additive effect of competing causes of death (see formulae 4.29 and 4.39) it might be advisable to fit an age stratified Cox model.

When mortality for other causes cannot be considered equal for the two groups, Brown's and Hakulinen's methods can be used, bearing in mind that the variance of d_{ki} differs from that specified by the binomial distribution. It is relatively easy to take this problem into account in the context of a generalized linear model such as that proposed by Hakulinen [39,40]. However, it seems more efficient to derive the likelihood from individual observations and not from data grouped by interval. This approach has been used by Pocock and coworkers [41], Buckley [42] and in the model presented in the first part of this chapter. Pocock assumes that the rate added to the baseline rate of the general population by the presence of the disease decreases exponentially with time. In contrast, Buckley considers the case where the distribution of net survival is exponential. The extension of his analysis to a proportional hazards model with baseline rate described by a step function is discussed by Esteve and co-workers [20] and summarized by the formulae (4.38), (4.39) and (4.40). This approach leads to a classical test based on the likelihood ratio principle analogous to that described for the Cox model. The strategy discussed for this latter model can be applied without change (see p. 268).

As an example, the method has been applied to colon cancer survival data from Geneva (page 244). Table 4.18 presents the test of the effect of sex on survival in three different contexts. In the first, the comparison is made ignoring mortality from other causes; in the second, the method described above is used and, in the third, cause-specific survival probabilities are compared. Sex has no significant effect regardless of the method used. Nevertheless, it is worth noting that the effect of sex is corrected in the right sense when competing causes are taken into account. The effect of age on net survival can also be evaluated by the likelihood ratio test. The logarithm of the likelihood of model (4.38) with ß=0 is calculated to be −1072.25, giving a χ^2 on two degrees of freedom equal to:

$$2[-1040.02 - (-1072.25)] = 64.46$$

Although the effect of age appears to be weaker for net survival, it still remains very high. The effect of age would have been incorrectly described if it had been

Table 4.18   The influence of age and sex on colon cancer survival in Geneva, Switzerland. (Incident cases 1970-1979)

Context	Estimate of β (Standard error)			Logarithm of the likelihood
	Sex males[a]	Age		
		65-74	75 +	
1) Crude survival[b]	0.101 (0.08)	0.621 (0.11)	0.986 (0.10)	− 4006.28
sex excluded	−	0.616 (0.11)	0.970 (0.10)	− 4007.07
2) Net survival[c]	0.048 (0.09)	0.593 (0.12)	0.916 (0.12)	− 1039.89
sex excluded	−	0.591 (0.12)	0.909 (0.12)	− 1040.02
3) Cause-specific survival[d]	0.005 (0.09)	0.613 (0.12)	0.934 (0.11)	− 3364.78
sex excluded	−	0.612 (0.12)	0.934 (0.11)	− 3364.78

[a] In each context, the second model contains age only in order to allow for the likelihood ratio test to be carried out.
[b] Proportional hazard models fitted by Cox's method with three months as the time unit.
[c] Proportional hazard model with a background rate constant for three-month intervals up to three years from diagnosis, six-month intervals up to four years and then an interval of one year and an interval of five years.
[d] The same models as for (b), but each death not recorded as due to cancer of the colon is censored at the date of death.

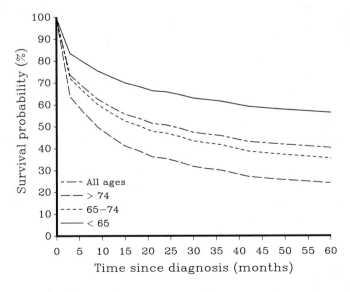

Figure 4.11   Relative survival of colon cancer cases diagnosed between 1970 and 1979 in Geneva, Switzerland, estimated by the method of maximum likelihood

studied for relative survival at five years and it would have been almost unnoticed using relative survival at ten years (Table 4.10). Figure 4.11 shows the net survival of the three age groups and of all groups calculated by the maximum likelihood method.

Bibliographical Notes

Chiang's now classic work [43] dedicated to stochastic processes in the field of human biology, provides a complete, systematic and integrated study of the application of probability theory to the concept of risk and survival which are essential in epidemiology. Although this work is usually reserved for statisticians, it contains many chapters which are relatively accessible mathematically. These sections mainly involve analysis of the life table and the mechanics of its construction, and the problem of competing risks. Chiang has written a manual for the World Health Organization on the life table which is more accessible to epidemiologists [44].

More detailed concepts and methods underlying survival analysis can be found in the more recent, fundamental work of Kalbfleisch and Prentice [26]. Although the concepts and methods are mainly described for mathematically-minded readers, the accompanying examples assist the non-statistician. Of particular note are the sections on parametric models (Weibull, exponential, log-normal, gamma) and the problems presented by the adequacy of the models fitted. Cox's proportional hazards model and its application are the subject of a substantial section in the book, especially with regard to time-dependent covariates. A review of the theory of competing risks and methods for the retrospective analysis of survival can also be found in this text.

The manual on survival analysis by Hill and co-workers is among the more practical texts for non-statisticians. Although it addresses clinical trials rather than epidemiology, this text is nevertheless useful for its detailed review of descriptive and comparative methods of survival study. Problems raised by tests of comparison have an important place in the book; an annex is entirely devoted to the principles underlying rank tests and the choice of the appropriate test. Parametric and semi-parametric models, the evaluation of goodness-of-fit, coding of variables, hierarchical tests and trend tests are treated with equal clarity.

The description of the life table in Pressat's text offers a more demographic view point [45]. Of historical interest, Berkson first proposed the concept of relative survival [19] and the classic article by Elveback presents somewhat didactically the principles behind the actuarial method [46]. The scientific publication on cancer registration published by the International Agency for Research on Cancer (IARC) considers the calculation of survival of incident cases [47].

Cancer registries can calculate survival using the computer program package developed by the Finnish Cancer Registry [48]. These programs enable users to estimate relative and observed survival curves and carry out comparative tests.

Clinicians will benefit from the article by Christensen describing the concepts underlying the Cox model in the context of clinical trials [49]. This article provides practical advice and many examples on how to conduct the analyses and interpret the results.

REFERENCES

[1] Denoix P, Amiel JL, Brulé G, et al. *La maladie cancéreuse.* Paris, J.-B. Baillière, 1968, Chap. V

[2] Walter SD, Stitt LW. Evaluating the survival of cancer cases detected by screening. *Stat Med* 1987 **6** : 885-900

[3] Kaplan EL, Meier P. Nonparametric estimation from incomplete observations. *J Am Stat Assoc* 1958 **53** : 457-64

[4] Glass DV. Graunt's life table. *Population (Paris)* 1937 **2** : 71-2

[5] Peto R, Pike MC, Armitage P et al. Organisation et analyse des essais thérapeutiques comparatifs comportant une longue surveillance des malades. *Rev Épidémiol Santé Publ* 1979 **273** : 171-257

[6] Greenwood M. *A report on the natural duration of cancer.* London, Ministry of Health, His Majesty's Stationery Office, 1926 (Reports on public health and medical subjects, n° 33)

[7] Rao CR. Linear statistical inference and its applications (2nd ed.). New York, John Wiley, 1973 pp. 385-8.

[8] Breslow N. Statistical methods for censored survival data. *Environ Health Perspect* 1979 **32** : 181-192

[9] Rothman KJ. Estimation of confidence limits for the cumulative probability of survival in life table analysis. *J Chron Dis* 1978 **31** : 557-60

[10] Anderson JR, Bernstein L, Pike MC. Approximate confidence intervals for probabilities of survival and quantiles in life-table analysis. Biometrics 1982 **38** : 407-16

[11] Emerson J. Nonparametric confidence intervals for the median in the presence of right censoring. *Biometrics* 1982 **38** : 17-27

[12] Brookmeyer R, Crowley J. A confidence interval for the median survival time. *Biometrics* 1982 **38** : 29-41

[13] Ederer F, Axtell LM, Cutler SJ. The relative survival rate : a statistical methodology. *Nat Cancer Inst Monogr* 1961 **6** : 101-120

[14] Hakulinen T. On long-term relative survival rates. *J Chron Dis* 1977 **30** : 431-43

[15] Reed LJ, Merrel M. A short method for constructing an abridged life table. *Am J Hyg* 1939 **30** : 33-62

[16] Hakulinen T. Cancer survival corrected for heterogeneity in patient withdrawal. *Biometrics* 1982 **38** : 933-942

[17] Ederer F, Heise H. *The effect of eliminating deaths from cancer on general population survival rates.* Methodological note n° 11, End Results Evaluation Section. National Cancer Institute, Aug. 1959

[18] Rothman KJ, Boice JD. *Epidemiologic analysis with a programmable calculator.* Washington, US Department of Health, Education, and Welfare, Public Health Service, National Institutes of Health, 1979

[19] Berkson J. The calculation of survival rates. *In* : W Walters, HK Gray, JT Priestley, (eds.) : *Carcinoma and other malignant lesions of the stomach.* Philadelphia, Saunders, 1942 pp. 467-84

[20] Estève J, Benhamou E, Croasdale M, Raymond L. Relative survival and the estimation of net survival : elements for further discussion. *Stat Med* 1990 **9** :529-38

[21] Breslow NE. Analysis of survival data under the proportional hazards model. *Int Stat Rev* 1975 **43** :45-58

[22] Andersen PK, Borch-Johnsen K, Deckert T et al. A Cox regression model for the relative mortality and its application to diabetes mellitus survival data. *Biometrics* 1985 **41** : 921-32

[23] Hill C, Laplanche A, Rezvani A. Comparison of the mortality of a cohort with the mortality of a reference population in a prognostic study. *Stat Med* 1985 **4** : 295-302

[24] Pocock SJ, Gore SM, Kerr GR. Long term survival analysis : the curability of breast cancer. *Stat Med* 1982 **1** : 93-104

[25] Cox DR. Regression models and life tables. *J R Statist Soc B* 1972 **34** : 187-220

[26] Kalbfleisch JD, Prentice RL. *The statistical analysis of failure time data.* New York, Wiley, 1980

[27] *In* Hill C, Com-Nougué C, Kramar A et al. *Analyse statistique des données de survie.* Paris, Médecine-Sciences Flammarion, 1990 pp. 159-168

[28] Peto R, Peto J. Asymptotically efficient rank invariant test procedures with discussion. *J R Statist Soc A* 1972 **135** : 185-207

[29] Gehan EA. A generalized Wilcoxon test for comparing arbitrarily singly-censored samples. *Biometrika* 1965 **52** : 203-23

[30] Breslow NE. A generalized Kruskal-Wallis test for comparing K samples subject to unequal patterns of censorship. *Biometrika* 1970 **57** : 579-94

[31] Peto R, Pike MC. Conservatism of the approximation $(0-E)^2/E$ in the logrank test for survival data or tumor incidence data. *Biometrics* 1973 **29** : 579-84

[32] Breslow NE, Crowley J. A large sample study of the life table and product limit estimates under random censorship. *Ann Stat* 1974 **2** : 437-53

[33] *In* C Hill, C Com-Nougué, A Kramar et al. *Analyse statistique des données de survie.* Paris, Médecine-Sciences Flammarion, 1990 pp. 68-73

[34] Raymond L, Gasser A, Levi F, Fioretta G. Taux de survie hospitaliers et épidémiologiques : résultats paradoxaux enregistrés à Genève. *Schweiz Krebs-Bull* 1988 **1** : 11-14

[35] Feinstein AR, Sosin DM, Wells CK. The Will Rogers phenomenon : stage migration and new diagnostic techniques as a source of misleading statistics for survival in cancer. *N Engl J Med* 1985 **312** : 1604-8

[36] Myers MH, Hawkey BF. *Cancer patient survival experience.* Bethesda, US Departement of Health and Human Services, 1980 NIH Publication 80-2148

[37] Hakulinen T. A comparison of nationwide cancer survival statistics in Finland and Norway. *World Health Stat Q* 1983 **36** : 35-46

[38] Brown CC. The statistical comparison of relative survival rates. *Biometrics* 1983 **39** : 941-8

[39] Hakulinen T, Tenkanen L, Abeywickrama K. Testing equality of relative survival patterns based on aggregated data. *Biometrics* 1987 **43** : 313-25

[40] Hakulinen T, Tenkanen L. Regression analysis of relative survival rates. *Appl Stat* 1987 **36** : 309-17

[41] Pocock, SJ, Gore SM, Kerr GR. Long term survival analysis : the curability of breast cancer. *Stat Med* 1982 **1** : 93-104

[42] Buckley JD. Additive and multiplicative models for relative survival rates. *Biometrics* 1984 **40** : 51-62

[43] Chin Long Chiang. *Introduction to stochastic processes in biostatistics.* New York, Wiley, 1968

[44] Chin Long Chiang. *Life table and mortality analysis.* Geneva, World Health Organization, 1979

[45] Pressat R. *L'analyse démographique, concepts, méthodes, résultats* (2e ed.). Paris, Presses Universitaires de France, 1969

[46] Elveback L. Estimation of survivorship in chronic disease : the « actuarial » method. *Amer Stat Ass* 1958 420-440

[47] Jensen OM, Parkin DM, MacLennan R, Muir CS, Skeet RG. *Cancer registration : principles and methods.* (IARC Scientific Publications No 95), Lyon, IARC, 1991

[48] Hakulinen T, Abeywickrama KL, Söderman B. A *computer program package for cancer survival studies.* Helsinki, Finnish Cancer Registry, 1987

[49] Christensen E. Multivariate survival analysis using Cox's regression model. *Hepatology*, 1987 **7** : 1346-1358

Appendix 1

Life table for Switzerland; 1978-1983
(source : Office fédéral de la statistique, Berne, 1985)

1 Age	2 Probability of death $\hat{q}_x$	3 Survival probability $\hat{p}_x$	4 Death rate $\hat{\lambda}_x$	5 Survivor function ℓ_x	6 Number of deaths d_x	7 Expectation of life $\overset{o}{e}_x$	8 Age
x							x
0	0.009487	0.990513		100000	949	72.40	0
1	0.000887	0.999113	0.003823	99051	88	72.09	1
2	0.000675	0.999325	0.000760	98963	66	71.16	2
3	0.000551	0.999449	0.000602	98897	55	70.20	3
4	0.000460	0.999540	0.000501	98842	45	69.24	4
5	0.000403	0.999597	0.000423	98797	40	68.27	5
6	0.000379	0.999621	0.000393	98757	38	67.30	6
7	0.000355	0.999645	0.000371	98719	35	66.33	7
8	0.000332	0.999668	0.000338	98684	32	65.35	8
9	0.000313	0.999687	0.000318	98652	31	64.37	9
10	0.000300	0.999700	0.000309	98621	30	63.39	10
11	0.000296	0.999704	0.000298	98591	29	62.41	11
12	0.000307	0.999693	0.000295	98562	30	61.43	12
13	0.000340	0.999660	0.000321	98532	34	60.45	13
14	0.000405	0.999595	0.000371	98498	40	59.47	14
15	0.000513	0.999487	0.000448	98458	50	58.49	15
16	0.000682	0.999318	0.000582	98408	67	57.52	16
17	0.000931	0.999069	0.000801	98341	92	56.56	17
18	0.001207	0.998793	0.001067	98249	118	55.61	18
19	0.001469	0.998531	0.001346	98131	145	54.68	19
20	0.001676	0.998324	0.001590	97986	164	53.76	20
21	0.001787	0.998213	0.001752	97822	175	52.85	21
22	0.001760	0.998240	0.001786	97647	171	51.94	22
23	0.001686	0.998314	0.001728	97476	165	51.03	23
24	0.001600	0.998400	0.001651	97311	156	50.12	24
25	0.001532	0.998468	0.001561	97155	148	49.20	25
26	0.001474	0.998526	0.001498	97007	143	48.27	26
27	0.001407	0.998593	0.001448	96864	137	47.34	27
28	0.001340	0.998660	0.001374	96727	129	46.41	28
29	0.001286	0.998714	0.001304	96598	124	45.47	29

1 Age x	2 Probability of death $\hat{q}_x$	3 Survival probability $\hat{p}_x$	4 Death rate $\hat{\lambda}_x$	5 Survivor function ℓ_x	6 Number of deaths d_x	7 Expectation of life $\overset{o}{e}_x$	8 Age x
30	0.001255	0.998745	0.001272	96474	122	44.53	30
31	0.001248	0.998752	0.001253	96352	120	43.58	31
32	0.001257	0.998743	0.001249	96232	121	42.64	32
33	0.001282	0.998718	0.001267	96111	123	41.69	33
34	0.001323	0.998677	0.001300	95988	127	40.74	34
35	0.001382	0.998618	0.001348	95861	132	39.80	35
36	0.001451	0.998549	0.001413	95729	139	38.85	36
37	0.001530	0.998478	0.001495	95590	147	37.91	37
38	0.001630	0.998370	0.001578	95443	155	36.97	38
39	0.001757	0.998243	0.001689	95288	168	36.02	39
40	0.001923	0.998077	0.001841	95120	183	35.09	40
41	0.002127	0.997873	0.002014	94937	201	34.15	41
42	0.002366	0.997634	0.002243	94736	225	33.23	42
43	0.002635	0.997365	0.002505	94511	249	32.30	43
44	0.002931	0.997069	0.002780	94262	276	31.39	44
45	0.003251	0.996749	0.003088	93986	305	30.48	45
46	0.003572	0.996428	0.003416	93681	335	29.58	46
47	0.003897	0.996103	0.003742	93346	364	28.68	47
48	0.004258	0.995742	0.004079	92982	396	27.79	48
49	0.004690	0.995310	0.004469	92586	434	26.91	49
50	0.005225	0.994775	0.004947	92152	481	26.03	50
51	0.005872	0.994128	0.005549	91671	539	25.17	51
52	0.006610	0.993390	0.006249	91132	602	24.31	52
53	0.007424	0.992576	0.007026	90530	672	23.47	53
54	0.008301	0.991699	0.007884	89858	746	22.64	54
55	0.009229	0.990771	0.008803	89112	823	21.83	55
56	0.010172	0.989828	0.009748	88289	898	21.03	56
57	0.011129	0.988861	0.010700	87391	973	20.24	57
58	0.012182	0.987818	0.011711	86418	1053	19.46	58
59	0.013356	0.986644	0.012826	85365	1140	18.69	59
60	0.014712	0.985288	0.014102	84225	1239	17.94	60
61	0.016236	0.983764	0.015566	82986	1347	17.20	61
62	0.017894	0.982106	0.017186	81639	1461	16.47	62
63	0.019706	0.980294	0.018953	80178	1580	15.77	63
64	0.021694	0.978306	0.020884	78598	1705	15.07	64
65	0.023879	0.976121	0.023028	76893	1837	14.40	65
66	0.026199	0.973801	0.025340	75056	1966	13.74	66
67	0.028641	0.971359	0.027767	73090	2093	13.09	67
68	0.031296	0.968704	0.030380	70997	2222	12.46	68
69	0.034256	0.965744	0.033267	68775	2356	11.85	69

1 Age x	2 Probability of death $\hat{q}_x$	3 Survival probability $\hat{p}_x$	4 Death rate $\hat{\lambda}_x$	5 Survivor function ℓ_x	6 Number of deaths d_x	7 Expectation of life $\overset{o}{e}_x$	8 Age x
70	0.037614	0.962386	0.036533	66419	2498	11.25	70
71	0.041271	0.958729	0.040190	63921	2638	10.67	71
72	0.045166	0.954834	0.044126	61283	2768	10.11	72
73	0.049446	0.950554	0.048389	58515	2894	9.56	73
74	0.054258	0.945742	0.053147	55621	3018	9.04	74
75	0.059752	0.940248	0.058576	52603	3143	8.53	75
76	0.065881	0.934119	0.064761	49460	3258	8.04	76
77	0.072548	0.927452	0.071618	46202	3352	7.57	77
78	0.079819	0.920181	0.079123	42850	3420	7.12	78
79	0.087762	0.912238	0.087383	39430	3461	6.69	79
80	0.096444	0.903556	0.096495	35969	3469	6.29	80
81	0.105845	0.894155	0.106497	32500	3440	5.91	81
82	0.115919	0.884081	0.117722	29060	3368	5.55	82
83	0.126306	0.873694	0.128832	25692	3245	5.21	83
84	0.137156	0.862844	0.140845	22447	3079	4.89	84
85	0.148622	0.851378	0.153833	19368	2879	4.59	85
86	0.160853	0.839147	0.167876	16489	2652	4.31	86
87	0.174001	0.825999	0.183060	13837	2408	4.03	87
88	0.187986	0.812014	0.199478	11429	2148	3.78	88
89	0.202840	0.797160	0.217228	9281	1883	3.54	89
90	0.218595	0.781405	0.236421	7398	1617	3.31	90
91	0.235280	0.764720	0.257173	5781	1360	3.10	91
92	0.252919	0.747081	0.279610	4421	1118	2.90	92
93	0.271533	0.728467	0.303869	3303	897	2.71	93
94	0.291138	0.708862	0.330099	2406	701	2.53	94
95	0.311742	0.688258	0.358459	1705	531	2.37	95
96	0.333347	0.666653	0.389123	1174	391	2.21	96
97	0.355943	0.644057	0.422278	783	279	2.06	97
98	0.379515	0.620485	0.458126	504	191	1.93	98
99	0.404031	0.595969	0.496885	313	127	1.80	99
100	0.429449	0.570551	0.538793	186	80	1.68	100
101	0.455714	0.544286	0.584104	106	48	1.58	101
102	0.482754	0.517246	0.633096	58	28	1.47	102
103	0.510481	0.489519	0.686067	30	15	1.37	103
104	0.538790	0.461210	0.743341	15	8	1.23	104
105	0.567559	0.432441	0.805267	7	4	1.07	105
106	0.596649	0.403351	0.872222	3	2	0.83	106
107	0.625905	0.374095	0.944617	1	1	0.50	107

Appendix 2

Using GLIM in descriptive epidemiology

The software GLIM[1] was specifically designed for fitting generalized linear models which are commonly used in the analysis of epidemiological data. It is therefore one of the most useful tools for carrying out epidemiological calculations

We should first recall the concept of the linear model. Suppose that Y is a normal variate with mean μ and variance σ^2 and that μ is linearly related to several covariates represented by the vector $\mathbf{z}$:

$$\mu = \boldsymbol{\beta}\mathbf{z} = \beta_1 z_1 + \ldots + \beta_p z_p$$

or

$$Y = \boldsymbol{\beta}\mathbf{z} + \varepsilon$$

where $\varepsilon \rightsquigarrow N(0, \sigma^2)$ is usually called the *error.* Suppose further that Y has been observed for several values of $\mathbf{z}$. The *response variable,* called also the *dependent variable* Y can therefore be represented by a vector of dimension n, the number of observations. Denoting Y_i as the ith observation corresponding to the value $\mathbf{z}_i$ of $\mathbf{z}$, the maximum likelihood method enables $\boldsymbol{\beta}$ to be estimated by minimizing the expression

$$L(\boldsymbol{\beta}) = \sum_{i=1}^{n} (Y_i - \boldsymbol{\beta}\mathbf{z}_i)^2$$

which is the negative of the log-likelihood.

GLIM provides estimates of the coordinates of $\boldsymbol{\beta}$, the variance-covariance of these estimates as well as fitted values ($\hat{Y}_i$) and residuals ($Y_i - \hat{Y}_i$).

GLIM is an interactive programme which can be run on either a personal computer or a mainframe and which is usually activated by simply typing GLIM on the keyboard. In order to introduce the reader to its use, the estimation of the parameters of the regression equation which was fitted to the data presented in table 3.3 (Chapter 3 page) is reproduced and commented upon below. Comments are framed and printed in italics; instructions given to the programme are printed in bold type, while output of the programme is printed in smaller character using the current typeface. As a rule an instruction is introduced by a '$' and remains activated until another $ character is input. With these conventions the dialogue between the computer and the user may be as follows :

GLIM

GLIM 3.77 update 2 (copyright)1985 Royal Statistical Society, London

---

[1] Generalised Linear Interactive Modelling, NAG Ltd, Wilkinson House, Jordan Hill Road, Oxford OX2 8DR, UK

> *After this welcome message the user is invited with a? to input a directive (a $ followed by a word). Directives are either a statement or a request for an action to be carried out. Their name can be abbreviated provided that it is unambiguous.*

? **$unit 11**

? **$data z y**

> *These directives state that there are 11 observations (n = 11) and that there are two values per unit in the input data (z and y)*

$DAT? **$read**

> *The above directive requests data to be read from the keyboard. They should be input as described in the directive **data**. The computer therefore expects 2 × 11 numbers as a series of z y pairs*

$REA? **0 0.65 0.1 1.21 0.2 1.36 0.3 1.77 0.4 2.55 0.5 2.63 0.6 1.21**

$REA? **0.7 3.22 0.8 2.50 0.9 4.23 1.0 2.34**

? **$look z y $**

> *This directive requests the output of the values of z and y. It is used here to check that the data have been input correctly.*

	Z	Y
1	0.0000	0.6500
2	0.1000	1.2100
3	0.2000	1.3600
4	0.3000	1.7700
5	0.4000	2.5500
6	0.5000	2.6300
7	0.6000	1.2100
8	0.7000	3.2200
9	0.8000	2.5000
10	0.9000	4.2300
11	1.0000	2.3400

? **$yvar y $err n fit**

> *The directive **yvar** enables the dependant variable to be specified, and **err** state that the error ε is normally distributed ('n' for normal). This complete the specification of the model. The estimation starts with the directive **fit** and initially produces the deviance and its d.f.*

deviance = 10.806

d.f. = 10

> *Since the argument of **fit** is empty, the request is for the adjustment of a constant mean ($Y = \beta \times 1 + \varepsilon$ where **1** is a vector with eleven coordinates equal to 1). In this case the estimate $\hat{\beta}$ of β is therefore $\overline{Y} = \sum\limits_{i=1}^{n} Y_i$ and the value of the negative of the maximum log-likelihood $L(\hat{\beta}) = \sum\limits_{i=1}^{n} (Y_i - \overline{Y})^2$, which is the minimum deviation from the observed data when fitted with this class of models, is called the **deviance**; when divided by σ^2, the deviance is distributed as χ^2 with **d. f.** degrees of freedom.*

? **\$disp e**

> *In order to display the estimates (e) the directive **disp**lay must be used. This latter directive automatically produces standard errors of estimates and the value of $L(\hat{\beta})$ /df, named the **scale parameter** which is here an estimate of σ^2.*

	estimate	s.e.	parameter
1	2.152	0.3134	1

scale parameter taken as 1.081

\$DIS ? **\$fit z \$disp e**

deviance = 4.8900

d.f. = 9

	estimate	s.e	parameter
1	0.9923	0.4158	1
2	2.319	0.7028	Z

scale parameter taken as 0.5433

> *The directive **fit z** requests the estimation of the linear model $\mu = \beta_0 + \beta_1 z$. Note that the constant **1** is always included in a model except if explicitly excluded (**fit z-1**). The estimates of the parameters of the regression equation are therefore $\hat{\beta}_0 = 0.9923,\ \hat{\beta}_1 = 2.319$ and $\hat{\sigma}^2 = 4.89/9 = 0.5433.$*

\$DIS ? **r**

> *The letter **r** is an argument of the directive **display**. When typed while display is still activated, it requests that the fitted values $(\hat{Y}_i)$ and the standardized residuals $(Y_i - \hat{Y}_i)/SE(Y_i)$ be output*

unit	observed	fitted	residual
1	0.6500	0.9923	-0.342
2	1.2100	1.2242	-0.014
3	1.3600	1.4561	-0.096
4	1.7700	1.6880	0.082
5	2.5500	1.9199	0.630
6	2.6300	2.1518	0.478
7	1.2100	2.3837	-1.174
8	3.2200	2.6156	0.604
9	2.5000	2.8475	-0.348
10	4.2300	3.0795	1.151
11	2.3400	3.3114	-0.971

$DIS? **$stop**

The generalized linear model differs from the above simple normal model in two respects, (i) the model now aims to describe a function of the mean and not the mean itself; (ii) the error is no longer distributed as a normal variate but belongs to a class of random variables which enable reliable estimation of linear models to be achieved. As pointed out often in this book, descriptive epidemiology collects data which are often distributed according to the Poisson distribution; in this context it is the logarithm of the mean which is modelled and the name *'Poisson regression'* is now commonly used to designate genralized linear modelling using Poisson distributed error and logarithmic transformation of the mean. We shall illustrate the principle of this method and its implementation in GLIM with the data of table 2.8, adjusting the model of equation 2.33 (see page...).

Suppose that the data are stored in a file named MHP.DAT and organized as shown below, where each line corresponds to a computer record :

8 8 36 54 53 96 115 145

10 6 7 18 17 25 35 37

22801 27291 26762 25899 19853 17431 15024 11961

13506 12480 11012 9887 7010 6845 6066 4492

A possible way of fitting the multiplicative model (2.33) to the above data is given below. Comments briefly introduce the directives.

GLIM

GLIM 3.77 update 2 (copyright)1985 Royal Statistical Society, London

> *Eight observations from each of two cancer registries.*

? **$unit 16**

> *Read the number of cases (k) in the file* MHP.DAT *which will be connected to the reading unit 1 after answering the file name request; then read the number of person-years (m). Note that* **dinput** *is used instead of* **read** *when reading from a file.*

? **$data k $dinput 1**

File name? **mhp.dat**

$DIN ? $data m $dinp 1 $

> *Create the variables AGE and REG (for registry) using the function %gl : this function creates a vector with values given by the first argument (here 8 and 2 because 1≤ age ≤ 8 and 1 ≤ reg ≤ 2). The second argument gives the number of repetitions of each value. Note that, if not specified otherwise, the dimension of a vector equals the number of units. The character ':' enables the activated directive to be repeated with other arguments (here the **calculate** directive).*

? $cal age=%gl(8,1) :reg=%gl(2,8) $loo reg age k m $

	REG	AGE	K	M
1	1.000	1.000	8.000	22801.
2	1.000	2.000	8.000	27291.
3	1.000	3.000	36.000	26762.
4	1.000	4.000	54.000	25899.
5	1.000	5.000	53.000	19853.
6	1.000	6.000	96.000	17431.
7	1.000	7.000	115.000	15024.
8	1.000	8.000	145.000	11961.
9	2.000	1.000	10.000	13506.
10	2.000	2.000	6.000	12480.
11	2.000	3.000	7.000	11012.
12	2.000	4.000	18.000	9887.
13	2.000	5.000	17.000	7010.
14	2.000	6.000	25.000	6845.
15	2.000	7.000	35.000	6066.
16	2.000	8.000	37.000	4492.

> *State, using **yvar**, that the response variable is the number of cases (k), state, using **err**, that the error distribution is the Poisson distribution and, using **offset,** that the origin of the response variable scale is shifted by log(m) (i.e., the mean μ is such that log(μ) = zero + βz).*

? $yvar k $err p $cal zero=%log(m) $offset zero

> *State that AGE and REG are categorical variables (factors). This directive requests the computer to create dummy variables for each level of the factors but one (i.e., 7 for AGE and 1 for REG).*

? $factor age 8 :reg 2 $

> *The successive fits enable the contribution of each factor to be assessed. Remember that the change in deviance is distributed as a χ^2 with df equal to the corresponding change in degrees of freedom.*

? $fit :+ age :+ reg $

    scaled deviance = 676.59 at cycle 4
            d.f. = 15

scaled deviance = 18.142 (change = −658.4) at cycle 3

d.f. = 8   (change = −7)

scaled deviance = 9.3920 (change = −8.750) at cycle 4

d.f. = 7   (change = −1)

? **$disp e r $**

	estimate	s.e.	parameter
1	-7.519	0.2374	1
2	-0.3572	0.3564	AGE(2)
3	0.8109	0.2808	AGE(3)
4	1.377	0.2636	AGE(4)
5	1.631	0.2644	AGE(5)
6	2.285	0.2527	AGE(6)
7	2.642	0.2495	AGE(7)
8	3.080	0.2472	AGE(8)
9	-0.2651	0.09168	REG(2)

scale parameter taken as 1.000

unit	observed	fitted	residual
1	8	12.376	-1.244
2	8	10.364	-0.734
3	36	32.683	0.580
4	54	55.690	-0.227
5	53	55.080	-0.280
6	96	92.987	0.312
7	115	114.526	0.044
8	145	141.293	0.312
9	10	5.624	1.845
10	6	3.636	1.240
11	7	10.317	-1.033
12	18	16.310	0.419
13	17	14.920	0.539
14	25	28.013	-0.569
15	35	35.474	-0.080
16	37	40.707	-0.581

The programme provides several statistics, values of which can be requested through the look directive. For example to get the classical goodness of fit χ^2 type :

? **$loo %x2 $**

9.892

Note that most statistics can also be calculated directly using system-built vectors storing the main results of the fit. For example the above χ^2 is obtained through %fv which stores the fitted values.

? **$cal (k-%fv)**2/%fv $**

    1.547

    0.5393

    0.3366

    0.05131

    0.07855

    0.09761

    0.001958

    0.09728

    3.405

    1.537

    1.066

    0.1752

    0.2900

    0.3240

    0.006321

    0.3376

> Note that the above values are the squares of the standardized residuals, $\dfrac{(Y_i - \hat{Y}_i)}{\sqrt{Y_i}}$ listed previously. The residuals could also be stored in a vector :

? **$cal r2=(k-%fv)**2/%fv $**

> The directive **table** is a powerful tabulation programme. It is used here in its simplest form to get the total of **r2** coordinates, that is the value of the goodness of fit χ^2.

? **$tab the r2 t $**

    9.892

? **$stop**

Before going to the next example of Poisson regression, we should remember that the estimates of the coordinates of β are the logarithms of the estimated relative rates; for example the relative rate of age-group 8 (70-74 years) compared with age-group 1 (35-39 years) is exp(3.08)=21.76. The incidence rate of this latter age-group is estimated as exp(−7.519)/5=10.85/100 000 (the estimated rate is divided by five because we input the populations instead of the person-years; see table 2.8); similarly the relative rate of Geneva (REG(2)) compared with Zaragoza is exp(−0.2651) = 0.767.

The method of Poisson regression is now applied to the data of table 2.13 (page), stored as previously in a file named HOMINCG.DAT. Only the data corresponding to age greater than 20 were used, since no case was observed before that age.

GLIM

GLIM 3.77 update 2 (copyright) 1985 Royal Statistical Society, London

> Thirteen age-groups and six cantons of Côte d'Or make 78 units of observation.

? **\$unit 78**

? **\$data k \$dinput 1**

File name? **homincg.dat**

\$DIN? **\$data m \$dinput 1**

> Create the variable AGE and PLACE (for canton). The first two arguments of the directive **look** select the output interval for the vectors looked at, 1 to 12 in the present example. Note that GLIM 3.77 retains only four meaningful letters to identify a variable (plac for place)

\$DIN? **\$cal age= %gl(13,6) :place= %gl(6,1) \$loo 1 12 place age k m \$**

	PLAC	AGE	K	M
1	1.000	1.000	0.000	52794.0
2	2.000	1.000	0.000	10073.0
3	3.000	1.000	0.000	8402.0
4	4.000	1.000	0.000	19034.0
5	5.000	1.000	1.000	9539.0
6	6.000	1.000	0.000	1186.0
7	1.000	2.000	0.000	54321.0
8	2.000	2.000	0.000	10499.0
9	3.000	2.000	0.000	7984.0
10	4.000	2.000	1.000	19009.0
11	5.000	2.000	0.000	7936.0
12	6.000	2.000	0.000	1345.0

> Specify the model and the factors to be used in the fit; then fit the multiplicative model.

? **\$yvar k \$err p \$cal zero= %log(m) \$offset zero**

? **\$factor age 13 plac 6**

\$FAC? **\$fit age+plac \$disp e \$**

scaled deviance = 68.198 at cycle 8

d.f. = 60

	estimate	s.e	parameter
1	-11.37	1.001	1
2	-0.006026	1.414	AGE(2)
3	-6.130	14.39	AGE(3)
4	1.806	1.118	AGE(4)
5	1.515	1.155	AGE(5)
6	2.730	1.049	AGE(6)
7	3.141	1.035	AGE(7)
8	3.901	1.021	AGE(8)
9	3.873	1.029	AGE(9)

10	4.491	1.014	AGE(10)
11	5.427	1.007	AGE(11)
12	5.466	1.010	AGE(12)
13	5.516	1.013	AGE(13)
14	-0.3498	0.2127	PLAC(2)
15	-0.5899	0.2198	PLAC(3)
16	-0.2367	0.1560	PLAC(4)
17	-0.3564	0.1902	PLAC(5)
18	-0.8039	0.4566	PLAC(6)

scale parameter taken as 1.000

> Note that the incidence rate estimate in age-group 3 is almost zero and has a very large standard error. Actually no case has been observed in this age-group and the incidence rate estimate should be zero. The next step is to assess the significance of the factor PLAC; to this end a model containing only the factor age is fitted to the data and the corresponding increase in deviance evaluated

?

? **$fit –plac $**

  scaled deviance = 80.781 (change = +12.58) at cycle 8

  d.f. = 65   (change = +5)

> This calculation confirms that the incidence differs in the various cantons of Côte d'Or. It is then possible to test whether this difference is mainly between the town of Dijon and the other cantons : a dummy variable is created which takes on the value 0 for Dijon and 1 for the other cantons; the best way to do this is to use the logical functions which are available in GLIM.

? **$cal other=(plac > 1) $fit age+other $disp e $**

  scaled deviance = 71.663 at cycle 8

  d.f. = 64

estimate s.e. parameter

	estimate	s.e	parameter
1	-11.36	1.001	1
2	-0.005996	1.414	AGE(2)
3	-6.097	14.18	AGE(3)
4	1.809	1.118	AGE(4)
5	1.515	1.155	AGE(5)
6	2.729	1.049	AGE(6)
7	3.136	1.035	AGE(7)
8	3.898	1.021	AGE(8)
9	3.867	1.029	AGE(9)
10	4.481	1.014	AGE(10)
11	5.417	1.007	AGE(11)
12	5.456	1.010	AGE(12)
13	5.508	1.013	AGE(13)
14	0.3700	-0.1214	OTHE

scale parameter taken as 1.000

> *The deviance is not increased significantly (71.66 − 68.20=3.46 for 4 degrees of freedom); this observation leads us to accept the homogeneity of incidence in the cantons other than Dijon. The relative rate for these regions compared with Dijon is estimated as exp(−0.37)=0.69; a confidence interval may be obtained as exp(−0.37±1.96*0.1214).*
>
> *The relationship between age and incidence rate can be modelled with a polynomial in order to describe the data with a more parsimonious model. The variable age is first centred, then the polynomial degree to be used is roughly evaluated.*

$cal x=age-6$

? **$cal x2=x*x :x3=x2*x :x4=x3*x $fit x+othe :+x :+x2 :+x3 :+x4 $**

    scaled deviance = 102.96 at cycle 4
              d.f. = 75
    scaled deviance = 102.96 (change = 0.00) at cycle 4
              d.f. = 75   (change = 0)
    scaled deviance = 91.70 (change = −11.261) at cycle 5
              d.f. = 74   (change = −1)
    scaled deviance = 88.98 (change = −2.73) at cycle 5
              d.f. = 73   (change = −1)
    scaled deviance = 87.58 (change = −1.40) at cycle 5
              d.f. = 72   (change = −1)

> *A third degree polynomial provides an acceptable model.......*

? **$fit −x4 $disp e $**

    scaled deviance = 88.98 (change = +1.40) at cycle 5
              d.f. = 73   (change = +1)

	estimate	s.e.	parameter
1	-8.916	0.1818	1
2	0.6368	0.05715	X
3	-0.3677	0.1213	OTHE
4	0.001819	0.01794	X2
5	-0.004087	0.002379	X3

    scale parameter taken as 1.000

> *.......which provides practically the same estimate of the relative rate as that obtained when age was modelled as a factor.*

? **$stop**

We shall consider as a last example the data from table 3.15 giving the trends in mortality from lung cancer among young adults in France Scotland and the USA. These data were stored in the computer as a file (TREND.DAT) with 18 records each containing two numbers, the number of cases (k) and the person-years in thousands (m). The records are sorted by country (USA, Scotland, France) and by time of death (1955 to 1984 by 6 groups of five years). The calculations which have been described on page... and in table 3.16 are reproduced below in detail.

GLIM

GLIM 3.77 update 2 (copyright)1985 Royal Statistical Society, London

---

Fitting a model for the USA.

? **$unit 6**

$data k m $dinput 1 $

File name? **trend.dat**

Create the variable time period (t).

? **$cal t=%gl(6,1) $loo t k m $**

	T	K	M
1	1.000	3762.	27599.
2	2.000	4900.	29249.
3	3.000	6147.	29859.
4	4.000	6318.	28416.
5	5.000	5638.	27590.
6	6.000	5413.	30569

Specify a model for a Poisson regression

? **$yvar k $err p $cal zero=%log(m) $offset zero $**

? **$cal t2=t*t $fit t+t2 $disp e $**

scaled deviance = 14.094 at cycle 3

d.f. = 3

	estimate	s.e.	parameter
1	-2.393	0.02757	1
2	0.4284	0.01696	T
3	-0.05299	0.002310	T2

scale parameter taken as 1.000

Wald's test based on the standard error of the T2 coefficient (−0.05299/0.002310=−22.9) shows that the quadratic term is strongly significant. The same evaluation can be made using the likelihood ratio test:

? **$fit −t2 $disp e $**

scaled deviance = 553.06 (change = +539.0) at cycle 3

d.f. = 4 (change = +1)

	estimate	s.e.	parameter
1	−1.857	0.01322	1
2	0.04836	0.003269	T

scale parameter taken as 1.000

> We shall now fit the same model expression using a different error distribution in considering that the logarithm of the incidence rate is normally distributed with a mean equal to the proposed expression and a variance proportional to the observed number of cases in each unit.

? **$cal y=%log(k/m) $yvar y $err n $cal w=k $weight w**
  – model changed

> Do not forget to set the origin back to zero. After having done so (**offset**), fit the quadratic model with the method of weighted least sqares.

? **$offset $fit t+t2 $disp e $**
  deviance = 14.042
      d.f. = 3

	estimate	s.e.	parameter
1	-2.393	0.05916	1
2	0.4283	0.03639	T
3	-0.05299	0.004965	T2

scale parameter taken as 4.681

> Fit the linear model by the same method.

? **$fit −t2 $**
  deviance = 547.19 (change = +533.1)
      d.f. = 4   (change = +1)
? **$disp e $**

	estimate	s.e.	parameter
1	−1.848	0.1622	1
2	0.04825	0.04053	T

scale parameter taken as 136.8

> Note the value of the standard error of the T coefficient, obtained when fitting this model by least squares and compare it with the same coefficient in the linear model fitted by Poisson regression.

> Fitting a model for Scotland.

? **$data k m $dinput 1 $**
? **$loo k m $**

	K	M
1	242.0	811.0
2	222.0	803.2
3	247.0	798.8
4	195.0	747.4
5	138.0	717.6
6	116.0	724.

> The method of least squares will be applied first, since it is the model which is activated.

? **\$cal y=%log(k/m) \$**

    – change to data affects model

> Do not forget to change the values stored in w before fitting....

? **\$cal w=k \$fit t+t2 \$**

    – change to data affects model

    deviance = 4.0117

        d.f. = 3

? **\$disp e \$**

	estimate	s.e.	parameter
1	−1.359	0.1395	1
2	0.1637	0.09516	T
3	−0.04125	0.01391	T2

    scale parameter taken as 1.337

> Note that the scale parameter is close to one and that the coefficient of the quadratic term is strongly significant, as confirmed by the calculation reported below, which is based on the Poisson distribution :

? **\$err p \$yvar k \$cal zero=%log(m) \$offset zero \$weight**

    – model changed

\$WEI?

> This last directive eliminates the weighting, which is irrelevant in the Poisson regression.

? **\$fit t+t2 \$**

    scaled deviance = 4.0565 at cycle 3

        d.f. = 3

? **\$disp e \$**

	estimate	s.e.	parameter
1	−1.359	0.1223	1
2	0.1622	0.08373	T
3	−0.04101	0.01224	T2

scale parameter taken as 1.000

? **$fit –t2 $**

scaled deviance = 15.495 (change = +11.44) at cycle 3

d.f. = 4 (change = +1)

? **$disp e $**

	estimate	s.e.	parameter
1	−1.012	0.06175	1
2	−0.1124	0.01754	T

scale parameter taken as 1.000

Fitting a model for France.

? **$data k m $dinput 1**

$DIN ? **$loo k m $**

	K	M
1	479.0	5878.
2	612.0	6586.
3	968.0	8333.
4	1265.0	8507.
5	1308.0	8032.
6	1349.0	7484.

– change to data affects model

? **$cal zero= %log(m) $fit t $disp e $**

scaled deviance = 14.875 at cycle 3

d.f. = 4

	estimate	s.e.	parameter
1	−2.641	0.03567	1
2	0.1627	0.008182	T

scale parameter taken as 1.000

? **$fit +t2 $**

scaled deviance = 6.4909 (change = −8.384) at cycle 3

d.f. = 3   (change = −1)

? **$disp e $**

	estimate	s.e.	parameter
1	−2.823	0.07334	1
2	0.2818	0.04219	T
3	−0.01589	0.005513	T2

scale parameter taken as 1.000

> *Now apply the least squares method :*

? **$cal y=%log(k/m) $err n $offsset $cal w=k $weight w**
   − − model changed
? **$yvar y $fit t $disp e $**
   − − model changed
   deviance = 15.015
      d.f. = 4

	estimate	s.e.	parameter
1	−2.640	0.07020	1
2	0.1627	0.01614	T

scale parameter taken as 3.754

? **$fit +t2 $**
   deviance = 6.5056 (change = −8.509)
      d.f. = 3   (change = −1)
? **$disp e $**

	estimate	s.e.	parameter
1	−2.822	0.1063	1
2	0.2816	0.06125	T
3	−0.01591	0.008032	T2

scale parameter taken as 2.169

> *Note that the reduction in deviance is identical for the two error models; However, the standard error of the coefficient of the quadratic term is greater in this second situation where the lack of fit is taken into consideration in the estimation of σ^2.*

? **$stop**

This brief description of the capabilities of GLIM for carrying out calculation in descriptive epidemiology may be supplemented by references [36] and [37] of Chapter 2. A new release of this software is now available and details can be found in :

Francis B J, Green M and Payne C P (eds) *The GLIM System : Release 4 Manual*, Oxford University Press, Oxford.

Subject index

PUBLICATIONS OF THE INTERNATIONAL AGENCY FOR RESEARCH ON CANCER

Scientific Publications Series

(Available from Oxford University Press through local bookshops)

No. 1 **Liver Cancer**
1971; 176 pages (*out of print*)

No. 2 **Oncogenesis and Herpesviruses**
Edited by P.M. Biggs, G. de-Thé and L.N. Payne
1972; 515 pages (*out of print*)

No. 3 *N*-**Nitroso Compounds: Analysis and Formation**
Edited by P. Bogovski, R. Preussman and E.A. Walker
1972; 140 pages (*out of print*)

No. 4 **Transplacental Carcinogenesis**
Edited by L. Tomatis and U. Mohr
1973; 181 pages (*out of print*)

No. 5/6 **Pathology of Tumours in Laboratory Animals, Volume 1, Tumours of the Rat**
Edited by V.S. Turusov
1973/1976; 533 pages (*out of print*)

No. 7 **Host Environment Interactions in the Etiology of Cancer in Man**
Edited by R. Doll and I. Vodopija
1973; 464 pages (*out of print*)

No. 8 **Biological Effects of Asbestos**
Edited by P. Bogovski, J.C. Gilson, V. Timbrell and J.C. Wagner
1973; 346 pages (*out of print*)

No. 9 *N*-**Nitroso Compounds in the Environment**
Edited by P. Bogovski and E.A. Walker
1974; 243 pages (*out of print*)

No. 10 **Chemical Carcinogenesis Essays**
Edited by R. Montesano and L. Tomatis
1974; 230 pages (*out of print*)

No. 11 **Oncogenesis and Herpesviruses II**
Edited by G. de-Thé, M.A. Epstein and H. zur Hausen
1975; Part I: 511 pages
Part II: 403 pages (*out of print*)

No. 12 **Screening Tests in Chemical Carcinogenesis**
Edited by R. Montesano, H. Bartsch and L. Tomatis
1976; 666 pages (*out of print*)

No. 13 **Environmental Pollution and Carcinogenic Risks**
Edited by C. Rosenfeld and W. Davis ,
1975; 441 pages (*out of print*)

No. 14 **Environmental *N*-Nitroso Compounds. Analysis and Formation**
Edited by E.A. Walker, P. Bogovski and L. Griciute
1976; 512 pages (*out of print*)

No. 15 **Cancer Incidence in Five Continents, Volume III**
Edited by J.A.H. Waterhouse, C. Muir, P. Correa and J. Powell
1976; 584 pages (*out of print*)

No. 16 **Air Pollution and Cancer in Man**
Edited by U. Mohr, D. Schmähl and L. Tomatis
1977; 328 pages (*out of print*)

No. 17 **Directory of On-going Research in Cancer Epidemiology 1977**
Edited by C.S. Muir and G. Wagner
1977; 599 pages (*out of print*)

No. 18 **Environmental Carcinogens. Selected Methods of Analysis. Volume 1: Analysis of Volatile Nitrosamines in Food**
Editor-in-Chief: H. Egan
1978; 212 pages (*out of print*)

No. 19 **Environmental Aspects of *N*-Nitroso Compounds**
Edited by E.A. Walker, M. Castegnaro, L. Griciute and R.E. Lyle
1978; 561 pages (*out of print*)

No. 20 **Nasopharyngeal Carcinoma: Etiology and Control**
Edited by G. de-Thé and Y. Ito
1978; 606 pages (*out of print*)

No. 21 **Cancer Registration and its Techniques**
Edited by R. MacLennan, C. Muir, R. Steinitz and A. Winkler
1978; 235 pages (*out of print*)

No. 22 **Environmental Carcinogens. Selected Methods of Analysis. Volume 2: Methods for the Measurement of Vinyl Chloride in Poly(vinyl chloride), Air, Water and Foodstuffs**
Editor-in-Chief: H. Egan
1978; 142 pages (*out of print*)

No. 23 **Pathology of Tumours in Laboratory Animals. Volume II: Tumours of the Mouse**
Editor-in-Chief: V.S. Turusov
1979; 669 pages (*out of print*)

No. 24 **Oncogenesis and Herpesviruses III**
Edited by G. de-Thé, W. Henle and F. Rapp
1978; Part I: 580 pages, Part II: 512 pages (*out of print*)

No. 25 **Carcinogenic Risk. Strategies for Intervention**
Edited by W. Davis and
C. Rosenfeld
1979; 280 pages (*out of print*)

No. 26 **Directory of On-going Research in Cancer Epidemiology 1978**
Edited by C.S. Muir and G. Wagner
1978; 550 pages (*out of print*)

No. 27 **Molecular and Cellular Aspects of Carcinogen Screening Tests**
Edited by R. Montesano,
H. Bartsch and L. Tomatis
1980; 372 pages £30.00

No. 28 **Directory of On-going Research in Cancer Epidemiology 1979**
Edited by C.S. Muir and G. Wagner
1979; 672 pages (*out of print*)

No. 29 **Environmental Carcinogens. Selected Methods of Analysis. Volume 3: Analysis of Polycyclic Aromatic Hydrocarbons in Environmental Samples**
Editor-in-Chief: H. Egan
1979; 240 pages (*out of print*)

No. 30 **Biological Effects of Mineral Fibres**
Editor-in-Chief: J.C. Wagner
1980; **Volume 1:** 494 pages **Volume 2:** 513 pages (*out of print*)

No. 31 *N*-**Nitroso Compounds: Analysis, Formation and Occurrence**
Edited by E.A. Walker, L. Griciute,
M. Castegnaro and M. Börzsönyi
1980; 835 pages (*out of print*)

No. 32 **Statistical Methods in Cancer Research. Volume 1. The Analysis of Case-control Studies**
By N.E. Breslow and N.E. Day
1980; 338 pages £18.00

No. 33 **Handling Chemical Carcinogens in the Laboratory**
Edited by R. Montesano *et al.*
1979; 32 pages (*out of print*)

No. 34 **Pathology of Tumours in Laboratory Animals. Volume III. Tumours of the Hamster**
Editor-in-Chief: V.S. Turusov
1982; 461 pages (*out of print*)

No. 35 **Directory of On-going Research in Cancer Epidemiology 1980**
Edited by C.S. Muir and G. Wagner
1980; 660 pages (*out of print*)

No. 36 **Cancer Mortality by Occupation and Social Class 1851-1971**
Edited by W.P.D. Logan
1982; 253 pages (*out of print*)

No. 37 **Laboratory Decontamination and Destruction of Aflatoxins B_1, B_2, G_1, G_2 in Laboratory Wastes**
Edited by M. Castegnaro *et al.*
1980; 56 pages (*out of print*)

No. 38 **Directory of On-going Research in Cancer Epidemiology 1981**
Edited by C.S. Muir and G. Wagner
1981; 696 pages (*out of print*)

No. 39 **Host Factors in Human Carcinogenesis**
Edited by H. Bartsch and
B. Armstrong
1982; 583 pages (*out of print*)

No. 40 **Environmental Carcinogens. Selected Methods of Analysis. Volume 4: Some Aromatic Amines and Azo Dyes in the General and Industrial Environment**
Edited by L. Fishbein,
M. Castegnaro, I.K. O'Neill and
H. Bartsch
1981; 347 pages (*out of print*)

No. 41 *N*-**Nitroso Compounds: Occurrence and Biological Effects**
Edited by H. Bartsch, I.K. O'Neill, M. Castegnaro and M. Okada
1982; 755 pages £50.00

No. 42 **Cancer Incidence in Five Continents, Volume IV**
Edited by J. Waterhouse, C. Muir, K. Shanmugaratnam and J. Powell
1982; 811 pages (*out of print*)

No. 43 **Laboratory Decontamination and Destruction of Carcinogens in Laboratory Wastes: Some** *N*-**Nitrosamines**
Edited by M. Castegnaro *et al.*
1982; 73 pages £7.50

No. 44 **Environmental Carcinogens. Selected Methods of Analysis. Volume 5: Some Mycotoxins**
Edited by L. Stoloff, M. Castegnaro, P. Scott, I.K. O'Neill and H. Bartsch
1983; 455 pages £32.50

No. 45 **Environmental Carcinogens. Selected Methods of Analysis. Volume 6:** *N*-**Nitroso Compounds**
Edited by R. Preussmann, I.K. O'Neill, G. Eisenbrand, B. Spiegelhalder and H. Bartsch
1983; 508 pages £32.50

No. 46 **Directory of On-going Research in Cancer Epidemiology 1982**
Edited by C.S. Muir and G. Wagner
1982; 722 pages (*out of print*)

No. 47 **Cancer Incidence in Singapore 1968-1977**
Edited by K. Shanmugaratnam, H.P. Lee and N.E. Day
1983; 171 pages (*out of print*)

No. 48 **Cancer Incidence in the USSR (2nd Revised Edition)**
Edited by N.P. Napalkov, G.F. Tserkovny, V.M. Merabishvili, D.M. Parkin, M. Smans and C.S. Muir
1983; 75 pages (*out of print*)

No. 49 **Laboratory Decontamination and Destruction of Carcinogens in Laboratory Wastes: Some Polycyclic Aromatic Hydrocarbons**
Edited by M. Castegnaro *et al.*
1983; 87 pages (*out of print*)

No. 50 **Directory of On-going Research in Cancer Epidemiology 1983**
Edited by C.S. Muir and G. Wagner
1983; 731 pages (*out of print*)

No. 51 **Modulators of Experimental Carcinogenesis**
Edited by V. Turusov and R. Montesano
1983; 307 pages (*out of print*)

No. 52 **Second Cancers in Relation to Radiation Treatment for Cervical Cancer: Results of a Cancer Registry Collaboration**
Edited by N.E. Day and J.C. Boice, Jr
1984; 207 pages (*out of print*)

No. 53 **Nickel in the Human Environment**
Editor-in-Chief: F.W. Sunderman, Jr
1984; 529 pages (*out of print*)

No. 54 **Laboratory Decontamination and Destruction of Carcinogens in Laboratory Wastes: Some Hydrazines**
Edited by M. Castegnaro *et al.*
1983; 87 pages (*out of print*)

No. 55 **Laboratory Decontamination and Destruction of Carcinogens in Laboratory Wastes: Some *N*-Nitrosamides**
Edited by M. Castegnaro *et al.*
1984; 66 pages (*out of print*)

No. 56 **Models, Mechanisms and Etiology of Tumour Promotion**
Edited by M. Börzsönyi, N.E. Day, K. Lapis and H. Yamasaki
1984; 532 pages (*out of print*)

No. 57 ***N*-Nitroso Compounds: Occurrence, Biological Effects and Relevance to Human Cancer**
Edited by I.K. O'Neill, R.C. von Borstel, C.T. Miller, J. Long and H. Bartsch
1984; 1013 pages (*out of print*)

No. 58 **Age-related Factors in Carcinogenesis**
Edited by A. Likhachev, V. Anisimov and R. Montesano
1985; 288 pages (*out of print*)

No. 59 **Monitoring Human Exposure to Carcinogenic and Mutagenic Agents**
Edited by A. Berlin, M. Draper, K. Hemminki and H. Vainio
1984; 457 pages (*out of print*)

No. 60 **Burkitt's Lymphoma: A Human Cancer Model**
Edited by G. Lenoir, G. O'Conor and C.L.M. Olweny
1985; 484 pages (*out of print*)

No. 61 **Laboratory Decontamination and Destruction of Carcinogens in Laboratory Wastes: Some Haloethers**
Edited by M. Castegnaro *et al.*
1985; 55 pages (*out of print*)

No. 62 **Directory of On-going Research in Cancer Epidemiology 1984**
Edited by C.S. Muir and G. Wagner
1984; 717 pages (*out of print*)

No. 63 **Virus-associated Cancers in Africa**
Edited by A.O. Williams, G.T. O'Conor, G.B. de-Thé and C.A. Johnson
1984; 773 pages (*out of print*)

No. 64 **Laboratory Decontamination and Destruction of Carcinogens in Laboratory Wastes: Some Aromatic Amines and 4-Nitrobiphenyl**
Edited by M. Castegnaro *et al.*
1985; 84 pages (*out of print*)

No. 65 **Interpretation of Negative Epidemiological Evidence for Carcinogenicity**
Edited by N.J. Wald and R. Doll
1985; 232 pages (*out of print*)

No. 66 **The Role of the Registry in Cancer Control**
Edited by D.M. Parkin, G. Wagner and C.S. Muir
1985; 152 pages £10.00

No. 67 **Transformation Assay of Established Cell Lines: Mechanisms and Application**
Edited by T. Kakunaga and H. Yamasaki
1985; 225 pages (*out of print*)

No. 68 **Environmental Carcinogens. Selected Methods of Analysis. Volume 7. Some Volatile Halogenated Hydrocarbons**
Edited by L. Fishbein and I.K. O'Neill
1985; 479 pages (*out of print*)

No. 69 **Directory of On-going Research in Cancer Epidemiology 1985**
Edited by C.S. Muir and G. Wagner
1985; 745 pages (*out of print*)

No. 70 **The Role of Cyclic Nucleic Acid Adducts in Carcinogenesis and Mutagenesis**
Edited by B. Singer and H. Bartsch
1986; 467 pages (*out of print*)

No. 71 **Environmental Carcinogens. Selected Methods of Analysis. Volume 8: Some Metals: As, Be, Cd, Cr, Ni, Pb, Se, Zn**
Edited by I.K. O'Neill, P. Schuller and L. Fishbein
1986; 485 pages (*out of print*)

No. 72 **Atlas of Cancer in Scotland, 1975–1980. Incidence and Epidemiological Perspective**
Edited by I. Kemp, P. Boyle, M. Smans and C.S. Muir
1985; 285 pages (*out of print*)

No. 73 **Laboratory Decontamination and Destruction of Carcinogens in Laboratory Wastes: Some Antineoplastic Agents**
Edited by M. Castegnaro *et al.*
1985; 163 pages £13.50

No. 74 **Tobacco: A Major International Health Hazard**
Edited by D. Zaridze and R. Peto
1986; 324 pages £24.00

No. 75 **Cancer Occurrence in Developing Countries**
Edited by D.M. Parkin
1986; 339 pages £24.00

No. 76 **Screening for Cancer of the Uterine Cervix**
Edited by M. Hakama, A.B. Miller and N.E. Day
1986; 315 pages £31.50

No. 77 **Hexachlorobenzene: Proceedings of an International Symposium**
Edited by C.R. Morris and J.R.P. Cabral
1986; 668 pages (*out of print*)

No. 78 **Carcinogenicity of Alkylating Cytostatic Drugs**
Edited by D. Schmähl and J.M. Kaldor
1986; 337 pages (*out of print*)

No. 79 **Statistical Methods in Cancer Research. Volume III: The Design and Analysis of Long-term Animal Experiments**
By J.J. Gart, D. Krewski, P.N. Lee, R.E. Tarone and J. Wahrendorf
1986; 213 pages £23.50

No. 80 **Directory of On-going Research in Cancer Epidemiology 1986**
Edited by C.S. Muir and G. Wagner
1986; 805 pages (*out of print*)

No. 81 **Environmental Carcinogens: Methods of Analysis and Exposure Measurement. Volume 9: Passive Smoking**
Edited by I.K. O'Neill,
K.D. Brunnemann, B. Dodet and D. Hoffmann
1987; 383 pages £37.00

No. 82 **Statistical Methods in Cancer Research. Volume II: The Design and Analysis of Cohort Studies**
By N.E. Breslow and N.E. Day
1987; 404 pages £25.00

No. 83 **Long-term and Short-term Assays for Carcinogens: A Critical Appraisal**
Edited by R. Montesano,
H. Bartsch, H. Vainio, J. Wilbourn and H. Yamasaki
1986; 575 pages £37.00

No. 84 **The Relevance of *N*-Nitroso Compounds to Human Cancer: Exposure and Mechanisms**
Edited by H. Bartsch, I.K. O'Neill and R. Schulte-Hermann
1987; 671 pages (*out of print*)

No. 85 **Environmental Carcinogens: Methods of Analysis and Exposure Measurement. Volume 10: Benzene and Alkylated Benzenes**
Edited by L. Fishbein and
I.K. O'Neill
1988; 327 pages £42.00

No. 86 **Directory of On-going Research in Cancer Epidemiology 1987**
Edited by D.M. Parkin and
J. Wahrendorf
1987; 676 pages (*out of print*)

No. 87 **International Incidence of Childhood Cancer**
Edited by D.M. Parkin, C.A. Stiller,
C.A. Bieber, G.J. Draper,
B. Terracini and J.L. Young
1988; 401 pages £35.00

No. 88 **Cancer Incidence in Five Continents Volume V**
Edited by C. Muir, J. Waterhouse, T. Mack, J. Powell and S. Whelan
1987; 1004 pages £58.00

No. 89 **Method for Detecting DNA Damaging Agents in Humans: Applications in Cancer Epidemiology and Prevention**
Edited by H. Bartsch, K. Hemminki and I.K. O'Neill
1988; 518 pages £50.00

No. 90 **Non-occupational Exposure to Mineral Fibres**
Edited by J. Bignon, J. Peto and R. Saracci
1989; 500 pages £52.50

No. 91 **Trends in Cancer Incidence in Singapore 1968–1982**
Edited by H.P. Lee , N.E. Day and K. Shanmugaratnam
1988; 160 pages (*out of print*)

No. 92 **Cell Differentiation, Genes and Cancer**
Edited by T. Kakunaga,
T. Sugimura, L. Tomatis and
H. Yamasaki
1988; 204 pages £29.00

No. 93 **Directory of On-going Research in Cancer Epidemiology 1988**
Edited by M. Coleman and
J. Wahrendorf
1988; 662 pages (*out of print*)

No. 94 **Human Papillomavirus and Cervical Cancer**
Edited by N. Muñoz, F.X. Bosch and O.M. Jensen
1989; 154 pages £22.50

No. 95 **Cancer Registration: Principles and Methods**
Edited by O.M. Jensen,
D.M. Parkin, R. MacLennan,
C.S. Muir and R. Skeet
1991; 288 pages £28.00

No. 96 **Perinatal and Multigeneration Carcinogenesis**
Edited by N.P. Napalkov,
J.M. Rice, L. Tomatis and
H. Yamasaki
1989; 436 pages £52.50

No. 97 **Occupational Exposure to Silica and Cancer Risk**
Edited by L. Simonato,
A.C. Fletcher, R. Saracci and
T. Thomas
1990; 124 pages £24.00

No. 98 **Cancer Incidence in Jewish Migrants to Israel, 1961–1981**
Edited by R. Steinitz, D.M. Parkin,
J.L. Young, C.A. Bieber and
L. Katz
1989; 320 pages £37.00

No. 99 **Pathology of Tumours in Laboratory Animals, Second Edition, Volume 1, Tumours of the Rat**
Edited by V.S. Turusov and
U. Mohr
740 pages £90.00

No. 100 **Cancer: Causes, Occurrence and Control**
Editor-in-Chief L. Tomatis
1990; 352 pages £25.50

No. 101 **Directory of On-going Research in Cancer Epidemiology 1989/90**
Edited by M. Coleman and
J. Wahrendorf
1989; 818 pages £42.00

No. 102 **Patterns of Cancer in Five Continents**
Edited by S.L. Whelan, D.M. Parkin & E. Masuyer
1990; 162 pages £26.50

No. 103 **Evaluating Effectiveness of Primary Prevention of Cancer**
Edited by M. Hakama, V. Beral, J.W. Cullen and D.M. Parkin
1990; 250 pages £34.00

No. 104 **Complex Mixtures and Cancer Risk**
Edited by H. Vainio, M. Sorsa and A.J. McMichael
1990; 442 pages £40.00

No. 105 **Relevance to Human Cancer of *N*-Nitroso Compounds, Tobacco Smoke and Mycotoxins**
Edited by I.K. O'Neill, J. Chen and H. Bartsch
1991; 614 pages £74.00

No. 106 **Atlas of Cancer Incidence in the Former German Democratic Republic**
Edited by W.H. Mehnert, M. Smans,
C.S. Muir, M. Möhner & D. Schön
1992; 384 pages £52.50

IARC MONOGRAPHS ON THE EVALUATION OF CARCINOGENIC RISKS TO HUMANS

(Available from booksellers through the network of WHO Sales Agents)

Volume 1 **Some Inorganic Substances, Chlorinated Hydrocarbons, Aromatic Amines, *N*-Nitroso Compounds, and Natural Products**
1972; 184 pages (*out of print*)

Volume 2 **Some Inorganic and Organometallic Compounds**
1973; 181 pages (*out of print*)

Volume 3 **Certain Polycyclic Aromatic Hydrocarbons and Heterocyclic Compounds**
1973; 271 pages (*out of print*)

Volume 4 **Some Aromatic Amines, Hydrazine and Related Substances, *N*-Nitroso Compounds and Miscellaneous Alkylating Agents**
1974; 286 pages Sw. fr. 18.–

Volume 5 **Some Organochlorine Pesticides**
1974; 241 pages (*out of print*)

Volume 6 **Sex Hormones**
1974; 243 pages (*out of print*)

Volume 7 **Some Anti-Thyroid and Related Substances, Nitrofurans and Industrial Chemicals**
1974; 326 pages (*out of print*)

Volume 8 **Some Aromatic Azo Compounds**
1975; 357 pages Sw. fr. 44.–

Volume 9 **Some Aziridines, *N*-, *S*- and *O*-Mustards and Selenium**
1975; 268 pages Sw.fr. 33.–

Volume 10 **Some Naturally Occurring Substances**
1976; 353 pages (*out of print*)

Volume 11 **Cadmium, Nickel, Some Epoxides, Miscellaneous Industrial Chemicals and General Considerations on Volatile Anaesthetics**
1976; 306 pages (*out of print*)

Volume 12 **Some Carbamates, Thiocarbamates and Carbazides**
1976; 282 pages Sw. fr. 41.-

Volume 13 **Some Miscellaneous Pharmaceutical Substances**
1977; 255 pages Sw. fr. 36.–

Volume 14 **Asbestos**
1977; 106 pages (*out of print*)

Volume 15 **Some Fumigants, The Herbicides 2,4-D and 2,4,5-T, Chlorinated Dibenzodioxins and Miscellaneous Industrial Chemicals**
1977; 354 pages (*out of print*)

Volume 16 **Some Aromatic Amines and Related Nitro Compounds - Hair Dyes, Colouring Agents and Miscellaneous Industrial Chemicals**
1978; 400 pages Sw. fr. 60.–

Volume 17 **Some *N*-Nitroso Compounds**
1978; 365 pages Sw. fr. 60.–

Volume 18 **Polychlorinated Biphenyls and Polybrominated Biphenyls**
1978; 140 pages Sw. fr. 24.–

Volume 19 **Some Monomers, Plastics and Synthetic Elastomers, and Acrolein**
1979; 513 pages (*out of print*)

Volume 20 **Some Halogenated Hydrocarbons**
1979; 609 pages (*out of print*)

Volume 21 **Sex Hormones (II)**
1979; 583 pages Sw. fr. 72.–

Volume 22 **Some Non-Nutritive Sweetening Agents**
1980; 208 pages Sw. fr. 30.–

Volume 23 **Some Metals and Metallic Compounds**
1980; 438 pages (*out of print*)

Volume 24 **Some Pharmaceutical Drugs**
1980; 337 pages Sw. fr. 48.–

Volume 25 **Wood, Leather and Some Associated Industries**
1981; 412 pages Sw. fr. 72.–

Volume 26 **Some Antineoplastic and Immunosuppressive Agents**
1981; 411 pages Sw. fr. 75.–

Volume 27 **Some Aromatic Amines, Anthraquinones and Nitroso Compounds, and Inorganic Fluorides Used in Drinking Water and Dental Preparations**
1982; 341 pages Sw. fr. 48.–

Volume 28 **The Rubber Industry**
1982; 486 pages Sw. fr. 84.–

Volume 29 **Some Industrial Chemicals and Dyestuffs**
1982; 416 pages Sw. fr. 72.–

Volume 30 **Miscellaneous Pesticides**
1983; 424 pages Sw. fr. 72.–

Volume 31 **Some Food Additives, Feed Additives and Naturally Occurring Substances**
1983; 314 pages Sw. fr. 66.–

Volume 32 **Polynuclear Aromatic Compounds, Part 1: Chemical, Environmental and Experimental Data**
1983; 477 pages Sw. fr. 88.–

Volume 33 **Polynuclear Aromatic Compounds, Part 2: Carbon Blacks, Mineral Oils and Some Nitroarenes**
1984; 245 pages (*out of print*)

Volume 34 **Polynuclear Aromatic Compounds, Part 3: Industrial Exposures in Aluminium Production, Coal Gasification, Coke Production, and Iron and Steel Founding**
1984; 219 pages Sw. fr. 53.–

Volume 35 **Polynuclear Aromatic Compounds, Part 4: Bitumens, Coal-tars and Derived Products, Shale-oils and Soots**
1985; 271 pages Sw. fr. 77.–

Volume 36 **Allyl Compounds, Aldehydes, Epoxides and Peroxides**
1985; 369 pages Sw. fr. 77.—

Volume 37 **Tobacco Habits Other than Smoking: Betel-quid and Areca-nut Chewing; and some Related Nitrosamines**
1985; 291 pages Sw. fr. 77.—

Volume 38 **Tobacco Smoking**
1986; 421 pages Sw. fr. 83.—

Volume 39 **Some Chemicals Used in Plastics and Elastomers**
1986; 403 pages Sw. fr. 83.—

Volume 40 **Some Naturally Occurring and Synthetic Food Components, Furocoumarins and Ultraviolet Radiation**
1986; 444 pages Sw. fr. 83.—

Volume 41 **Some Halogenated Hydrocarbons and Pesticide Exposures**
1986; 434 pages Sw. fr. 83.—

Volume 42 **Silica and Some Silicates**
1987; 289 pages Sw. fr. 72.

Volume 43 **Man-Made Mineral Fibres and Radon**
1988; 300 pages Sw. fr. 72.—

Volume 44 **Alcohol Drinking**
1988; 416 pages Sw. fr. 83.

Volume 45 **Occupational Exposures in Petroleum Refining; Crude Oil and Major Petroleum Fuels**
1989; 322 pages Sw. fr. 72.—

Volume 46 **Diesel and Gasoline Engine Exhausts and Some Nitroarenes**
1989; 458 pages Sw. fr. 83.—

Volume 47 **Some Organic Solvents, Resin Monomers and Related Compounds, Pigments and Occupational Exposures in Paint Manufacture and Painting**
1989; 535 pages Sw. fr. 94.—

Volume 48 **Some Flame Retardants and Textile Chemicals, and Exposures in the Textile Manufacturing Industry**
1990; 345 pages Sw. fr. 72.—

Volume 49 **Chromium, Nickel and Welding**
1990; 677 pages Sw. fr. 105.—

Volume 50 **Pharmaceutical Drugs**
1990; 415 pages Sw. fr. 93.—

Volume 51 **Coffee, Tea, Mate, Methylxanthines and Methylglyoxal**
1991; 513 pages Sw. fr. 88.—

Volume 52 **Chlorinated Drinking-water; Chlorination By-products; Some Other Halogenated Compounds; Cobalt and Cobalt Compounds**
1991; 544 pages Sw. fr. 88.—

Volume 53 **Occupational Exposures in Insecticide Application and some Pesticides**
1991; 612 pages Sw. fr. 105.—

Volume 54 **Occupational Exposures to Mists and Vapours from Strong Inorganic Acids; and Other Industrial Chemicals**
1992; 336 pages Sw. fr. 72.—

Volume 55 **Solar and Ultraviolet Radiation**
1992; 316 pages Sw. fr. 65.—

Volume 56 **Some Naturally Occurring Substances: Food Items and Constituents, Heterocyclic Aromatic Amines and Mycotoxins**
1993; 600 pages Sw. fr. 95.—

Volume 57 **Occupational Exposures of Hairdressers and Barbers and Personal Use of Hair Colourants; Some Hair Dyes, Cosmetic Colourants, Industrial Dyestuffs and Aromatic Amines**
1993; 428 pages Sw. fr. 75.—

Volume 58 **Beryllium, Cadmium, Mercury and Exposures in the Glass Manufacturing Industry**
1993; 426 pages Sw. fr. 75.—

Volume 59 **Hepatitis Viruses**
1994; 286 pages Sw. fr. 65.—

Volume 60 **Some Industrial Chemicals**
1994; 560 pages Sw. fr. 90.—

Supplement No. 1
Chemicals and Industrial Processes Associated with Cancer in Humans (IARC Monographs, Volumes 1 to 20)
1979; 71 pages (*out of print*)

Supplement No. 2
Long-term and Short-term Screening Assays for Carcinogens: A Critical Appraisal
1980; 426 pages Sw. fr. 40.—

Supplement No. 3
Cross Index of Synonyms and Trade Names in Volumes 1 to 26
1982; 199 pages (*out of print*)

Supplement No. 4
Chemicals, Industrial Processes and Industries Associated with Cancer in Humans (IARC Monographs, Volumes 1 to 29)
1982; 292 pages (*out of print*)

Supplement No. 5
Cross Index of Synonyms and Trade Names in Volumes 1 to 36
1985; 259 pages (*out of print*)

Supplement No. 6
Genetic and Related Effects: An Updating of Selected IARC Monographs from Volumes 1 to 42
1987; 729 pages Sw. fr. 80.—

Supplement No. 7
Overall Evaluations of Carcinogenicity: An Updating of IARC Monographs Volumes 1-42
1987; 440 pages Sw. fr. 65.—

Supplement No. 8
Cross Index of Synonyms and Trade Names in Volumes 1 to 46
1990; 346 pages Sw. fr. 60.—

IARC TECHNICAL REPORTS*

No. 1 Cancer in Costa Rica
Edited by R. Sierra,
R. Barrantes, G. Muñoz Leiva, D.M.
Parkin, C.A. Bieber and
N. Muñoz Calero
1988; 124 pages Sw. fr. 30.-

**No. 2 SEARCH: A Computer
Package to Assist the Statistical
Analysis of Case-control Studies**
Edited by G.J. Macfarlane,
P. Boyle and P. Maisonneuve
1991; 80 pages (*out of print*)

**No. 3 Cancer Registration in the
European Economic Community**
Edited by M.P. Coleman and
E. Démaret
1988; 188 pages Sw. fr. 30.-

**No. 4 Diet, Hormones and Cancer:
Methodological Issues for
Prospective Studies**
Edited by E. Riboli and
R. Saracci
1988; 156 pages Sw. fr. 30.-

No. 5 Cancer in the Philippines
Edited by A.V. Laudico,
D. Esteban and D.M. Parkin
1989; 186 pages Sw. fr. 30.-

**No. 6 La genèse du Centre
International de Recherche sur le
Cancer**
Par R. Sohier et A.G.B. Sutherland
1990; 104 pages Sw. fr. 30.-

**No. 7 Epidémiologie du cancer dans
les pays de langue latine**
1990; 310 pages Sw. fr. 30.-

**No. 8 Comparative Study of Anti-
smoking Legislation in Countries of
the European Economic Community**
Edited by A. Sasco, P. Dalla Vorgia
and P. Van der Elst
1992; 82 pages Sw. fr. 30.-

**No. 9 Epidemiologie du cancer dans
les pays de langue latine**
1991 346 pages Sw. fr. 30.-

**No. 11 Nitroso Compounds:
Biological Mechanisms, Exposures
and Cancer Etiology**
Edited by I.K. O'Neill & H. Bartsch
1992; 149 pages Sw. fr. 30.-

**No. 12 Epidémiologie du cancer dans
les pays de langue latine**
1992; 375 pages Sw. fr. 30.-

**No. 13 Health, Solar UV Radiation
and Environmental Change**
By A. Kricker, B.K. Armstrong, M.E.
Jones and R.C. Burton
1993; 216 pages Sw.fr. 30.–

**No. 14 Epidémiologie du cancer dans
les pays de langue latine**
1993; 385 pages Sw. fr. 30.-

**No. 15 Cancer in the African
Population of Bulawayo, Zimbabwe,
1963–1977: Incidence, Time Trends
and Risk Factors**
By M.E.G. Skinner, D.M. Parkin, A.P.
Vizcaino and A. Ndhlovu
1993; 123 pages Sw. fr. 30.-

**No. 16 Cancer in Thailand,
1988–1991**
By V. Vatanasapt, N. Martin, H.
Sriplung, K. Vindavijak, S. Sontipong,
S. Sriamporn, D.M. Parkin and J.
Ferlay
1993; 164 pages Sw. fr. 30.-

**No. 18 Intervention Trials for Cancer
Prevention**
By E. Buiatti
1994; 52 pages Sw. fr. 30.-

**No. 19 Comparability and Quality
Control in Cancer Registration**
By D.M. Parkin, V.W. Chen, J. Ferlay,
J. Galceran, H.H. Storm and S.L.
Whelan
1994; 110 pages plus diskette
Sw. fr. 40.-

**No. 20 Epidémiologie du cancer dans
les pays de langue latine**
1994; 346 pages Sw. fr. 30.-

**No. 21 ICD Conversion Programs for
Cancer**
By J. Ferlay
1994; 24 pages plus diskette
Sw. fr. 30.-

DIRECTORY OF AGENTS BEING TESTED FOR CARCINOGENICITY (Until Vol. 13 Information Bulletin on the Survey of Chemicals Being Tested for Carcinogenicity)*

No. 8 Edited by M.-J. Ghess,
H. Bartsch and L. Tomatis
1979; 604 pages Sw. fr. 40.-

No. 9 Edited by M.-J. Ghess,
J.D. Wilbourn, H. Bartsch and
L. Tomatis
1981; 294 pages Sw. fr. 41.-

No. 10 Edited by M.-J. Ghess,
J.D. Wilbourn and H. Bartsch
1982; 362 pages Sw. fr. 42.-

No. 11 Edited by M.-J. Ghess,
J.D. Wilbourn, H. Vainio and
H. Bartsch
1984; 362 pages Sw. fr. 50.-

No. 12 Edited by M.-J. Ghess,
J.D. Wilbourn, A. Tossavainen and H.
Vainio
1986; 385 pages Sw. fr. 50.-

No. 13 Edited by M.-J. Ghess,
J.D. Wilbourn and A. Aitio 1988; 404
pages Sw. fr. 43.-

No. 14 Edited by M.-J. Ghess,
J.D. Wilbourn and H. Vainio
1990; 370 pages Sw. fr. 45.-

No. 15 Edited by M.-J. Ghess, J.D.
Wilbourn and H. Vainio
1992; 318 pages Sw. fr. 45.-

No. 16 Edited by M.-J. Ghess, J.D.
Wilbourn and H. Vainio
1994; 294 pages Sw. fr. 50.-

NON-SERIAL PUBLICATIONS

Alcool et Cancer†
By A. Tuyns (in French only)
1978; 42 pages Fr. fr. 35.-

**Cancer Morbidity and Causes of
Death Among Danish Brewery
Workers†**
By O.M. Jensen
1980; 143 pages Fr. fr. 75.-

**Directory of Computer Systems Used
in Cancer Registries†**
By H.R. Menck and D.M. Parkin
1986; 236 pages Fr. fr. 50.-

**Facts and Figures of Cancer in the
European Community***
Edited by J. Estève, A. Kricker, J.
Ferlay and D.M. Parkin
1993; 52 pages Sw. fr. 10.-

* Available from booksellers through the network of WHO Sales agents.

† Available directly from IARC

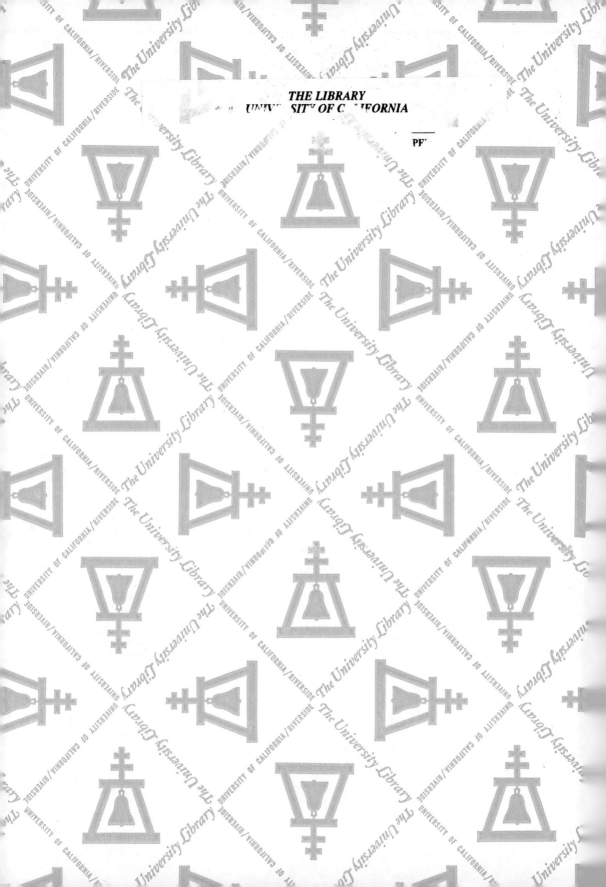